Applied Probability and Statistics (Conti

BHAT · Elements of Applied Stocl
BOX and DRAPER · Evolutionar〉   d
for Process Improvement
BROWNLEE · Statistical Theory a   d
Engineering, *Second Edition*
CHAKRAVARTI, LAHA and RC ....ok of Methods of
Applied Statistics, Vol. II
CHERNOFF and MOSES · Elementary Decision Theory
CHIANG · Introduction to Stochastic Processes in Biostatistics
CLELLAND, deCANI, BROWN, BURSK, and MURRAY · Basic
Statistics with Business Applications, *Second Edition*
COCHRAN · Sampling Techniques, *Second Edition*
COCHRAN and COX · Experimental Designs, *Second Edition*
COX · Planning of Experiments
COX and MILLER · The Theory of Stochastic Processes
DANIEL and WOOD · Fitting Equations to Data
DAVID · Order Statistics
DEMING · Sample Design in Business Research
DODGE and ROMIG · Sampling Inspection Tables, *Second Edition*
DRAPER and SMITH · Applied Regression Analysis
DUNN and CLARK · Applied Statistics: Analysis of Variance and
Regression
ELANDT-JOHNSON · Probability Models and Statistical Methods
in Genetics
FLEISS · Statistical Methods for Rates and Proportions
GOLDBERGER · Econometric Theory
GUTTMAN, WILKS and HUNTER · Introductory Engineering
Statistics, *Second Edition*
HAHN and SHAPIRO · Statistical Models in Engineering
HALD · Statistical Tables and Formulas
HALD · Statistical Theory with Engineering Applications
HOEL · Elementary Statistics, *Third Edition*
HOLLANDER and WOLFE · Nonparametric Statistical Methods
HUANG · Regression and Econometric Methods
JOHNSON and KOTZ · Distributions in Statistics
             Discrete Distributions
             Continuous Univariate Distributions-1
             Continuous Univariate Distributions-2
             Continuous Multivariate Distributions
JOHNSON and LEONE · Statistics and Experimental Design: In
Engineering and the Physical Sciences, Volumes I and II
LANCASTER · The Chi Squared Distribution
LANCASTER · An Introduction to Medical Statistics
LEWIS · Stochastic Point Processes
MILTON · Rank Order Probabilities: Two-Sample Normal Shift
Alternatives
OTNES and ENOCHSON · Digital Time Series Analysis
RAO and MITRA · Generalized Inverse of Matrices and Its Appli-
cations
SARD and WEINTRAUB · A Book of Splines
SARHAN and GREENBERG · Contributions to Order Statistics

continued on back

An Introduction to
Medical Statistics

A WILEY PUBLICATION IN APPLIED STATISTICS

An Introduction to Medical Statistics

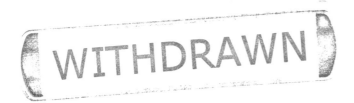

H. O. LANCASTER

Professor of Mathematical Statistics
University of Sydney, Australia

John Wiley & Sons
New York · London · Sydney · Toronto

To the memory of
J. H. L. Cumpston, Epidemiologist,
and
C. H. Wickens, Statistician

Library of Congress Cataloging in Publication Data:

Lancaster, Henry Oliver, 1913–
    An introduction to medical statistics.

    (Wiley series in probability and mathematical statistics) (A Wiley publication in applied statistics)
    "A Wiley-Interscience publication."
    Bibliography: p.
    1. Medical statistics.   I. Title.   [DNLM: 1. Medicine.   2. Statistics.   HA29 L244i 1973]

RA409.L35   610'.21'2   73–11323
ISBN 0-471-51250-8

Printed in the United States of America

10 9 8 7 6 5 4 3 2 1

Preface

This introduction to medical statistics has been written to assist medical students, graduates, and scientists to obtain a degree of familiarity with the many applications of statistical methods to medical problems. The first eight chapters follow the lines of a course in medical statistics, which the author had given to students in a postgraduate diploma in hygiene which had covered the systematization of observations, as well as the use and interpretation of official statistics. The author's aims then and now have been to provide an elementary review of vital statistics and the application of statistical methods to the understanding of clinical and laboratory medicine, and to suggest that there are many more applications of statistical, computing, and mathematical methods to the science and practice of medicine.

Although it must be recognized that medical statistics is an application of general statistical theory to medical problems, many important and interesting problems in medical science and practice can be stated and solved with the use of quite elementary mathematics. Therefore, we have used only elementary mathematical methods in the treatment of the first eleven chapters, with the exception of Section IX.3, in which we introduce a discussion of the integral equation of population growth. In Chapter XII, more mathematical formalism is necessary for the introduction of the multinomial, Poisson, χ^2, and t distributions, although it did not seem to be appropriate to prove theorems on distribution. Those sections which have a heavier mathematical content have been distinguished by an asterisk; they are Sections IX.3, XII.1, XVI.1 and XVI.2. A good deal can be done with only a few standard distributions.

No adequate account of *medical* statistics can neglect the numerous documentary sources of data on the members of the human population. With the development of the modern centralized states, such sources have become more numerous and extensive. In the early chapters, therefore, only a minimum of mathematical methodology is introduced, sufficient for the computation of rates, means, and standard deviations and for the construction of the life tables. Even in the interpretation of the mortality rates, however, some attention has to be paid to sampling problems; thus the binomial and normal distributions are introduced in Chapter IV.

Epidemiological ideas are introduced into the discussion of the death rates, but a detailed treatment is left until the later chapters. There is also a short chapter on genetical theory and special related topics.

The second part of the book begins with a few introductory notions on scientific method and inference. Then additional statistical distributions are introduced and the methods are applied to various medical problems, such as laboratory methods, clinical trials, follow-up studies and epidemiological surveys.

Detailed frequency tables are presented in Chapter I, and rules are laid down for their effective use. A number of observed or empirical frequency distributions appear in Chapters I and II, which later provide useful examples for practice in computation and graphical methods. Some of the examples introduce topics that are discussed in more detail in later chapters.

Chapter III presents general methods for the description of frequency distributions. Means, medians, standard deviations, and other descriptive measures are carefully defined and applied to data. Since the need for a theory of samples drawn from populations has now become apparent, elementary distribution theory is outlined in Chapter IV; in particular, the normal and binomial distributions are described. In Chapter V we mention medical aspects of the census and of other official statistics, including morbidity statistics. In the notes to Chapter V, attention is drawn to the various national systems of vital statistics and also to the work of the international bodies and their agencies, particularly the International Statistical Institute, the League of Nations, and the United Nations. Some relevant journal sources are also listed. In the general bibliography at the end of the book, many references to the works of these international agencies are furnished, and they are indexed by subject in the appropriate chapters.

Chapter VI serves to define the death rates and to describe the methods for their computation. The uses of the generation or cohort death rates and the standardized death rates are duly emphasized.

Chapter VII describes the theory of the life table and an abridged method for the construction of such tables. No attention is paid to the problem of graduation of the life tables, which so often clouds the description of their construction.

Chapter VIII is perhaps the central chapter of the book. Here the methods of Chapters VI and VII are used to interpret the progress of the death rates, principally by age, sex, and cause, as it has been observed in the developed countries (particularly Australia, England and Wales, Sweden, and the United States). However, statistical study of mortality is a very large field, and we can summarize it only partially. Therefore, an ample bibliography is provided in the notes to Chapter VIII.

In Chapter IX, the fertility and reproduction rates are defined. Next we deal with the effects of changes in mortality and fertility on the age and sex structure of the human populations, in what is essentially an elementary discussion of the integral equation of population growth. Some social consequences of the changes in mortality are also deduced.

Some elementary statistics are applied to genetical theory in Chapter X. Pedigrees, dominant and recessive autosomal inheritance, and sex-linked inheritance are discussed. Remarks are made on twinning and also on the sex ratio in sibships. In addition, reasons are given for believing that the dysgenic effects of the improvements in mortality up to the present time may have been overstressed by some authors.

Chapter XI deals with some topics in the methodology of science, of which statistical inference is but a part.

In Chapter XII, the hypergeometric, Poisson, χ^2, and t distributions are defined, and the uses of various tests of significance are explained.

Chapter XIII presents some general theory of calibration and the control of laboratory procedures, examples being chosen from common hematological procedures.

Clinical trials and observations are described in Chapter XIV, and the very special economic, legal, and ethical problems involved are briefly treated.

In Chapter XV we sample the many applications of numerical and statistical methods to medical problems which might be considered to be operations research. The possibilities of computers are mentioned, but no attempt is made to describe the mechanics of their use.

The theory of stochastic processes is mentioned in Chapter XVI, and its relevance to such biological problems as Brownian movement, the genetic constitution of populations, epidemics, and the importance of population size for the maintenance of epidemics, is pointed out. The discussion of the epidemiology of congenital malformations due to rubella is thus concluded.

In Chapter XVII we apply elementary set theory to the problems of taxonomy, diagnosis, and information retrieval.

Chapter XVIII contains a few remarks on the history of medical statistics and a guide to reference books, texts, and review articles relevant to the aims of this book. Some remarks are also made on the special features of medical statistics.

There follows a rather lengthy bibliography. This has been made necessary by the desire to make the book an introduction to a great diversity of topics and by the consideration that some of these topics, notably mortality, have many different facets. We wish also to encourage the use of the series published by the United Nations, the World Health Organization, and the U.S. National Center for Health Statistics.

I thank Drs. D. Shanks and J. W. Wrench, the editor of the *Mathematics of Computation* and the American Mathematical Society for permission to reprint the digits of the expansion of π as random sampling numbers.

I thank Mr. W. Brass of the London School of Hygiene and Dr. D. G. S. Christie, lately of the same School, for reading Chapters I to VIII in another version and for advice on presentation during my stay at the London School of Hygiene in 1969. I have to thank the librarians of the University of Sydney, Miss M. Rolleston of the Australian Medical Association, and Mr. F. J. Packer of the School of Public Health and Tropical Medicine, Sydney, for assistance with references. Mr. M. Thuner has drawn the diagrams. In my Department of Mathematical Statistics Dr. E. A. Eyland has read the text and helped to clear up some obscurities, and Mr. G. H. Cooney has assisted by reading certain sections. I have to thank Miss K. Yamamoto, Miss P. Thompson, Mrs. M. Buncombe, and especially Mrs. I. Ryan and Mrs. E. I. Adler for typing and other assistance.

H. O. LANCASTER

Sydney, Australia
March 1973

Contents

CHAPTER | PAGE

I. METHODS OF TABULATION   1

    1. Frequency Tables, 1
    2. The Principles of Classification, 8
    3. The Construction of Frequency and Contingency Tables, 10
      Notes, 11

II. THE GRAPHICAL REPRESENTATION OF DATA   13

    1. Coordinate Systems, 13
    2. Types of Graphical Representation, 16
    3. Principles for the Construction of Statistical Diagrams, 18
    4. Relations Between Variables, 20
      Exercises, 23
      Notes, 25

III. EMPIRICAL FREQUENCY DISTRIBUTIONS   26

    1. Introductory, 26
    2. Cumulative Frequency Distributions, 28
    3. The Mode, 31
    4. Extreme Values and the Range, 31
    5. The Median and Other Order Statistics, 32
    6. The Arithmetic Mean or Average, 32
    7. The Harmonic and Geometric Means, 34
    8. Dispersion Measured by Order Statistics, 35

9. The Mean Deviation, 35
10. The Standard Deviation and Variance, 35
11. Some Miscellaneous Properties of Empirical Distributions, 39
    Exercises, 39
    Notes, 41

IV. SAMPLING DISTRIBUTIONS   42

1. Introductory, 42
2. Permutations, 42
3. Combinations, 43
4. The Binomial Theorem, 44
5. Elementary Probability Theory, 46
6. The Binomial Distribution, 47
7. The Normal Curve, 51
8. The Normal Approximation to the Binomial Distribution, 53
    Exercises, 54
    Notes, 55

V. MEDICAL ASPECTS OF THE CENSUS AND OFFICIAL STATISTICS   56

1. Introductory, 56
2. Medical Information from the Census, 57
3. Other Official Sources of Medical Statistical Information, 60
4. Morbidity Statistics, 61
    Notes, 64

VI. MEASUREMENT OF MORTALITY   68

1. Introductory, 68
2. Definitions of Death, 71
3. The Populations at Risk, 73
4. The Age-Specific Death Rates, 74
5. The Relation Between m_x and q_x, 74
6. The Standard Error of m_x, 75
7. The Analysis of the Age-Specific Death Rates, 76
8. The Crude Death Rate, 77
9. Standardization of the Death Rates: Direct Method, 79
10. Standardization of the Death Rates: The Indirect Method, 81
11. Forecasting the Mortality Rates, 83
    Exercises, 83

VII. THE LIFE TABLE   87

1. The Purposes of the Life Table, 87
2. Select Life Tables or Mortality Studies, 88
3. The Fundamental Assumptions of the Life Table, 89
4. The Life-Table Functions, 89
5. Construction of the Life Table, 91
6. Description of the Life-Table Functions, 92
   Exercises, 95
   Notes, 99

VIII. MORTALITY IN HUMAN POPULATIONS   100

1. Introductory, 100
2. Infant Mortality, 100
3. The Mortality of Childhood, 102
4. The Mortality of Young Adult Life, 103
5. The Mortality of Adult Life, 104
6. The Mortality of Old Age, 104
7. Mortality from Tuberculosis, 105
8. Mortality from Lung Cancer, 111
9. Mortality from Other Cancers, 112
10. Mortality from Violent and Accidental Causes, 114
11. Causes of the Declines in Mortality, 115
    Exercises, 118
    Notes, 122

IX. FERTILITY AND POPULATION DYNAMICS   128

1. Definitions and Introductory, 128
2. Gross and Net Reproduction Rates, 131
*3. The Integral Equation of Population Growth, 134
4. Mortality and Population Increase, 142
5. Aging of the Populations, 143
6. Other Social Aspects of the Declines of Mortality, 146
   Exercises, 148
   Notes, 149

* Indicates section having heavy mathematical content.

X. STATISTICAL ASPECTS OF HUMAN GENETICS   151

1. Genetic Models, 151
2. Commentary on the Models, 154
3. Equilibrium of the Genotypes in a Population, 156
4. Pedigrees and Genealogical Records, 159
5. Dominant Inheritance, 160
6. Recessive Inheritance, 162
7. Sex-Linked Inheritance, 165
8. The Sex Ratio in Sibships, 165
9. Twinning, 167
10. Evolutionary Aspects of the Declines in Mortality Rates, 169
    Exercises, 171
    Notes, 172

XI. PROBLEMS OF INFERENCE   174

1. Scientific Method, 174
2. The Null Hypothesis, 176
3. The Alternative Hypothesis, 177
4. The Critical Region, 177
5. The Power of a Test, 179
6. Multiple Comparisons, 180
7. Estimation, 181
8. Estimation and Tests of Significance, 182

XII. FURTHER DISTRIBUTION THEORY   183

*1. Random Variables, 183
2. Conditional Probability, 185
3. The Poisson Distribution, 186
4. The Multinomial Distribution, 188
5. The Distribution of χ^2, 189
6. Contingency Tables, 195
7. Student's t Test, 197
8. The Bivariate Normal Distribution, 198
9. Regression in Mathematical Models, 200
    Exercises, 202
    Notes, 209

XIII. THE CONTROL OF LABORATORY MEASUREMENTS   210

1. Precision and Accuracy, 210
2. Counting Experiments, 213
3. The Control of Routine Measurements, 216
    Exercises, 217
    Notes, 218

XIV. CLINICAL TRIALS AND OBSERVATIONS   220

1. Introductory, 220
2. Conduct of the Clinical Trial, 222
3. Design of Experiment, 225
4. Special Points of Technique, 225
5. Alternatives to the Clinical Trial, 227
6. Ethics of Clinical Trials, 227
7. Clinical and Epidemiological Observations, 228
    Notes, 230

XV. SPECIAL TECHNIQUES   232

1. Operations Research, 232
2. The Use of Computers, 233
3. Simulation, 234
4. The Use of Card Systems in Clinical Research, 236
5. Cancer Registries, 238
6. Hospital Records, 239
7. Investigation of an Unexpected Epidemic, 240
8. Interpretations of Surveys, 241
    Notes, 243

XVI. STATISTICAL EPIDEMIOLOGY   244

*1. Stochastic Processes, 244
*2. Population Size and Epidemics, 245
3. Epidemic Behavior, 248
4. Rubella Epidemics and Congenital Defects, 249
    Notes, 250

XVII. PROBLEMS OF CLASSIFICATION   252

1. Introductory, 252
2. Elementary Set Theory, 252
3. The Taxonomy and Diagnosis of Diseases, 255
4. Information Retrieval, 258
    Notes, 258

XVIII. MEDICAL STATISTICS   259

1. The History of Medical Statistics, 259
2. General References to Medical Statistics, 261
3. The Scope of Medical Statistics, 262

BIBLIOGRAPHY   264

APPENDIX   291

AUTHOR INDEX   299

SUBJECT INDEX   300

CHAPTER I

Methods of Tabulation

1. FREQUENCY TABLES

An important task of the statistician is to display numerical observations in a way that allows conclusions to be drawn from them. It is often possible to derive important conclusions by the appropriate arrangement of the data in a frequency table; that is, the observations are classified and the numbers in the classes are recorded and presented in the form of a table.

Example i. In 1941 N. M. Gregg of Sydney had reported the occurrence of some 75 cases of congenital cataract in infants; inquiring of the mothers' health, he had found that each woman had suffered from an attack of rubella during pregnancy. The importance of this astute observation was widely acclaimed. Some epidemiologists believed that the virus of rubella was acting in a new way and that mutation had occurred, for previously rubella had appeared in clinical medicine as a mild disease, important only in the differential diagnosis of the skin eruptions of the acute fevers and lacking major complications. Such a hypothesis of a new strain could not be directly tested and possibly falsified, as a similar hypothesis could in veterinary science; however, doubts could be cast on it by a historical study, using readily available documentary evidence, as we now proceed to show.

It was observed in the *Reports of the Statistician* on the Australian Censuses of 1911, 1921, and 1933 that there were excessive numbers of deaf-mute persons in Australia at ages suggesting that they had been born between 1898 and 1901. The figures for New South Wales are given in Table I.1. The numbers in 1911 at ages 10 to 14 years are larger than those in the neighboring age groups. The statistician in the *Report on the Census of 1911* believed these figures to be explicable by a more complete enumeration of the deaf-mutes once they begun to attend school, since before the age of approximately 6, affected children had been thought to be mentally defective rather than deaf. When the results of the Census of 1921 appeared, this explanation was no longer tenable, for the excessive numbers of deaf-mutes now appeared at ages 20 to 24 years. With good reason, the statistician then cited the high rate of infections in the infancy of these children as a possible cause, for postnatal measles and meningitis were well-known causes of deafness. In 1933 although it was not the subject of comment by the statistician, these excessive numbers had become evident at ages 30 to 34 years; thus 1898 can be determined as the earliest

Table I.1

THE DEAF-MUTES IN NEW SOUTH WALES AS ENUMERATED AT THREE CENSUSES

Age Group	1911 Census		1921 Census		1933 Census	
	Males	Females	Males	Females	Males	Females
0–	8	8	7	10	7	4
5–	34	25	39	33	57	38
10–	(54)	(57)	43	43	56	33
15–	35	29	30	27	68	73
20–	36	29	(69)	(46)	49	49
25–	34	26	36	23	44	25
30–	24	30	35	32	(78)	(62)
35–	35	22	35	27	44	27
40–	14	22	22	25	31	28
45–	19	13	25	25	28	24
50–	13	15	9	17	29	18
55–	8	6	13	11	18	22
60–	11	7	12	14	15	14
65+	4	16	21	29	14	25
Unclassified	1	5	0	3	1	1
Total	330	310	396	365	539	443

Data from *Statistician's Report* on the Australian Census of 1933.

possible year of birth of the affected group. The 1911 figures enable us to fix 1901 as the latest possible year, because children born later would not have reached the age of 10 by 1911. Now the problem was to obtain more data. Fortunately, in the admission book of the New South Wales Institution for the Deaf, Dumb and Blind, the dates of birth and the sex of all admissions were available. The dates of birth could then be arranged in a frequency table, as in Table I.2. It is clear that an unusually large number of the infants who had been born in 1899 were later admitted to the

Institution. The numbers of births of such infants were: 15 for 1898, 70 for 1899, and 16 for 1900, whereas 16 could be taken to be an average or expected number at that time. Excessive numbers of births of deaf-mutes also occurred in 1916, 1924–1925, 1938, 1940, 1941, and 1943. The "epidemic" nature of these births can be brought out by a classification of the births

Table I.2

BIRTHS OF THE DEAF IN NEW SOUTH WALES

Year	\multicolumn{10}{c}{Total Births}
	0	1	2	3	4	5	6	7	8	9
188-	5	16	13	10	8	12	11	17	12	14
189-	8	8	10	12	10	11	16	12	15	70
190-	16	7	8	13	14	8	11	13	13	12
191-	15	16	13	16	21	16	32	19	13	11
192-	19	14	17	18	27	29	14	11	12	15
193-	23	17	11	10	19	15	19	21	33	14
194-	25	91	15	31	14	19	17	15	25	13
195-	14	19	21	22	16	20	14	13	13	11

	\multicolumn{10}{c}{Rubella Births}
193-[a]	—	—	—	—	—	—	—	2	4	3
194-	7	59	7	12	3	1	2	1	0	0
195-	2	1	1	1	0	3	2	3	1	1

Data from the *Brit. Med. J.*, **2** (1951), 1429–1432; **1** (1964), 1046. The first three digits of the year are given in the first column and the final digit above the table.
[a] Owing to the form of recording, perhaps the numbers of rubella births should be considered as minimum figures for 1941 and preceding years; for until rubella had been established as a cause of congenital deafness, the referring physician would not have made the diagnosis.

by month (see Table I.3). Clearly, in years when their number is high, the births take the form of an epidemic wave, centered on April and May. Indeed, for the 1899 births, an epidemic of rubella is known to have occurred in Sydney in and around October 1898. Data for the presumed rubella epidemic of 1915 are scanty, although it is known that rubella was epidemic in Australia during World War I. A clinical history of a rubella-deaf person born in 1924 is available (see Lancaster, 1951a), and Table I.2 gives cases diagnosed by the physician referring cases to the Institution in the more recent years. It is clear that a simple display of the births in an institution for the deaf has made a strong case that rubella has caused congenital malformations in the past. We return to this topic in Chapter XVI.

Table I.3

BIRTHS OF THE DEAF IN NEW SOUTH WALES BY MONTH

	Year				
Month	1899	1916	1938	1941[a]	1917–1937
January	1	1	2	12	23
February	5	0	0	11	32
March	2	4	8	30	33
April	8	1	3	18	31
May	8	3	5	14	29
June	8	9	2	5	25
July	14	6	3	4	34
August	12	2	2	4	32
September	6	4	4	2	34
October	1	1	3	1	31
November	3	1	0	2	32
December	2	0	1	1	23
Total	70	32	33	104	359

Data from *Brit. Med. J.*, **2** (1951) 1429–1432.
[a] Also July–December, 1940: 0, 3, 3, 2, 2, 6.

Example ii. Sometimes the observations can take only a restricted class of values; for example, the integers 0, 1, 2, 3, ... Table I.4 gives the result of a complete count over the whole 400 squares of the hemocytometer. Here it is evident that the mean cell count per small hemocytometer square is of interest, for this value will give us the red blood cell count. The cells on the whole 400 small squares can be counted and averaged. Of course, it is common clinical practice to count the cells over 80 small squares and multiply by 10,000 to obtain the red cell count per cubic centimeter. The grand total can be obtained by a simple addition, and division by the number of small squares gives the mean.

It is more instructive, however, to proceed in an alternative manner. The counts recorded are 0, 1, 2, ...; thus the small squares can be classified. The number of cells, x say, occurs with a frequency f_x. Each x can now be multiplied by the frequency f_x with which it occurs, and the products xf_x

can be summed to yield a *grand total* from which the *arithmetic* mean can be obtained (by division by the number of small hemocytometer squares). In Table I.4 we used a useful check on the arithmetic based on the following equation:

$$(1) \qquad (x + 1)f_x = xf_x + f_x$$

and on the fact that the sum of the terms on the left is equal to the sum of the two sums of the terms on the right; namely,

$$(2) \qquad \sum (x + 1)f_x = \sum xf_x + \sum f_x,$$

where $\sum$, the Greek capital S, is a sign for summation. The identity (2) can be proved by writing out the two sides of (1) in the three columns with $x = 0$, $x = 1$, ..., and summing each column to give the identity (2).

Variables such as the cell count per square, taking values, 0, 1, 2, ..., form an important class of *discrete* variables.

Table I.4

A COMPLETE ENUMERATION OF RED CELLS OVER THE
SQUARES OF A HEMOCYTOMETER

Cells/Small Square, x	Observed Frequencies and Products		
	f_x	$x \times f_x$	$(x + 1) \times f_x$
0	11	0	11
1	36	36	72
2	76	152	228
3	80	240	320
4	74	296	370
5	58	290	348
6	38	228	266
7	17	119	136
8	6	48	54
9	3	27	30
10	0	0	0
11	1	11	12
Total	400	1447	1847

Computation check: $\sum (x + 1)f_x = \sum xf_x + \sum f_x$
$$1847 = 1447 + 400.$$

Example   iii. Some variables, in principle taking any value within certain limits, are said to be *continuous*. Heights and weights are good examples. Usually, however, the recorded values are restricted in number by the nature of the measuring apparatus. Table I.5 is a frequency table of the heights of boys aged 4 years. These measurements had been made to the nearest

Table I.5

HEIGHTS[a] OF 222 BOYS AGED 4 YEARS

Height (in.)	Number of Boys
35–	1
36–	2
37–	4
38–	12
39–	16
40–	39
41–	51
42–	53
43–	23
44–	11
45–	8
46–	1
47–	0
48–	0
49–	1

[a] 38– is to be interpreted as 37.875–38.875 in.

quarter-inch and then, for convenience of computation, heights (measured as 38, 38.25, 38.50, and 38.75 in.), are recorded in the table as 38– in. If the measuring has been accurate, the smallest height that can enter the class is 37.875 in. and the largest is 38.875 in.; thus the midpoint of the class is 38.375 in. A routine for the computation of the means was given in Table I.4, and descriptive measures of such frequency distributions appear in Chapter III.

Example   iv. Table I.6 presents a frequency distribution of the hemoglobin values of certain Papuan native laborers working under unfavorable conditions in 1945. We note a tendency for them to be grouped about a central value of 10.5 g of hemoglobin per 100 ml of blood.

Table I.6

HEMOGLOBIN VALUES OF 878 PAPUAN
LABORERS

Hemoglobin (to nearest 0.5 g/100 ml)	Frequency
5.0	1
5.5	1
6.0	5
6.5	13
7.0	22
7.5	26
8.0	42
8.5	71
9.0	68
9.5	83
10.0	105
10.5	105
11.0	92
11.5	77
12.0	60
12.5	42
13.0	31
13.5	19
14.0	10
14.5	2
15.0	1
15.5	1
16.0	0
16.5	0
17.0	0
17.5	1

Example v. In 1889 A. Geissler reported the distribution of the sexes in sibships or families enumerated at the Census in Saxony. We discuss these data in Chapter X. In Table I.7 we have data relating to two types of sibships—those which include eight and those numbering nine, from which the last child has been removed.

Table I.7

THE SEX RATIO IN SIBSHIPS

Number of Males	Number of Sibships before the Ninth Birth	Relative Frequency	Number of Sibships after the Eighth Birth	Relative Frequency
8	264	686	342	637
7	1,655	4,299	2,092	3,897
6	4,948	12,854	6,678	12,440
5	8,498	22,076	11,929	22,222
4	10,263	26,661	14,959	27,867
3	7,603	19,751	10,649	19,838
2	3,951	10,264	5,331	9,931
1	1,152	2,993	1,485	2,766
0	161	418	215	401
Total	38,495	100,000	53,680	100,000

Data from A. Geissler, Z. Königl. Sächs. Statist. Bur. (1889), 1–24.

2. THE PRINCIPLES OF CLASSIFICATION

The tables in Section I.1 have been formed by a classification of individuals according to the values of certain variables, such as date of birth and size of family. Variables can be *qualitative* (e.g., sex, marital status, religion, occupation, and nationality); in this case, they are usually referred to as *attributes*. Other variables are *quantitative* and are recorded as the result of a measurement or a count. Usually there is no difficulty in forming a classification from counting data: thus the number of children to a marriage can take values 0, 1, 2, ..., and this yields a natural classification. Similarly, the small squares of a hemocytometer can be classified by the number of red cells falling on them. These are examples of *discrete* variables.

Continuous variables do not give a classification directly, since it is possible that no two heights, say, are the same. However, arbitrary classes can be formed by dividing the domain of possible values into *class intervals* (e.g., heights taken to the nearest centimeter). The possible heights are all classifiable in principle, since the probability of obtaining a height of exactly 151.5 cm or any other such height ending in .5 is zero. Special devices can often be adopted to avoid the recording of such a measurement.

The differences between quantitative and qualitative are not absolute, and some qualities can be made quantitative by suitable definitions (e.g., sensations of color, sensations of comfort under varying meteorological conditions). Thus also, the criterion for classification after a clinical trial may be death or survival up to a period of, say, five years from the initiation of treatment. However, mere survival may be held not to be an adequate criterion of the effectiveness of treatment, and it may be thought desirable to devise a scoring system that gives weight to the condition of the survivors, as well. For comparative purposes, we might construct a scale that gives a score of zero to perfect recovery, rather more to survival with mild symptoms, more to survival with severer symptoms, and still more to death before the termination of the five years. Within this framework, a treatment can be considered to be better if it has a lower mean score than a second treatment.

A good classification, of course, should be according to an attribute of interest or importance. The classes should be distinctly defined, to indicate to investigators what properties any individual in the class will possess, and they should be *mutually exclusive*, to ensure that no individual will be assignable to two classes. Every individual should be assignable to a class; that is, the classification should be *exhaustive*. Sometimes, a criterion of interest will not apply to all individuals in the population; in such cases, it is necessary to have a residual class, perhaps labeled "others" or "result unknown." Much of the foregoing discussion can be formalized profitably by the introduction of the notation of set theory, which is deferred to Chapter XVII.

In general, the choice of a good criterion or criteria depends on the physical or social context rather than on statistical theory.

For a quantitative classification, the following conditions must be met:

1. *The class intervals must be exactly defined.*
2. *It must be shown how intermediate values have been avoided.* If, for example, in a survey of heights, observers may have measured to the nearest inch, it must be indicated how a height measured as, say, 40.5 in., has been classified.
3. *The class intervals can be specified by the end points or by the midpoints.*
4. *Care should be taken to make the original measurements in the same units used for classification in the table.* Thus if heights are taken to the nearest centimeter and the table has a classification by inches, some 1-in. intervals will include three midpoints of the centimeter classes, others only two. The same type of difficulty arises if we read hemoglobin values as a percentage of a standard but make up the table with grams of hemoglobin. Furthermore, all observers should use the same conventions, such as measuring to the nearest inch, in order to avoid the uncertainty about the

class boundaries that arises if some observers measure to the nearest inch, others to the nearest half-inch.

5. *Class intervals should be equal.* Usually this is practicable, but there may be a long tail, which may necessitate some pooling. Care must be taken in reading such frequency tables, for if classes are pooled, a false impression of increased frequency may be created.

6. *The table should be self-contained, so that it can be understood without reference to the text.* On occasion, it is possible and desirable to add explanatory footnotes.

Similar considerations apply to the classification by several criteria simultaneously to form *contingency tables.*

It should be noted that the marginal numbers do not determine the contents of a two-way table; thus it is necessary to give the whole array or set of entries and not merely the marginal frequencies.

Example   i. Suppose we have a table of two rows and two columns and the total in each row and each column is 10. It is easily shown that the entry in any given cell can take any value, 0, 1, 2, ..., 10; once it is given, however, the whole table is determined for the contents of the other cells can be obtained by subtraction.

The aims of a frequency table are as follows:

1. To summarize material in a minimum of space with minimum of words.

2. To arrange the observations to allow computations, such as the calculation of the mean and, standard deviation, to be readily performed on them. Time is often wasted by carrying out these computations on ungrouped data.

3. To measure correlation or association in contingency tables.

3.   THE CONSTRUCTION OF FREQUENCY AND CONTINGENCY TABLES

Perhaps all the individuals of a population have been measured—for example, we may know the heights of boys aged 4 years in a given area at a specific epoch. It would be possible to record all these heights and present them as a table giving each height. This would be neither economical of space nor informative, since in order to draw conclusions or to make a summary, we would have to read each result and hold it in the mind. The alternative is to classify the heights and record the numbers in each class. Thus the results would look like the following tabulation:

Class (in.)	Number of Boys
35–	1
36–	11
37–	1111
38–	̶H̶H̶ ̶H̶H̶ 11
39–	̶H̶H̶ ̶H̶H̶ ̶H̶H̶ 1
	…

In this table, each stroke represents the presence of one boy in the class. In work of this kind, it is conventional but not essential to record the fifth member of every set of five as a sloping stroke, which facilitates the counting of groups of five. Another method is to type the details of each individual and to cut up the typescript and sort the slips representing individuals. A further elaboration is to record the results on cardboard. In some cases, quite small pieces of 5 × 3 cm will suffice. One-dimensional frequency tables are then readily constructed by a sort, or classification, on a single attribute. Two-dimensional tables can be constructed by subdividing the members in each of the classes, defined by one attribute, by a sorting according to the second attribute. When it is possible to know beforehand what data will be available, specially designed cards can be used. These are very useful if the information is to be punched onto "tape" for feeding into an automatic processing machine.

The design of record cards is often unduly elaborate. Workers who feel that new features will be suggested by the inquiry as it proceeds often allow for all possibilities and thus obtain too much information for processing. Difficulties in interpretation will also be caused if the hypotheses to be tested are not listed beforehand; these difficulties are treated later under the heading of multiple comparisons.

4. NOTES

Norman MacAlister Gregg (1892–1966) was a leading children's opththalmologist in Sydney, Australia. His findings—that many cases of congenital cataract had been caused by rubella infections *in utero*—were given in Gregg (1941) and recalled in Gregg (1956); they caused worldwide interest. However, it was Swan, Tostevin, Moore, Mayo, and Black (1943), who first reported congenital deafness due to maternal rubella; these authors and Gregg (1941) reported congenital heart defects. Previously, rubella had been regarded as an unimportant disease of childhood (Aycocks and Ingalls, 1946). Clinicians had been aware that rubella had died out in Australia in former years, but the importance of this observation had not been realized. We defer to Chapter XVI a full discussion of the epidemiology of deaf-mutism.

Many examples can be found in the medical literature of the efficient display of the results of observations or experiments, the *Observations* of John Graunt (1662) being classical. Of the textbooks, we especially mention Bradford Hill (1961), Mills (1955), and Yule and Kendall (1940 and other editions).

CHAPTER II

The Graphical Representation of Data

1. COORDINATE SYSTEMS

It is necessary first to consider the conventions by which points on a plane can be represented by pairs of numbers, usually pairs of distances or a distance and an angle.

In the commonly used Cartesian system, a point O is taken to be the *origin*, and two *axes* are drawn through it at right angles. These axes are commonly designated $X'OX$ and $Y'OY$. Displacements are measured along the axes from the origin; on the X-axis, the distances from the origin are taken to be positive when measured in the OX direction, and negative in the OX' direction; similarly, distances can be measured on the Y-axis. The position of a general point P in the plane then can be given by a pair of distances; its *coordinates*, to be written (x, y), are obtained by drawing through P straight lines parallel to the axes. A point on the X-axis will have coordinates of the form $(x, 0)$, x being its distance from the origin O, and a point on the Y-axis will have coordinates of the form $(0, y)$.

We now make the convention that all points at a distance x units from the Y-axis are to have the same first coordinate or *abscissa* as the point on the X-axis at a distance x from the origin; furthermore, the second coordinate or *ordinate* is to be set equal to the distance of the point from the X-axis. Thus a general point P is denoted by the pair of coordinates (x, y): x is the *abscissa* and y is the *ordinate* of the point. Given a point P, the coordinates can be determined by drawing lines parallel to the two axes, as in Figure II.1, and measuring the distances along them to the axes.

Conversely, given a pair of coordinates (x, y), a point P is uniquely determined. In one common convention, the positive X-axis is toward the right, the positive Y-axis vertically upward, the negative X-axis to the left, and the negative Y-axis downward. The quadrants are numbered in a counterclockwise direction commencing at the first, for which both coordinates have positive value. The ordinates of points on the X-axis are all zeroes; the abscissas of points on the Y-axis are all zeroes. The origin thus is given by $(0, 0)$. The choice of the scales of measurement are arbitrary. The

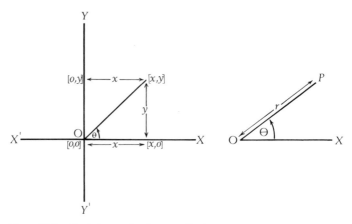

Figure II.1.   Cartesian and polar coordinates.

determination of the coordinates of a point is greatly aided if the paper used is ruled to give a *grid*. The Cartesian system thus uses a rectangular grid.

A second system of coordinates employs the distance from an origin or pole O and an angle measured from a fixed direction. To use this system, we need a bit of elementary trigonometry. Suppose that A, B, and C are the vertices of a triangle, that C is a right angle, and that the lengths of the sides opposite to the vertices are a, b, and c, as in Figure II.2; then we can write

(1) $$c^2 = a^2 + b^2.$$

Suppose now that the angle at the vertex A is θ. We define the sine and the cosine of the angle θ as follows:

(2) $$\sin \theta = \frac{a}{c},$$

$$\cos \theta = \frac{b}{c};$$

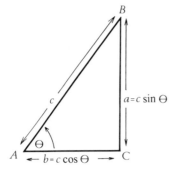

Figure II.2.   Relations in the triangle.

and consequently we have

(3)
$$\cos^2 \theta + \sin^2 \theta = \frac{a^2 + b^2}{c^2} = 1.$$

Hence $\cos \theta$ and $\sin \theta$ are never greater than unity in absolute value. We define

(4)
$$\tan \theta = \frac{a}{b} = \frac{\sin \theta}{\cos \theta}.$$

The definitions for the functions $\sin \theta$, $\cos \theta$, and $\tan \theta$ can be extended for negative values of θ or for values of θ greater than a right angle. We need especially the values of $\tan \theta$ for angles greater than 90° and less than 180°; we can note without proof that

(5)
$$\sin(180° - \theta) = \sin \theta,$$
$$\cos(180° - \theta) = -\cos \theta,$$
$$\tan(180° - \theta) = -\tan \theta.$$

Any point in the plane can now be determined as follows. Let O be chosen as the origin or pole and OX as a fixed direction. If P is any point, P is determined by its distance from the origin and by the angle θ between the lines OP and OX, the angle being measured in a counterclockwise direction. Conversely, given any (r, θ), we can draw a circle of radius r with the origin as center and mark out that radius OP which makes an

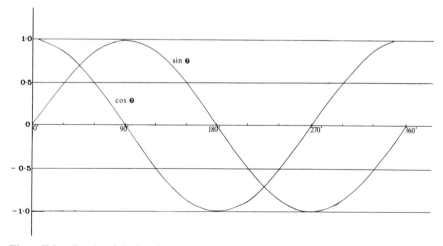

Figure II.3.   Graphs of $\sin \theta$ and $\cos \theta$.

angle θ with the line OX. The coordinates and the polar coordinates of a general point P are related by

$$x = r \cos \theta, \qquad r^2 = x^2 + y^2$$

(6)

$$y = r \sin \theta, \qquad \tan \theta = \frac{y}{x}.$$

We could trace the relation between $\sin \theta$, $\cos \theta$, and θ by the following device. If we put $c = 1$ in Figure II.2, then $a = \sin \theta$ and $b = \cos \theta$. We could then give θ various values and measure off a and b. It is evident that $\sin \theta$ increases and $\cos \theta$ decreases as θ increases from 0 to 90°. We have plotted the relations in Figure II.3.

2. TYPES OF GRAPHICAL REPRESENTATION

The Cartesian system is more commonly used in graphical representation in the form of bar diagrams, histograms, frequency polygons, spot diagrams, and contour diagrams. The polar coordinate system serves in the form of the cyclic diagram and the pie diagrams.

1. **The bar diagram.** The bar graph is useful in plotting values y of the "dependent" variable against the "independent" variable; for example, numbers of deaths y, against the age x years, $x = 0$, 1, 2, ... The convention here is clear—mortality is regarded as depending on age rather than the reverse; on occasion, the distinction between dependent and independent variables is more difficult to make. Bar diagrams are especially appropriate when the variable is qualitative or discrete. One such example is given as Figure II.4, where frequencies of counts of red cells on the hemocytometer are plotted against the count.

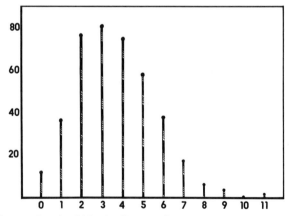

Figure II.4.   Frequencies of red blood cell counts (bar diagram; for numbers see Table I.4).

2. **The histogram.** It may happen that the variable being studied can take any value over a given range; such a variable is said to be continuous. Not all such values can be recorded; thus heights will be measured to the nearest millimeter, to the nearest centimeter, and so on. These measuring rules lead to a number of classes, and the *class frequencies* (i.e., the number of observations within the class), can be displayed as a histogram in which the values of the variable are represented by abscissa. Hence the classes and the number of observations falling into the class are shown by an interval and by an area of a rectangle raised on the interval, respectively. If measurement is to the nearest centimeter, "160 cm" means that the height measured is between 159.5 cm and 160.5 cm. Therefore, if the centimeter is represented by a unit length on the axis, the frequency, y say, is represented by a rectangle y units in height (the horizontal and vertical units chosen may be unequal). It may be desirable to combine or pool classes, say two classes. Suppose the number of observations in those two classes are z_1 and z_2 and their sum is z. Unpooled, the class frequencies are represented by heights of z_1 and z_2 units, respectively; pooled, the combined class frequency is represented by a height of $\frac{1}{2}z = \frac{1}{2}(z_1 + z_2)$ units (see Figure II.5), and the area is z or $z_1 + z_2$, which shows that the representation is consistent. The distributions of heights, weights, and hemoglobin values are appropriately represented by histograms rather than by bars, since the variable in each case is continuous.

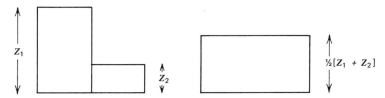

Figure II.5.   Conventions in the histogram. The area, but not the height, remains constant with the pooling of the classes.

3. **The frequency polygon.** A frequency polygon is usually obtained by erecting bars proportional in height to the class frequencies at the centers of the class intervals and then joining the top points. The lines joining the top points constitute the frequency polygon. Alternatively, if we are given a histogram, a frequency polygon is obtained by joining the midpoints of the uppermost side of the rectangles. Although this type of curve is defective from certain points of view, sometimes it is more convenient to compare two frequency distributions by drawing the two frequency polygons, than to erect the sets of bars and to compare their heights.

4. **Spot diagrams.** There are two variables in the spot diagrams, and frequency is indicated by the number of points plotted. For example, we may have observations of heights and weights of adult male Scotsmen, each man being represented by a dot.

5. **Contour diagrams.** If the dots are very numerous in the spot diagrams, it is sometimes convenient to indicate areas of approximately equal density of observations by means of contours.

6. **Cyclic diagrams.** If the time of day or the time of year be considered to be the independent variable, it is sometimes convenient (as in the first case), to plot the hour as the angle and the dependent variable as the radius length, 24 hr being represented by 360° (i.e., 1 hr by 15°). This is especially appropriate for plotting the incidence of births (see Figure II.6) or street accidents against the hour or the incidence of disease against time of year.

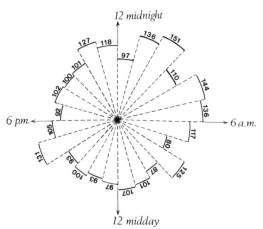

Figure II.6.   Births by hour of day (cyclic diagram). Original data cited in Exercise XII.3.

7. **The pie diagram.** The radius is kept constant in the pie diagram, and the variables considered may be qualitative. The frequency or amount is shown proportional to the angle and thus to the area. The different qualities are indicated by shading or other suitable device. Pie diagrams are useful only in popularizations.

3.   PRINCIPLES FOR THE CONSTRUCTION OF STATISTICAL DIAGRAMS

General principles may be laid down for the construction of diagrams; the first rules apply especially to graphs drawn on a Cartesian grid. The diagram should be readable from left to right, the abscissa should be increasing as a point moves along the axis toward the right, and the ordinate should be increasing as a point moves vertically upward. Wherever practical, the zero line of the vertical scale should be shown. If this is not practical or desirable, however, a convention, such as a break in the diagram, should be used to indicate that the values of the variable are not proportional to the distances vertically as measured from the baseline. The axes, or zero lines, where applicable should be clearly distinguished from other coordinate lines (i.e., other lines on the grid). If time is the independent variable, measured as the abscissa, there will be, of course, no zero line in annual series. Often, however, time zero is defined naturally—as, for example, the time of birth or operation or entry into a clinical trial. If the curve represents a plotting of percentages against time, for example, it is usually desirable to distinguish by heavy ruling the 100% line as well as the zero line. It is advisable not to show more coordinate lines than are necessary to guide the eye. In applied work, as a rule, a diagram is useful in calling to mind general conclusions; it is not used as a source of numerical information, such as is conveyed by a nomograph or a mathematical curve expressing exact relations between two variables such as volume and pressure. The scale of the diagram should be indicated by suitable markings on the axes or at the bottom of the diagram. It may be desirable to include numerical data in the diagram; thus the vertices of a frequency polygon can be distinguished by writing in the coordinate pair having abscissa equal to the value of the independent variable and ordinate equal to the frequency. For example, in a bar diagram showing the number of boys in sibships of eight (see Figure II.7) we have (x, y), where x is the number of boys and y is the frequency of sibships with x boys. If it is not possible to give such numerical data without crowding the diagram, they should be supplied in tables. All lettering and all figures in a diagram should be set to be read from the bottom or from the right-hand side of the page. The title of the diagram should be fully descriptive, and it should be possible to read the diagram without reference to the text. If the data displayed come from another source, this should be noted in the *legend* or in descriptive remarks at the base of the diagram. The legend should include any necessary explanatory material.

If the vertical scale of the grid is *logarithmic*, the positions of the powers of 10 should be clearly displayed and a power of 10 (e.g., 1, 10, 100, ..., should be chosen as the base). (If the vertical scale is logarithmic and the horizontal scale is the usual arithmetic scale, the grid is termed *semilogarithmic*. In such a grid, the value of the variable can be read directly from the vertical scale. Since equal ratios between values of the variables appear as equal differences between the ordinates, these *grids* are sometimes referred to as *ratio charts*.)

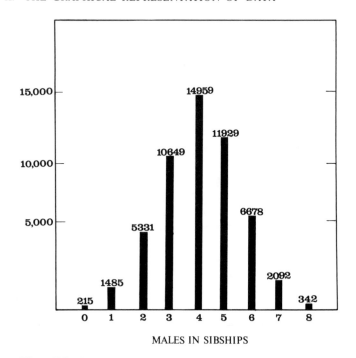

MALES IN SIBSHIPS

Figure II.7.   Sex ratios in sibships (data of Table I.7).

4.   RELATIONS BETWEEN VARIABLES

Any line drawn on a Cartesian graph represents a relation between the coordinates. Let us consider the simplest cases. A straight line through the origin corresponds to the relation (or equation)

(1) $y = mx.$

Let us consider any point P on the line with coordinates x and y, as in Figure II.1. If a perpendicular is dropped onto the X-axis, we have $\tan \theta = y/x$, which is equal to m by (1); therefore, θ is constant for every pair of points (x, y) obeying the equation. The line joining every such point to the origin is thus the same, and the origin itself lies on the line. Conversely, any straight line through the origin can be represented by (1), since for any point (x, y) on the line, $y/x = \tan \theta = m$ (m is usually called the *slope* of the line). If m takes the value zero, y is equal to zero to every value of x; thus the equation $y = 0$ corresponds to the X-axis. Similarly, $x = 0$ corresponds to the Y-axis.

The equation

(2) $y = mx + c$

can be treated similarly. Here $m = (y - c)/x$ is the tangent of the slope of the line passing through the $(0, c)$ and the point (x, y); therefore, every point (x, y) obeying (2) lies on the same straight line. Conversely, every point lying on a line with slope $m = \tan \theta$ which passes through the point $(0, c)$ satisfies (2) (see Figure II.8).

The relation $y = c$ is a straight line parallel to the X-axis, $x = a$ is a straight line parallel to the Y-axis. The slopes of these lines are zero and infinity, respectively. The relation

$$(3) \qquad\qquad ax + by + d = 0$$

is called a *linear equation* in x and y because, if x and y are thought of as lengths, only their linear dimension comes into the equation. For example, if s and e are constants, $x^2 + x + y + s = 0$ is not a linear relation, since x^2 appears in it, moreover, $xy = e$ is not linear, since x^2 and xy correspond

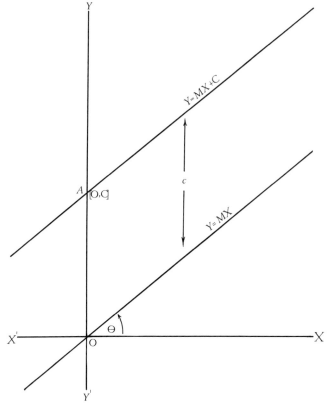

Figure II.8.   A straight line in a Cartesian grid. All lines $y = mx + c$ have the same slope and $\tan \theta = m$. The line OA is the intercept and has length c.

to areas—that is, to the products of linear measurements or lengths. Every linear equation of the form (3) can be brought into the standard form of a linear equations if b is not zero by setting

(4) $$m = -\frac{a}{b} \quad \text{and} \quad c = -\frac{d}{b}.$$

A variable y is said to be a *function* of x if for every value of x there is a rule for determining y. In all applied work, the value of y so determined is unique. In (2) and (3), y is a function of x, and since the equation is linear, y is said to be a *linear function* of x.

If the abscissa x represents time, the graph of a function y plotted against x will show the changes of y with time. Let us imagine two distinct times x_1 and x_2:

(5) $$\frac{\text{increase in } y \text{ from time } x_1 \text{ to time } x_2}{\text{time } x_2 - \text{time } x_1}$$

$$= \frac{y_2 - y_1}{x_2 - x_1} = \frac{mx_2 + c - (mx_1 + c)}{x_2 - x_1}$$

$$= \frac{m(x_2 - x_1)}{x_2 - x_1} = m.$$

Constant slope thus corresponds to constant rate.

In biological applications, the rate of increase often depends on the size. Thus the growth of human or bacterial populations is to be related to the size of the population at the time of measurement. If $f(x)$ is the size of population, we have

(6) $$\frac{f(x + \Delta) - f(x)}{f(x)} \frac{1}{\Delta} = \frac{1}{f(x)} \frac{f(x + \Delta) - f(x)}{\Delta}$$

as the rate of the proportional change in size in a time Δ between times, x and $(x + \Delta)$, per unit of time.

We know from the theory of the calculus that as the time interval Δ becomes small, if the second expression on the right of (6) becomes independent of Δ, it can be written as the differential coefficient. Then the relative rate of increase can be written in the following form:

(7) $$\frac{1}{f(x)} \frac{d}{dx} f(x) = \frac{1}{y} \frac{dy}{dz} = \frac{d}{dx} \log y.$$

It would be convenient to graph y against x in such a way that constant proportional rate of increase corresponds to constant slope. However, this would give us

(8)
$$\frac{1}{y}\frac{dy}{dx} = k,$$

where k is a constant, and the general mathematical theory gives the following solution:

(9)
$$\log y = kx + q.$$

Thus, for the vertical scale, $\log y$ rather than y would be plotted. Grids are readily available commercially from which one can read the actual value, rather than the logarithm, of the independent variable. They are termed *semilogarithmic*. The use of semilogarithmic grids is particularly appropriate in the plotting of population size against time or the mortality rate against age.

EXERCISES

(In later chapters, the exercises provide examples of various computations, such as of the mean and standard deviation, and illustrate other points. There is, therefore, some duplication here.)

1. The heights of 489 girls aged 5 years last birthday were measured to the nearest inch and recorded as follows: 36 in., 1; 37 in., 2; 38 in., 0; 39 in., 12; 40 in., 15; 41 in., 36; 42 in., 90; 43 in., 97; 44 in., 104; 45 in., 68; 46 in., 29; 47 in., 21; 48 in., 9; 49 in., 3; 50 in., 2; 51 in., 0; 52 in., 0; 53 in., 0. Plot the findings as a histogram. Compute the mean height.

2. Heights of 1052 women were recorded to the nearest inch, and the results were recorded for each of the heights 53 in., 54., ..., 70 in., as follows: 2, 1, 2; 6, 18, 35, 80, 135; 163, 183, 163, 115, 78; 41, 16, 8, 4, 2. (These results are given more briefly than those of Exercise 1. The use of the semicolon after frequencies at the 55, 60, 65, and 70 in. enables the student to identify readily the heights corresponding to each frequency.) Construct a histogram and calculate the mean height.

3. The deaths from scarlatina in successive groups of 50 cases were recorded by J. Brownlee, *J. Roy. Sanit. Inst.* (1913), as follows:

1	3	1	2	1	1	0	2	2	2
0	0	3	7	3	2	1	3	1	1
2	3	3	3	2	3	2	0	3	1
0	1	2	2	1	2	4	1	1	2
1	1	1	3	3	3	1	2	4	
3	0	4	3	2	0	4	2	5	
1	2	4	1	3	2	0	0	7	
3	1	1	4	4	6	3	1	4	
3	5	3	3	2	2	3	1	2	
0	4	2	3	1	2	2	1	1	

Form a frequency table from the data, giving the number of groups containing 0, 1, 2, ..., 7 deaths. Compute the mean number of deaths per group of 50 cases, and verify that the mean case fatality for the whole set of cases can be determined.

4. Sedimentation rates of the fall in one hour of the red cell mass were recorded to the nearest millimeter, and the numbers of persons recorded as having falls of 1, 2, 3, ..., were as follows: 206, 488, 446, 236, 138; 69, 49, 27, 29, 24; 12, 5, 4, 2, 6; 4, 3, 4, 3. Total: 1755. Compute the mean fall. Plot the results as a histogram. Data from Walsh et al. (1953).

5. The weights of women in a certain survey were taken to the nearest pound. A frequency table was formed as follows:

Weight (lb)	Number of Women
71–80	1
81–90	35
91–100	248
101–110	654
111–120	1142
121–130	1031
131–140	763
141–150	523
151–160	330
161–170	221
171–180	143
181–190	86
191–200	58
201–210	27
211–220	11
221–230	4
231–240	8

What are the class limits or boundaries between the classes?

6. The heights of boys aged 15.5 years were measured to the nearest inch. The observed frequencies of heights 57, 58, ..., 72 in., were 2, 3, 5, 16; 27, 35, 62, 52, 38; 24, 13, 12, 2, 1; 0, 1, respectively. Calculate the mean.

7. Chest circumferences of Scottish soldiers, measured to the nearest inch, are recorded for 33, 34, ..., 48 in., as follows: 3, 19, 81; 189, 409, 753, 1062, 1082; 935, 646, 313, 168, 50; 18, 3, 1 in. Calculate the mean.

8. The lengths of *Trypanosomes* measured to the nearest micron were 11, 12, ..., 26, and the frequencies of these classes were 32, 103, 239, 624, 1187; 1650, 1883, 1930, 1638, 1130; 737, 427, 221, 110, 57; 32. Calculate the mean.

9. If values depending on time are given for fixed epochs or times, values calculated for intermediate values of the time, variable according to some law, are said to be interpolated. Suppose that at time 1 the value is 4, and at time 5 the value is 64. If the increase per unit of time is constant, the series will be 4, 19, 34, 49, 64. If we assume that the ratio between successive terms is constant, we obtain 4, 8, 16, 32, 64.

Verify that if we interpolate three values between 4 and 64, assuming a uniform increase or constant difference, we obtain the series 4, 19, 34, 49, 64; but if we assume that the ratio between successive terms is constant, we obtain 4, 8, 16, 32, 64. In general, the values interpolated by the ratio method lie below the values obtained by the constant difference method. It can be said that linear interpolation (i.e., by constant difference) gives higher values for mean populations than the more appropriate ratio method. Often, the difference between the results of the two methods is negligible because, for example, populations at say ages, 10–19 years, do not increase very rapidly in the decade between censuses.

NOTES

The principles of the graphical display of data have been set out in the texts of Mills (1935), Arkin and Colton (1940), Schmid (1954), and Brinton (1914, 1939), and by Bradford Hill (1971) in the special medical context.

According to Royston (1956), William Playfair (1759–1823) was the first writer to use graphical methods to display economic or demographic data. Fitzpatrick (1962), Funkhouser (1937), and Funkhouser and Walker (1935) have given excellent historical accounts of the development of graphical methods. An attempt was made in the United States in the early years of this century to lay down standards for the construction of graphs. W. C. Brinton played a leading part in the committees formed (Brinton, 1915).

Graphs can also be used to carry out various computations (e.g., to compute ratios, to estimate surface area, to solve quadratic or other equations); this field of application is called *nomography*, and we refer the reader to Adams (1950), Davis (1962), Levens (1948), and Allcock, Jones, and Michel (1963) for further details.

The theory of the mathematical representation of straight line, circles, or other geometrical figures is treated in the elementary textbooks on the calculus and coordinate geometry.

Besides the theory of the types of graphs already considered, there is now an extensive mathematical discipline, known as graph theory, which treats the configurations obtained by joining points (e.g., network theory in radio or in nervous networks, airline routes, family trees). This theory is finding many applications in other branches of mathematics and in physics and biology, as well.

CHAPTER III

Empirical Frequency Distributions

1. INTRODUCTORY

In Chapter I, we studied a number of samples from (or subsets of) various existent or empirical populations. Here we are considering general properties of such samples and populations, and we use the term, *population* in a wider sense than in common language, in which it refers to a collection of individuals. In statistics, the collection of heights of individuals can be called a "population of heights." Sometimes the populations are existent, as the heights of boys aged 4 years at any given epoch; at other times, the population is potential, as is, for example, the population of blood counts that could be carried out on a given individual.

The frequencies of classes in subsets of the population can be examined; these can be termed *empirical frequency distributions.* If it is possible to examine every member of an actual population and to record the results, the list that is obtained is called a *census.* When it is not practicable or desirable to carry out a census, a *sample survey* is performed, in which only a part of the population is examined.

There are various techniques for making sample surveys in such way that the sample enables good estimates to be obtained of the properties of the parent population. In *simple random sampling,* every combination of individuals of the same size has an equal chance of appearing as the sample. To draw a sample of size n from a population of size N, we proceed as follows. We assign a number 1, 2, ..., N to the individuals in the population and arrange a drawing of n *random sampling numbers* to determine which n of the total population is to enter the sample. These lists of random numbers have been constructed so that there is an equal chance of being drawn for each of the numbers, 1 to 10, 1 to 100, 1 to 1000, ... If $N = 10$, we could number the individuals 1, 2, ..., 10 in any order.

If $n = 2$, we look up a list of random sampling numbers and read, beginning at a predetermined point; when we find that 5 and 8 are to be chosen, we examine the corresponding individuals. If we drew 5, 5, we would continue until we obtained a number different from 5 for the second place.

Similarly, if $N = 100$, we might be given 23, 57, 91, and 04 as our random sampling numbers and the corresponding individuals numbered 4, 23, 57, and 91 form our *sample*.

Once again, repetitions may occur; we accept any number the first time it appears and ignore it at later drawings. For $N = 1000$ we would use random sampling numbers 231, 510, 001, and so on. We interpret 000 as 1000. If N is not a power of 10, it will be not greater than some power of 10 in our tables 10, $10^2 = 100$, $10^3 = 1000$, and so on. If $N > 10^3$, say, but $N < 10^4$, we might select the random sampling numbers in groups of four and ignore any sets of four digits that gave zero or a number greater than N.

In some cases we are interested in how the character $\mathscr{B}$ varies in different classes of the population determined by a criterion $\mathscr{A}$, which might be income or geographical site, for example. We can, therefore, divide the population into *strata* and carry out simple random sampling within the *strata*. Thus the set of N individuals U may have been classified by the criterion $\mathscr{A}$ into classes $A_1, A_2, \ldots, A_m$, $U = A_1 \cup A_2 \cup, \ldots, \cup A_m$, the numbers in the classes being $N_1, N_2, \ldots, N_m$. Samples of sizes $n_1, n_2, \ldots, n_m$ then can be constructed, and these samples can be examined for the criterion $\mathscr{B}$.

Another variation is *cluster sampling*, which is an obvious convenience in sampling households if they are not too far distant from one another. A city can be partitioned into blocks in order to perform a random sampling experiment in which all the blocks have an equal chance of entering the survey. Within the chosen blocks, every household is examined.

Of the other devices or designs that are available for sample surveys of populations, some ensure that a statement can be made about the total population by an examination of a subset of it; however, the probability methods are distinguished from all others by the following properties: (1) they are *unbiased* in the sense that if the procedure were repeatedly carried out, the overall mean would approximate to the true mean; and (2) a statement can be made about their accuracy (e.g., how the estimated values would cluster about the true values).

Example i. The blood-type gene frequencies are of importance in the study of human origins. Most gene frequency estimates have been made on volunteer blood donors or recruits to the army or to industry. This is not a probability sampling method; usually it has been assumed, probably with truth, that the donors do represent the population adequately.

Example ii. If the tuberculosis rate is estimated in a population by means of a survey for which individuals volunteer, a biased view may well result because of a tendency for the relatives of people who have the disease to volunteer.

Example   iii. Although it is obviously possible to measure the heights of school children, such means have usually been found to be unreliable for the first year of school life. This is because the better developed children are more likely to be sent to school at relatively earlier ages.

2. CUMULATIVE FREQUENCY DISTRIBUTIONS

In the consideration of a population of measurements, we shall usually expect to know something about typical values or *centers of location* and about the variation of the individuals around the typical values. This variation can be measured by *measures of dispersion*. We proceed now to describe centers of location and measures of dispersion, after a brief description of the cumulative frequencies.

Table I.5 presents a frequency distribution of the numbers of individuals in the sample who have given heights or heights within given ranges.

Table III.1

CUMULATIVE FREQUENCIES OF HEIGHTS
OF BOYS

Heights (in.)	Cumulative[a] Frequencies of Boys
34.875	0
35.875	1
36.875	3
37.875	7
38.875	19
39.875	35
40.875	74
41.875	125
42.875	178
43.875	201
44.875	212
45.875	220
46.875	221
49.875	222

[a] By definition, the cumulative frequency is the number of boys whose heights do not exceed the stated values (34.875 in., etc.).

Equally well, the numbers of individuals whose height is not greater than certain values could have been given. We note that no individual has a height less than 34.875 in., one has a height less than 35.875 in., three have a height less than 36.975 in., seven have a height less than 37.875 in., and so on. These cumulative frequencies are simply the sums, $1 = 1$, $1 + 2 = 3$, $1 + 2 + 4 = 7$, $1 + 2 + 4 + 12 = 19$, and so on (see Table III.1). Similarly from Table I.4 the cumulative frequencies for the counts of 0, 1, 2, 3, ..., are 11, 47, 123, 203, 277, 335, 373, 390, 396, 399, 399, and 400; 11 squares have a zero count, 47 have a count not greater than 1, 123 have a count not more than 2, and so on. The cumulative frequencies can be written in the form

(1) $$F_0 = f_0, F_1 = f_0 + f_1, F_2 = f_0 + f_1 + f_2, \ldots$$

It is evident also that

(2) $$f_0 = F_0, f_1 = F_1 - F_0, f_2 = F_2 - F_1, \ldots$$

The cumulative frequency may be plotted against the values of the variable, as in Figure III.1, where we have plotted the cumulative frequencies of the

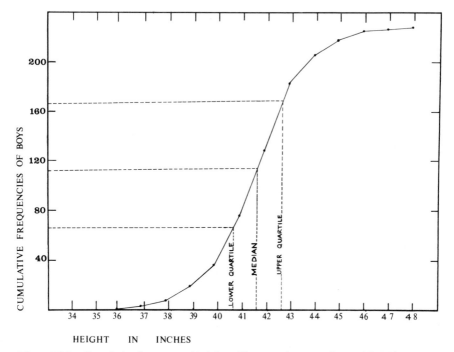

Figure III.1.   Cumulative frequency of heights of boys aged 4 years. (See Table I.5.)

heights of boys against the height. As an approximation, it is customary to treat the heights as if they occurred equally spaced between the two end points of the class interval, and this is equivalent to joining the successive points (x, F_x) and $(x + 1, F_{x+1})$ by a straight line in each case. Now the increase between x and $x + 1$ is equal to $F_{x+1} - F_x = f_{x+1}$; thus the slope of the cumulative frequency curve is equal to the class frequency.

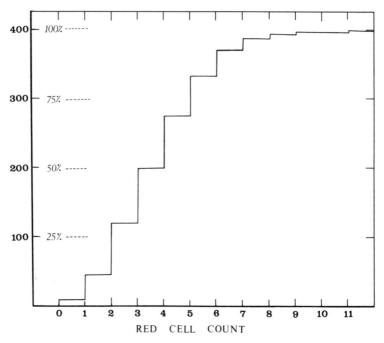

Figure III.2. Cumulative frequencies of red blood cell counts per hemocytometer square. (See Fig. II.4 and Table I.4.)

The cumulative frequency curves are always nondecreasing in height as we pass in the positive direction. At first the curve is rather flat, next the slope usually increases to a maximum corresponding to the mode. Ultimately the slope decreases, the curve finally becoming flat when all the frequency is exhausted; it is often said that the curve is S-shaped or *sigmoid*. If the variable is discrete, the curve has a staircase appearance, characterized by jumps equal to the frequencies at certain points, although there is no increase between these discrete points. This is evident in Figure III.2, where the cumulative frequencies of Table I.4 are plotted.

3. THE MODE

The *mode* is defined as the most numerous class in a frequency distribution. Thus in the frequency distribution of Table I.4 of counts over the 400 squares of a hemocytometer, the commonest count is 3 cells, 80 squares having this count; 76 squares have a count of 2 cells and 74 a count of 4 cells. By definition, in this observed or empirical distribution, the mode is 3 cells per hemocytometer square. Since the modal frequency is only slightly greater than the two other neighboring frequencies, we should not be surprised to obtain a mode of 2 or 4, in another sample. Similarly, in the heights of boys, we find in Table I.5, a mode in the 42-in. class. If the data of Table I.5 or similar data are plotted in the form of a histogram, the mode can be identified as the class with the greatest height. If the number of observations were very large, the class intervals could be made shorter, and finally we could refer to the midpoint of the modal class as the mode, without appreciable error. Since very large numbers of observations are required for such an argument to be valid, the mode is little used in practice. In using the foregoing argument on finer subclassifications, we have made assumptions that appear to be true for many types of biological measurements; namely, that samples behave as if they were elements of a very large population in which the numbers falling into fine classes behave in a regular manner (i.e., the numbers in the classes do not "jump about," or $f_x, f_{x+1}, f_{x+2}, \ldots$, form an orderly sequence). In fact, it seems to be almost the rule that f begins at zero, increases to a mode, and decreases regularly to zero. Usually, this is assumed when the term "continuous variable" is used. If an observed distribution has more than one mode or more than one class, more numerous than its neighbors, a *mixture* of distributions is usually suspected.

4. EXTREME VALUES AND THE RANGE

The largest and smallest values in a population might be taken as indicating the location of the populations (i.e., of the size of a typical member). For example, we might give the heights of the tallest and the shortest members of the population of Scotland and compare these heights with those of the tallest and shortest in England in order to compare the general populations of heights. Experience suggests that such *extreme values* may not be characteristic of the population and that they are subject to chance variations that are not sufficiently reduced by taking large samples. The difference between the greatest and least is known as the *range*. The extreme values and the range are of limited value in describing populations.

5. THE MEDIAN AND OTHER ORDER STATISTICS

The *median* is the "middle" value of the variable; we can better define it as the value assumed by the middle observation or individual when the individuals are ranked. Thus if there is an odd number of members $(2m + 1)$ in the population and if the members are arranged in increasing order of magnitude of the variable, the $(m + 1)$th member clearly has m members with a smaller value and m with a larger value. If there are $2m$ members in the population, it is conventional to take a point midway between the mth value and the $(m + 1)$th as the median value. There may be more than one member with the median value. Thus in the blood counting example, all members from the 114th to the 203rd have the same value, namely, three cells. If the distribution is given as a graph in the cumulative frequency form, the computation of the median is simple. A horizontal line is drawn midway between the total height and the base, and from the point at which it meets the cumulative curve, a perpendicular is dropped to a point or *foot* on the base-line. This point is the median, since half the members have a value less than that represented by the foot of the perpendicular. We can generalize the notion of a median to a *percentile* or *quantile*. The p *percentile* is defined to be that value of the variable such that exactly $p\%$ of the members have values less than it. The 50 percentile is the median. The 25 percentile is the *lower quartile*. The 75 percentile is the *upper quartile*. The quartiles and other order statistics can also be determined as the abscissa of the point at which the cumulative curve attains 25% of its total height 75%, ... The difference between the upper and lower quartiles is the *interquartile range*; half this distance—the *semiinterquartile range*—is often used as a measure of dispersion.

6. THE ARITHMETIC MEAN OR AVERAGE

If we have N observations $x_1, x_2, \ldots, x_N$, the *arithmetic mean* or, more simply, the *mean*, is defined as

$$(1) \qquad \bar{x} = \frac{x_1 + x_2 + \cdots + x_N}{N},$$

where the mean is indicated by a bar above the letter used for the observations (a common statistical convention). The mean can be computed as implied by (1), but often the data have been or can be grouped; in such cases, it is necessary only to multiply the number in each class by the typical measurement of the class and sum. Often a simplification of the arithmetic is possible. From (1) we can write

(2)
$$\bar{x} = a + \frac{(x_1 - a) + (x_2 - a) + \cdots + (x_N - a)}{N}$$

and the numbers $(x_1 - a)$, $(x_2 - a)$, may be quite small numbers and easy to manipulate. In (2), a is said to be an *arbitrary origin*, in contrast to the "natural" origin at zero. A combination of grouping and the use of the arbitrary origin may greatly simplify the arithmetic.

Example i. Four red blood cell counts on the same subject have yielded 530, 538, 512, and 519. The total is 2099 for the four counts, and the mean is $2099/4 = 524.75$. Suppose we take the arbitary origin to be 520; the distances of the counts from the arbitrary origin are $+10$, $+18$, -8, and -1, a total of 19. We also have $19/4 = 4.75$, and once again the mean $= 520 + 4.75 = 524.75$.

Example ii. We show in Table III.2 the computation of the mean, in microns, of the lengths of *Trypanosomes*. Since the original measurements were made "to the nearest micron," 12 means 11.5 to 12.5. The class "12, 13" contains individuals measured as 12 and as 13 μ. This combined class, therefore, covers the interval 11.5 to 13.5, and the midpoint is 12.5 μ. The arbitrary origin, which is taken to be the midpoint of the class 22, 23, is thus 22.5 μ. The working unit is 2 μ. The classes (24, 25), (26, 27) are then scored as $+1$ and $+2$ working units from the arbitary origin; (20, 21) is scored as -1, (18, 19), as -2, and so on. Our computations are now all in working units until the final step is reached. The table gives the class in the first column, the frequency f_x in the second, the distance x from the arbitrary origin in the third, the product xf_x in the fourth, and finally the $(x + 1)$ in the fifth column and the product $(x + 1)f_{x+1}$ in the sixth column. Since $f_x + xf_x = (x + 1)f_x$, the total of the sixth column is equal to the sum of the totals for the second and fourth columns. The total of the frequencies is obtained by simple addition. In the fourth and sixth columns, the totals of the negative and positive quantities have been taken separately, and the total has been determined by subtracting the sum of the negative entries from the sum of the positive entries. The check is $1000 + 291 = 1291$. A feature of this check is that the actual arithmetic details are different in obtaining the two sums. If the totals cannot be so reconciled, the same check can be applied to each row until the error is determined. A general formula for the computation of the mean is as follows:

true mean $=$ (arbitrary origin) $+$ (mean of the deviations) $\times$ (scale factor). Therefore, the mean length of the *Trypanosomes* is $22.5 + 0.291 \times 2 = 23.082$ μ.

Table III.2

CALCULATION OF THE ARITHMETIC MEAN

Lengths[a] of Trypanosomes (μ)	Frequency, f_x	Distance x from Arbitrary Origin (working units)	Product xf_x	$x + 1$	Product $(x + 1)f_x$
12, 13	9	−5	−45	−4	−36
14, 15	38	−4	−152	−3	−114
16, 17	83	−3	−249	−2	−166
18, 19	134	−2	−268	−1	−134
20, 21	134	−1	−134	0	0
22, 23	127	0	0	1	127
24, 25	135	1	135	2	270
26, 27	140	2	280	3	420
28, 29	112	3	336	4	448
30, 31	60	4	240	5	300
32, 33	22	5	110	6	132
34, 35	4	6	24	7	28
36, 37	2	7	14	8	16
Totals	1000	—	−848		−450
			+1139		1741
			291		1291

[a] Data from K. Pearson, *Biometrika*, **10** (1914), 129.
[a] Measurements are to the nearest micron. Classes have been pooled so that 12, 13 includes all these measurements from 11.5 to 13.5 and the midpoint of the class is 12.5. The working units are 2 μ.

Working mean = 0.291 workings units = 0.582 μ from arbitrary origin.

Mean = 22.5 + 0.582 = 23.082 μ.

Check. $1291 = \sum (x + 1)f_x = \sum xf_x + \sum f_x = 291 + 1000 = 1291$.

7. THE HARMONIC AND GEOMETRIC MEANS

The *harmonic mean* is the reciprocal of the mean of the reciprocals. It is defined by

(1)
$$H = \frac{N}{1/x_1 + 1/x_2 + \cdots + 1/x_N},$$

where x_1, x_2, ..., x_N are the N values in the population and H is the harmonic mean. The harmonic mean cannot be defined if any x_i is zero.

The *geometric mean*, the Nth root of the product of the N values, is given by

(2) $$G = (x_1 x_2 \cdots x_N)^{1/N}.$$

If all the observations are positive, G cannot exceed the arithmetic mean $\bar{x} = \sum x_i/N$. The geometric mean is zero if any x_i is zero. We can rewrite (2) as follows:

(3) $$\log G = \frac{\log x_1 + \log x_2 + \cdots + \log x_N}{N},$$

and

(4) $$G = \text{antilog} \frac{\sum \log x_i}{N}.$$

8. DISPERSION MEASURED BY ORDER STATISTICS

The *range* (i.e., the difference between greatest and least) is a possible measure of the dispersion. Range is usually rejected on mathematical grounds, because it takes insufficient notice of the great bulk of the observations in most distributions. On biological grounds, it is unsatisfactory because the extreme observations are often abnormal; for example, sporadic cases of dwarfism and gigantism would interfere with estimates of the dispersion of heights based on the extreme values. Rather more satisfactory is the semi-interquartile range mentioned in Section III.5. The *semiinterquartile* range is very close in most common continuous distributions to the *probable error*, which is defined as the distance from the mean that divides the distribution into two equal parts. In fact, the only distinction between them arises because in the distribution the mean may not coincide with the median.

9. THE MEAN DEVIATION

It might be thought that the deviations about the mean would give a simple measure of dispersion; however, if x_1, x_2, ..., x_N are the observations with mean $\bar{x}$ the sum of the deviations is

$$(x_1 - \bar{x}) + (x_2 - \bar{x}) + \cdots + (x_N - \bar{x}) = x_1 + x_2 + \cdots + x_N - N\bar{x} = 0,$$

from the definition of the mean; and this will hold for every population. To avoid this difficulty, the deviations can always be taken with the positive sign and averaged; thus we have

(1) $$\text{mean deviation} = \frac{|x_1 - \bar{x}| + |x_2 - \bar{x}| + \cdots + |x_N - \bar{x}|}{N},$$

where the enclosure of an expression in vertical bars is to be read as *the absolute value* of the expression. Thus if a is a positive number, $|a| = a$ and $|-a| = a$ (e.g., $|3| = 3$ and $|-3| = 3$). The *mean deviation* is a good measure of dispersion, which has a clear intuitive meaning; but the presence of the "absolute signs" leads to difficulties in the mathematical analysis of distributions. An alternative device, which abolishes the negative signs, is the taking of squares, since b^2 is zero or positive for every real quantity b; or, more briefly, b^2 is *nonnegative* for every real quantity b. This leads us to the most important measure of dispersion, the *standard deviation*. Let us note here the equivalence of the words *deviation* and *error* in statistical theory. "Error" was a term introduced from astronomy, when astronomers were making many readings on the position of a star, and these readings were not all the same. In general, an astronomer would prefer the mean of the observations as closest to the true value of the position. Then, of course, the deviations could be thought of as errors. The biologist is in a different position. If he is examining a population of *Trypanosomes* or human femora, he does not expect every length to be the same. He is thinking of deviations about some center of location for the lengths.

10.   THE STANDARD DEVIATION AND VARIANCE

The *variance* of N observations is defined by

$$(1) \qquad V = \frac{(x_1 - \bar{x})^2 + (x_2 - \bar{x})^2 + \cdots + (x_N - \bar{x})^2}{N - 1}.$$

It is advisable to use $N - 1$ as the divisor in (1), although the divisor N would be appropriate in theoretically given distributions. In elementary work, and especially when V is being estimated from the observations, $N - 1$ is always to be preferred.

The *standard deviation* s of a set of N observations is defined to be the square root of the variance; thus we have

$$(2) \qquad s = \sqrt{V}, \qquad s^2 = V.$$

The standard deviation is found in practice to be the most useful measure of dispersion.

The proportion of observations more distant from the mean than k standard deviations (k s.d.) is at most equal to $= 1/k^2$, since each observation more than k standard deviations contributes at least $(k \text{ s.d.})^2$ to the sum in (1). If more than N/k^2 were at such distances, the sum in the numerator would exceed $N/k^2 \times (k \text{ s.d.})^2$, and $V > 1$, which would falsify the arithmetic already carried out. However, stricter inequalities than this are possible in theoretically given distributions. In empirical distributions of not more than a few thousand observations, almost all the observations fall within a range of 6 s.d., and this is a useful check on arithmetical computations.

Equation 1 is not convenient for computation. Therefore, let us derive some equivalent formulas.

$$(2) \qquad \sum (x_i - \bar{x})^2 = \sum x_i^2 - \bar{x} \sum x_i = \sum x_i^2 - \frac{(\sum x_i)^2}{N}.$$

For proof, we could write the sum on the left as

$$x_1^2 - 2x_1\bar{x} + \bar{x}^2 + x_2^2 - 2x_2\bar{x} + \bar{x}^2 + \cdots + x_N^2 - 2x_N\bar{x} + \bar{x}^2$$
$$= x_1^2 + x_2^2 + \cdots + x_N^2 - 2\bar{x}x_1 - 2\bar{x}x_2 - \cdots - 2\bar{x}x_N + \bar{x}^2 + \bar{x}^2$$
$$+ \cdots + \bar{x}^2$$
$$= \sum x_i^2 - 2\bar{x} \sum x_i + N\bar{x}^2 = \sum x_i^2 - 2\bar{x} \sum x_i + \bar{x} \sum x_i$$
$$= \sum x_i^2 - \bar{x} \sum x_i,$$

which yields the second expression in (2). This in turn yields the final expression of (2) if we replace $\bar{x}$ by $\sum x_i/N$.

Example i. Suppose we have counts of 18, 18, 22, 11, 17, 19; $N = 6$; $\sum x_i = 18 + 18 + 22 + 11 + 17 + 19 = 105$; $\sum x_i^2 = 324 + 324 + 484 + 121 + 289 + 361 = 1903$; $\bar{x} = \sum x_i/6 = 17.5$; $\sum (x_i - \bar{x})^2 = 1903 - 1837.5 = 65.5$, where $1837.5 = 17.5 \times 105$, $V =$ variance $= 65.5/5 = 13.1$; standard deviation (s.d.) $= \sqrt{V} = \sqrt{13.1} = 3.62$.

We could carry out this computation also by considering the deviations y_i from 20, namely, $-2, -2, +2, -9, -3, -1$; $N = 6$; $\sum y_i = -15$; $\sum y_i^2 = 4 + 4 + 4 + 81 + 9 + 1 = 103$; $\sum (y_i - \bar{y})^2 = 103 - (-15)^2/6 = 103 - 37.5 = 65.5$, as before. Indeed, it is obvious that if $y_i = x_i - 20$, $\bar{y} = \bar{x} - 20$, and $(y_i - \bar{y}) = (x_i - \bar{x})$. If many of the x's coincide, the computation of (2) can be considerably shortened. Let us suppose that the x's take values $z_1, z_2, z_3, \ldots, z_m$, with frequencies $f_1, f_2, \ldots, f_m$. Then

$$\sum x_i^2 = x_1^2 + x_2^2 + \cdots + x_N^2 = f_1 z_1^2 + f_2 z_2^2 + \cdots + f_m z_m^2$$

and

$$\sum_{i=1}^{i=N} x_i = f_1 z_1 + f_2 z_2 + \cdots + f_m z_m = \sum_{k=1}^{k=m} f_k z_k,$$

for in both these summations, instead of adding all x's that take the same value z, we need merely to multiply the value z by the frequency with which it occurs. The same applies to the summation of the values of z^2.

An extension of this method serves in the computation of the means and standard deviation of heights, whereby the heights are grouped into classes and all the observations in a class are treated as if they possessed the central value of the class. The mean of the *Trypanosomes* was computed on this principle in Table III.2.

Example   ii. The standard deviation of the lengths of *Trypanosomes* is computed in Table III.3. For brevity, we have omitted the original class titles that appear as the first column of Table III.2.

Table III.3[a]

CALCULATION OF THE STANDARD DEVIATION

Frequency	Distance x from Arbitrary Origin (working units)	Computation and Checks				
		xf_x	x^2f_x	$x + 1$	$(x + 1)f_x$	$(x + 1)^2f_x$
9	−5	−45	225	−4		144
38	−4	−152	608	−3	−114	342
83	−3	−249	747	−2	−166	332
134	−2	−268	536	−1	−134	134
134	−1	−134	134	0	0	0
127	0	0	0	1	127	127
135	1	135	135	2	270	540
140	2	280	560	3	420	1260
112	3	336	1008	4	448	1792
60	4	240	960	5	300	1500
22	5	110	550	6	132	792
4	6	24	144	7	28	196
2	7	14	98	8	16	128
1000	—	−848	5705	—	−450	7287
		+1139			1741	
		291			1291	

[a] Additional details in Table III.2.

Checks: $1291 = \sum (x + 1)f_x = \sum xf_x + \sum f_x = 291 + 1000 = 1291$
$7287 = \sum (x + 1)^2f_x = \sum x^2f_x + 2 \sum xf_x + \sum f_x = 5705$
$+ 582 + 1000 = 7287.$

11. SOME MISCELLANEOUS PROPERTIES OF EMPIRICAL DISTRIBUTIONS

In elementary work and also in much applied work, the properties of empirical distributions are summarized adequately by the descriptive measures already mentioned in this chapter. For completeness, we add a few more.

The rth *moment about the origin* is defined by

$$(1) \qquad \mu_r' = \sum_{i=1}^{N} \frac{x_i^r}{N} = \sum_{j=1}^{m} \frac{z_j^r f_j}{N},$$

where we have used the convention that if the x's are not all distinct, they take values $z_1, z_2, \ldots, z_m$, having frequencies $f_1, f_2, \ldots, f_m$. The rth *moment about the mean* μ_r is defined by

$$(2) \qquad \mu_r = \sum_{i=1}^{N} \frac{(x_i - \bar{x})^r}{N} = \sum_{j=1}^{m} \frac{(z_j - \bar{z})^r f_j}{N},$$

in which the moments about the origin are written with a prime, those about the mean without a prime (another common statistical convention). We may notice that μ_2 is defined with divisor N, rather than $N - 1$, as in our previous definition of the variance. The computations of the moments can be carried through as in Tables III.2 and III.3 for grouped or ungrouped data.

The *coefficient of variation* is defined as the ratio of the standard deviation to the mean, expressed as a percentage. It has relevance only for positive quantities. For example, we might ask whether the lengths of elephants are more variable than the lengths of mice, and it seems reasonable to reduce the variability to a dimensionless number by dividing the standard deviation by the mean. It may be noted that the coefficient of variation has a close relationship to the standard deviation of the logarithm of the variable.

1. Use a table of random sampling numbers in the following applications:

(a) To give a sample of 5 from a population of 100.
(b) To give a sample of 5 from a population of 50.
(c) To give a sample of 5 from a population of 1500.

2. A population of 1000 is divided into three strata of 100, 300, and 600. Draw a sample of 5% in the first stratum, 2% in the second stratum, and 1% in the third stratum, with the aid of random sampling numbers.

3. Suppose that clusters are formed of groups of five individuals, numbered 1, 2, 3, 4, 5; 6, 7, 8, 9, 10; ...; 96, 97, 98, 99, 100, and so on. Draw a set of four clusters by the use of random sampling numbers and write down the individuals which are contained in them. (*Hint.* Number the clusters 1, 2, ..., 20 and draw a set of four of these. Cluster 1 contains 1, 2, 3, 4 and 5; cluster 7 contains 31, 32, 33, 34, and 35, and so on.) This example imitates the procedure of sampling city blocks with five houses to the block. There would be less travel in collecting information from individuals in blocks than there would be with simple random sampling.

4. Draw cumulative frequency curves of some of the distributions of Exercises 1, 2, 5, 6, 7, and 8 of Chapter II. Mark off the median (50% point) and the upper and lower quartiles (75 and 25% points).

5. Determine the extreme values and the ranges of the distributions mentioned in Exercise 4. If there is an open-ended terminal class in cases of the other class intervals all having been the same length, it seems reasonable to score the extreme value as though it was at one-half a class interval from the inner boundary of the terminal class.

6. Verify that the range is approximately 6 s.d. for distributions for which you have computed both range and s.d.

7. Determine the median of the observations 11, 15, 17, 18, 19, 25, and 27 cm. Determine the median of 11, 15, 17, 18, 19, and 31 cm.

8. Give examples to show that the median is unaffected by adding any quantity onto the terminal values in a series of readings.

9. Compute the median for the observations of Table III.1. (Since there are 222 observations, we must take the mean of the 111th and 112th observations.) We find that 74 readings are less than 40.875 in. and 125 readings are less than 41.875 in. Assume that the observations are equally spaced from 40.875 to 41.875 in. and find the position of observation 111.5 (i.e., the mean of the 111th and 112th observations) as $40.875 + (111.5 - 74)/(125 - 74)$ in.

10. If there are m objects in one class with a mean of A and n objects in a second class with a mean of B, prove that the mean of the $N = m + n$ objects is $(mA + nB)/N$. More generally, if there are n_j objects in the jth class, where the mean is A_j and $n_1 + n_2 + \cdots + n_k = N$, the mean of the N objects is given by $(n_1 A_1 + n_2 A_2 + \cdots + n_k A_k)/N$.

11. The frequencies of trypanosomes of *Glossina morsitans* having lengths (to the nearest micron) of 15, 16, 17, ..., 35 μ were as follows: 6; 4, 27, 57, 94, 49; 37, 22, 14, 13, 11; 19, 25, 23, 29, 27; 18, 13, 7, 3, 2. Draw a histogram of this distribution and note that there are well developed modes at 19 and 29 μ. [Data of Sir David Bruce cited by K. Pearson, *Biometrika*, **10** (1914–1915), 85–143.]

12. Define the mean, mode, and median of a distribution, and the variance, the standard deviation, and the semiinterquartile range. If you were requested to describe the heights of boys aged 9 years, what procedures would you adopt and

what measures would you compute to indicate the general location and spread of the heights? What difficulty would you meet if you used institutional data to measure the growth rate of boys (e.g., if you collected data on the heights of boys of varying age at a point of time)?

NOTES

Cumulative frequency curves deserve more frequent use than they obtain.

In some empirical distributions, such as the distribution of cloud cover, measured as the proportion of time in which the sun is obscured by cloud, there are two modes, which appear at or near 0 and 1.

In a wide class of distributions, the mean, median, and mode appear in that order, and the following equation holds approximately

$$2(\text{median} - \text{mean}) = \text{mode} - \text{median}.$$

In symmetrical distributions, the mean is equal to the median, and this common value usually coincides with the mode.

The mean deviation is often defined as the mean of the absolute deviations from the median. This mean deviation measured from the median is less than the mean deviation measured from any other point.

Standard deviation and standard error are synonymous terms. However, standard error is often used as a shortened statement of "standard error of the mean," and care must be taken to ascertain from the context which is the usage.

In calculations using an arbitrary origin, all the computations should be carried through in arbitrary or working units until the standard deviation has been obtained.

CHAPTER IV

Sampling Distributions

1. INTRODUCTORY

In Chapter III, we described the properties of empirical distributions as given. When considering the mathematical models that give rise to observed distributions, we must develop some elementary probability theory, emphasizing probabilities defined for discrete values of the variable.

2. PERMUTATIONS

For any positive integer n, we define

$$(1) \qquad n! = 1.\,2.\,3.\,\ldots.\,n$$

where $n!$ is to be read as *factorial n*. The function factorial n obeys a recurrence formula,

$$(2) \qquad (n+1)! = (n+1)n!,$$

which follows easily from the definition, since $(n + 1)! = 1.\,2.\,\ldots.\,n.$ $(n + 1) = n!\,(n + 1)$, as required in the formula. The relation $1! = 1 \cdot 0!$ appears in a natural way in some formulas (given later), and it is convenient to note that (2) suggests that $0!$ should be set equal to 1, since $1! = 1 \cdot 0!$.

Suppose there are n distinguishable objects, labeled 1, 2, 3, ..., n. Then any arrangement of r of the objects is an *r-permutation* of them. Thus we can place r of the objects in r places numbered 1, 2, ..., r, $r \leq n$. The number of ways this can be done is written ^nP_r, and we can also write $^nP_1 = n$, since if there are n objects, any one of them can be arranged in a single position; there are precisely n possibilities. If there are two positions to be filled, the first object can be chosen in n ways and then, corresponding to each choice, the second position can be filled in $n - 1$ ways. Thus we have $^nP_2 = n(n - 1)$. This process can be continued; after k places have been filled, there remain $n - k$ objects, and any one of these can be chosen, giving

$$(3) \qquad ^nP_{k+1} = (n-k)\,{}^nP_k.$$

Applying this formula and beginning with the known $^nP_1 = n$, we obtain $^nP_2 = (n - 1)^nP_1 = n(n - 1)$, $^nP_3 = (n - 2)^nP_2 = n(n - 1)(n - 2)$ and generally

(4)
$$^nP_r = n(n - 1)(n - 2) \cdots (n - r + 1)$$

$$= \frac{n!}{(n - r)!}$$

In particular, $^nP_n = n!$. Many authors restrict the use of the term *permutation* to arrangements of all n objects. In all other cases, the phrases 1-permutations, 2-permutations, ..., r-permutations, ... are used.

Example. The 2-permutations of ABC are AB, AC, BA, BC, CA, and CB.

Permutations are frequently encountered. Thus in testing the palatability of food, in measuring the intensity of pain, and in attempting to ascertain many other qualities of objects presented to a judge, the judge may be able to arrange his preferences in order without being able to grade them quantitatively. If n objects are presented to the judge and he records his preferences in a form of the style 4132, he has given a permutation. Another judge gives an order of preference 4123. The consistency of such orderings by the judges is a test of whether the judges are measuring on objective standards. The measurement of the consistency of such orderings is sometimes carried out by the *rank correlation coefficient*.

3. COMBINATIONS

An *r-combination* is a choice of r objects from among n distinguishable objects. This is typified by the choice of r of n numbered balls from an urn and the placing of them in a bag in which there is no ordering of the balls.

Example. The 2-combinations of ABC are AB, AC, and BC. To every r-combination of n objects, there correspond precisely $r!$ r-permutations of the n objects. For if we choose our r-combination, the objects in it can be ordered in $r!$ ways to give $r!$ distinct permutations. Conversely, all r-permutations can be grouped in classes, each class containing a particular r-combination of the objects, and the objects being ordered in all possible $r!$ ways.

Hence we can write

(1)
$$^nP_r = r!\,^nC_r$$

(2)
$$^nC_r = \frac{^nP_r}{r!} = \frac{n!}{[r!\,(n - r)!]}.$$

From (2) it follows that

(3) $$^nC_r = {}^nC_{n-r}.$$

It is otherwise evident that to every r-combination taken from a set of n objects, there corresponds an $(n - r)$-combination of those objects remaining. Note that $^nC_n = 1$, since the whole set of n objects can be selected in only one way. We define $^nC_0 = 1$. (There is, indeed, only one way of not selecting any object.) The symbols ^nC_r obey the following *recurrence relation*:

(4) $$^{n+1}C_r = {}^nC_r + {}^nC_{r-1},$$

for the r-combinations of $n + 1$ objects can be divided into two classes— those which do not contain a given object, b say, and those which do. The first class contains ^nC_r, since they are r-combinations of the n objects not containing b. The second class consists of all those r-combinations which contain b and to which have been added $r - 1$ of the remaining n objects. We can now calculate all the numbers of combinations using the recurrence formula (4) as in Table IV.1. The first column consists of units, since $^nC_0 = 1$. In addition, $^1C_1 = 1$. Every other entry is now made by adding the element immediately above to the element above and one step to the left. Thus $^2C_1 = 1 + 1 = 2$; $^5C_2 = 6 + 4 = 10$, and so on. The array of numbers is usually referred to as Pascal's triangle (see Section IV.4).

Table IV.1

TABLE OF COMBINATIONS (PASCAL'S TRIANGLE)

Number of Distinguishable Objects, n	Number of r-Combinations of n Distinguishable Objects, ^nC_r for Eight Values of r							
	0	1	2	3	4	5	6	7
1	1	1						
2	1	2	1					
3	1	3	3	1				
4	1	4	6	4	1			
5	1	5	10	10	5	1		
6	1	6	15	20	15	6	1	
7	1	7	21	35	35	21	7	1

4. THE BINOMIAL THEOREM

We call $(a + b)$ a binomial expression because it contains precisely two terms. We wish to express the *powers of* $(a + b)$, namely, $(a + b)^n$, in terms of the powers of a and b and their products. We note that

(1) $(a + b)^1 = a + b,$ by definition;

(2) $(a + b)^2 = a^2 + 2ab + b^2,$

since we can carry out the multiplication in an elementary way

$$
\begin{array}{l}
a + b \\
a + b \\
\hline
a^2 + ab \\
 + ba + b^2 \\
\hline
a^2 + 2ab + b^2.
\end{array}
$$

We see that (1) and (2) can be rewritten as

(3) $(a + b)^1 = a + b = {}^1C_1 a + {}^1C_0 b$

and

(4) $(a + b)^2 = a^2 + 2ab + b^2 = {}^2C_2 a^2 + {}^2C_1 ab + {}^2C_0 b^2,$

respectively. Equations 3 and 4 can be generalized as a theorem.

Binomial theorem.

(5) $(a + b)^n = {}^nC_n a^n b^0 + {}^nC_{n-1} a^{n-1} b + \cdots + {}^nC_0 a^0 b^n,$ $a^0 = 1 = b^0$

with the general term ${}^nC_k a^{n-k} b^k.$

Proof. We saw that the theorem is true for $n = 1$ and $n = 2$ in (3) and (4). We assume the theorem to be true for $n = k$, and we prove that it must be true for $n = k + 1$. By hypothesis, we write

$$(a + b)^k = {}^kC_k a^k + {}^kC_{k-1} a^{k-1} b + {}^kC_{k-2} a^{k-2} b^2 + \cdots + {}^kC_0 b^k.$$

We multiply both sides by a and then by b and add the results to obtain

$$
\begin{aligned}
a(a + b)^k &= {}^kC_k a^{k+1} + {}^kC_{k-1} a^k b + {}^kC_{k-2} a^{k-1} b + \cdots \\
b(a + b)^k &= \cdots {}^kC_k a^k b + {}^kC_{k-1} a^{k-1} b^2 + \cdots \\
(a + b)^{k+1} &= (a + b)(a + b)^k = {}^kC_k a^{k+1} + [{}^kC_{k-1} + {}^kC_k] a^k b \\
&\quad + [{}^kC_{k-2} + {}^kC_{k-1}] a^{k-1} b^2 + \cdots \\
&= {}^{k+1}C_{k+1} a^{k+1} + {}^{k+1}C_k a^k b + {}^{k+1}C_{k-1} a^{k-1} b^2 + \cdots,
\end{aligned}
$$

since the coefficient of $a^{k+1-s} b^s$ is of the form

$$[{}^kC_{k-s} + {}^kC_{k-s-1}] = {}^{k+1}C_{k-s}$$

by (4) of Section IV.3.

The theorem is true for $n = k = 1$, and it is therefore true for $n = k + 1 = 2$. Thus it is true for $k = 2$ and also for $n = k + 1 = 2 + 1 = 3$, and, by the principle of mathematical induction, for every value of k. This method of proof is called *mathematical induction*; the principle was first clearly enunciated by Blaise Pascal (1623–1662), after whom the triangular array of numbers in Table IV.1 is called the *Pascal triangle*. Notice that if we set $a = b = 1$ in (5) we obtain

(6) $$2^n = (1 + 1)^n = {}^nC_n + {}^nC_{n-1} + \cdots + {}^nC_0.$$

In words, the sum of all combinations that can be formed from n objects is 2^n. This is otherwise evident, since each object can either appear in a combination or not appear. If we set $a = t$, $b = 1$, we obtain from (5) a *generating function* for ${}^nC_k$, for ${}^nC_k$ is the coefficient of t^k, namely:

(7) $$(1 + t)^n.$$

Example. The combinations of A, B, and C are the empty set, $\emptyset$, A, B, AB, C, AC, BC, and ABC, or otherwise $\emptyset$; A, B, C; AB, AC, BC; ABC, that is, one 0-combination, three 1-combinations, three 2-combinations, and one 3-combination, giving a total of eight different combinations. However, we can see that A can appear or not appear, and similarly for B and C; thus the total number of combinations is $2 \times 2 \times 2 = 8$.

5. ELEMENTARY PROBABILITY THEORY

For our purposes here, we adopt the common frequency interpretation of probability. A familiar *random variable* is the result of the toss of a coin. When a coin is tossed, it may fall heads or tails. At the time of tossing, it is not known whether the coin will appear as a head or a tail. Presumably if we knew the initial conditions of the motion of the coin at the time of tossing, as well as the conditions of the air and other physical conditions, we could say that the event was determined. But in the absence of such knowledge we do not know which face will appear. We might ask in what proportion of times in a long series of tosses a head will result. Since there seems to be little prior reason for believing that heads will fall either more or less frequently than tails, we assign probabilities, $\frac{1}{2}$ to heads and $\frac{1}{2}$ to tails. We expect to see about half the tosses in a long series to result in heads. Heads and tails are said to be *equally likely*. Similar consideration leads to a general definition of probability in models of such events.

Definition. *If an experiment can occur in n equally likely ways and if m of them are favorable to an event, the probability of the event is defined to be m/n.*

Example i. A toss of a coin can result in a head or a tail. There are thus two results to the toss; $n = 2$. A head can occur in precisely one way; $m = 1$. The probability of a head is thus $\frac{1}{2}$.

Example ii. When a die is thrown, one of the faces—marked 1, 2, 3, 4, 5, or 6—will be observed. There are six equally likely cases. Of these 1, 3, and 5 are odd numbers, and the probability of an odd number resulting thus is $\frac{3}{6} = \frac{1}{2}$. The probability of any given score such as 5 is $\frac{1}{6}$, since it occurs in one of the six equally likely ways.

Events occurring as the result of an experiment are said to be *mutually exclusive* if the occurrence of any two events together is impossible. Thus in throwing a die, a 3 and a 4 cannot appear simultaneously; they are mutually exclusive events. Similarly, the appearances of a 3 and an even number are mutually exclusive.

A set of events, which could occur as the result of an experiment, is said to be *exhaustive* if the union of all the members includes all possible events. Thus the events, odd and even, are exhaustive for the toss of a die. The event "odd" and the event "4" are not *exhaustive*, since they do not cover the events 2 and 6.

Theorem.   *The probability of the union of two mutually exclusive events is the sum of the probabilities of the two events.*

Proof.   If there are n equally likely possibilities, m_1 will be favorable to the first event and m_2 will be favorable to the second. Moreover, these $m_1 + m_2 = m$ possibilities are all distinct, since the events are mutually exclusive. The probability that either event occurs is thus m/n. The required statement is $m/n = m_1/n + m_2/n$.

Corollary.   *The sum of the probabilities of a set of mutually exclusive and exhaustive events is unity.*

Proof.   We have that, for the union of the set of mutually exclusive and exhaustive events, $m_1 + m_2 + \cdots + m_k = n$.

Random variables X and Y are said to be *mutually independent*—or, as it is usually written, *independent*—if the probability of X taking any particular value is unaffected by Y having already assumed a particular value.

6. THE BINOMIAL DISTRIBUTION

Variables occur in mathematics apart from any reference to probability. For example, we may have a variable x that can take any one of a set of values such, as the interval between zero and unity, any of the set of the positive integers, and so on. *Random variables* are functions that take such values according to the result of a random experiment or random process. Thus if X is a random variable that takes the values "heads" or "tails" with equal probabilities at a given trial, it takes precisely one of these values as the result of a random process—namely, tossing the coin by hand—when it cannot be known whether the toss will result in a head or a tail. It is convenient sometimes to say that X takes the values 1 or 0 in this example, interpreting 1 as one head and 0 as no head and, thus, as a tail. We may wish to compute the probability of 2 heads, 1 head, or no head when two coins are tossed independently. We write $\mathscr{P}$ for the phrase "the probability that" and include in parentheses words such as "2 heads" as an abbreviation for "two heads should occur" or, more formally, "$X = 2$" or even "$X = 2, Y = 3$."

(1)
$$\begin{aligned}
\mathscr{P}(2 \text{ heads}) &= \mathscr{P}(X_1 = 1, X_2 = 1) \\
&= \mathscr{P}(X_1 = 1)\mathscr{P}(X_2 = 1), \quad \text{from the independence} \\
&= \tfrac{1}{2} \cdot \tfrac{1}{2} = \tfrac{1}{4}
\end{aligned}$$

(2)
$$\begin{aligned}
\mathscr{P}(2 \text{ tails}) &= \mathscr{P}(X_1 = 0, X_2 = 0) \\
&= \mathscr{P}(X_1 = 0)\mathscr{P}(X_2 = 0), \quad \text{from the independence} \\
&= \tfrac{1}{2} \cdot \tfrac{1}{2} = \tfrac{1}{4}
\end{aligned}$$

(3)
$$\begin{aligned}
\mathscr{P}(1 \text{ head}) &= \mathscr{P}(X_1 = 1, X_2 = 0) + \mathscr{P}(X_1 = 0, X_2 = 1) \\
&= \tfrac{1}{4} + \tfrac{1}{4} = \tfrac{1}{2}.
\end{aligned}$$

We can generalize this computation by supposing that the probabilities are not equal to $\tfrac{1}{2}$ but take some general value, p; for example, the probability of throwing a "five" with a true die is $\tfrac{1}{6}$. With two independent throws

(4) $\mathscr{P}(X_1 = 5, X_2 = 5) = \mathscr{P}(X_1 = 5)\mathscr{P}(X_2 = 5) \quad$ by the independence
$$= \tfrac{1}{6} \cdot \tfrac{1}{6} = \tfrac{1}{36},$$

(5) $\mathscr{P}(X_1 \neq 5, X_2 \neq 5) = \mathscr{P}(X_1 \neq 5)\mathscr{P}(X_2 \neq 5)$
$$= \tfrac{5}{6} \cdot \tfrac{5}{6} = \tfrac{25}{36},$$

(6) $\mathscr{P}(\text{precisely one throw of 5}) = \mathscr{P}(X_1 = 5)\mathscr{P}(X_2 \neq 5)$
$$+ \mathscr{P}(X_1 \neq 5)\mathscr{P}(X_2 = 5),$$
$$= 2 \cdot \tfrac{1}{6} \cdot \tfrac{5}{6} = \tfrac{10}{36},$$

and we could replace $\tfrac{1}{6}$ and $\tfrac{5}{6}$ with any numbers, p and q such that $p \geq 0$, $q \geq 0$, and $p + q = 1$. We could also write $X \in A$, X takes a value in the set A, instead of $X = a$, a number. Often $X \in A$ is referred to as a *success*. To facilitate these computations, we could write

$$(pt + q)$$

as a generating function of the probabilities of the event A happening or not happening at a single trial, if we interpret $pt + q$ as $pt^1 + qt^0$. The power of t is to be interpreted as the number of times A has occurred. We consider pt^1 to be "the probability of the event A happening once is p" and $q \equiv qt^0$ as "the probability of the event A not happening." The two events are mutually exclusive and exhaustive, $p + q = 1$.

Now suppose that we carry out two independent trials with the result that the probability of the event A in the first trial and the event A in the second trial is just the product of the two probabilities; the probabilities of 2 successes, 1 success, or 0 success are given then by the coefficient of t^2, t, and 1 in the expansion of $(pt + q)^2$. This is true because $(pt + q)^2$ can be obtained by the following elementary multiplication:

$$
\begin{array}{r}
pt + q \\
pt + q \\
\hline
p^2 t^2 + pqt \\
+ qpt + q^2 \\
\hline
p^2 t^2 + 2pqt + q^2,
\end{array}
$$

and the coefficient of t^2 is p^2

$$
= \mathscr{P}(X_1 \in A)\mathscr{P}(X_2 \in A) = \mathscr{P}(X_1 \in A, X_2 \in A)
$$
$$
= \mathscr{P}(\text{two successes}).
$$

Similarly, the coefficient of t^0 is q^2 and $q^2 = q \cdot q = \mathscr{P}(X_1 \in \bar{A})\mathscr{P}(X_2 \in \bar{A}) = \mathscr{P}(X_1 \in \bar{A}, X_2 \in \bar{A}) = \mathscr{P}(\text{no success})$. The $2pq$ is identified as $pq + qp = \mathscr{P}(X_1 \in A, X_2 \in \bar{A}) + \mathscr{P}(X_1 \in \bar{A}, X_2 \in A) = \mathscr{P}(\text{one success})$.

Note that $\bar{A}$ is the complement of A. In other words, A and $\bar{A}$ are exhaustive and mutually exclusive. See Section XVII.2.

Binomial probability theorem.   *Let n observations be made on a variable X, and call them X_1, X_2, ..., X_n. Suppose that the n experiments are independent and carried out so that $X_1 \in A$ with probability p, $X_2 \in A$ with probability, p, ... Then the probabilities that on n occasions $X \in A$, on $(n - 1)$ occasions $X \in A$, on $(n - 2)$ occasions $X \in A$, ..., on no occasion $X \in A$, are given by the coefficients of t^n, t^{n-1}, ..., 1, in $(pt + q)^n$.*

   Proof.   The theorem is true for $n = 1$. If it is true for $n = k$, we have to prove it true for $n = k + 1$. It is thus given that

$$
(pt + q)^k = {}^kC_k p^k t^k + {}^kC_{k-1} p^{k-1} q t^{k-1} + \cdots + {}^kC_0 q^k.
$$

We say that s successes can occur after $k + 1$ experiments if s successes had occurred at the first k trials and no success occurred at the $(k + 1)$th trial, or if $s - 1$ successes had occurred at the first k trials and 1 success occurred at the $(k + 1)$th trial. The coefficient of t^s is thus to be the coefficient of t^s in $(pt + q)^k$ multiplied by q plus the coefficient of t^{s-1} in $(pt + q)^k$ multiplied by p. Now this sum is obtained if we multiply the expansion of $(pt + q)^k$ by $(pt + q)$, for we have

$$(pt + q)^k = \cdots + {}^kC_s p^s q^{k-s} t^s + {}^kC_{s-1} p^{s-1} q^{k-s+1} t^{s-1} + \cdots$$
$$q(pt + q)^k = \cdots + {}^kC_s p^s q^{k-s+1} t^s + \cdots$$
$$pt(pt + q)^k = \cdots + {}^kC_{s-1} p^s q^{k-s+1} t^s + \cdots$$

$$
\begin{aligned}
(pt + q)^k &= \cdots + ({}^kC_s + {}^kC_{s-1}) p^s q^{k-s+1} t^s + \cdots \\
&= \cdots + {}^{k+1}C_s p^s q^{k-s+1} t^s + \\
&= \cdots \text{ general term of } (pt + q)^{k+1} \ldots.
\end{aligned}
$$

If the theorem is true for $n = k$, it is true for $n = k + 1$. But since it is already true for $n = 1$, it is true for $n = 2$, $n = 3$, ...; thus it is generally true.

Example i. Twin births are of two types—binovular and monovular. Twins are of the sex types, MM, MF (or FM), and FF or 2M, 1M, and 0M types. The MF (or FM) types are readily identified and must be of the binovular type. Let us look at the binovular type and suppose that the probability of a twin being a male is p. We assume that the sex of first twin is independent of the sex of the second twin, and thus, by the binomial probability theorem, we have probabilities of 2M, 1M, and 0M in the proportions p^2, $2pq$, and q^2. If p is close to $\frac{1}{2}$, say $p = \frac{1}{2} + d$, $2pq = 2(\frac{1}{2} + d)(\frac{1}{2} - d) = 2(\frac{1}{4} - d^2) = \frac{1}{2} - 2d^2$, and d^2 is so small that it can be neglected, with the result that $2pq$ is close to $\frac{1}{2}$. We return to this topic in Section X.9.

Example ii. If the probability of a child being a boy is p, the probabilities of n boys, $(n - 1)$ boys, ..., 0 boy in a sibship of n are the coefficients of t^n, t^{n-1}, ..., in the expansion of $(pt + q)^n$, if we make the assumptions (1) p is constant within a family, (2) the sex at each birth is independent of that at the others, and (3) p does not vary between families. We discuss this example again in Section X.8.

Example iii. Let us suppose that a male and a female are selected at random in a population. The contribution of each parent to a zygote in the next generation is a dominant D with probability p. The probability that the zygote will receive 2, 1, or 0 dominants is given by the terms of the binomial distribution with generating function $(pt + q)^2$, and the result follows. We discuss this example again in Section X.3.

Example iv. The probability of surviving a given disease can sometimes be deduced from past experience to be p. If we have n patients, the probability of $n, n - 1, \ldots, 0$ survivors are the coefficients of t^s of the binomial $(pt + q)^n$, $s = n, n - 1, \ldots, 0$. If $p = 0.8$, and $n = 10$, we have the survivals given by the coefficients in the expansion, $(0.1074t^{10} + 0.2684t^9 + 0.3020t^8 + 0.2013t^7 + 0.0881t^6 + 0.0264t^5 + 0.0055t^4 + 0.0008t^3 + 0.0001t^2)$. The most probable result is 8 survivals, but we should not be surprised to see any number, 6 to 10, and even 5 survivors would occur with a probability 0.0264 (i.e., in 2.64 % of groups of 10).

7. THE NORMAL CURVE

We define the *exponential function*, e^x, or exp x as it is more conveniently written for printing purposes, by the following equation:

$$(1) \qquad e^x \equiv \exp x = 1 + \frac{x}{1!} + \frac{x^2}{2!} + \frac{x^3}{3!} + \cdots + \frac{x^n}{n!} + \cdots$$

It can be verified that this function has the remarkable property

$$(2) \qquad e^x e^y = e^{x+y},$$

or equivalently

$$(3) \qquad \exp x \exp y = \exp(x + y).$$

Indeed, the exponential function can be defined as that infinite sum in powers of x which gives a general solution to (3) with the coefficient of x equal to unity. We note that $\exp 0 \equiv e^0 = 1$. exp 1 is written simply as e and has the value $2 \cdot 7182818 \ldots$, we can write

$$(4) \qquad e = 1 + \frac{1}{1!} + \frac{1}{2!} + \frac{1}{3!} + \cdots$$
$$= 1 + 1 + 0 \cdot 5 + 0 \cdot 16666\dot{6} + 0 \cdot 04166\dot{6} + \cdots,$$

and it is easily proved that the terms drop off so rapidly in absolute value that the sum has the determined irrational value $2 \cdot 7182818 \ldots$ Furthermore, it is easy to show that for any fixed value of x, the sum of the series for exp x can be determined exactly (the sum *converges* in the sense that for a given η the finite sums of n terms of the series for n greater than a fixed value n_0 all differ by less than η). The value of exp x is always positive. It is small if x is large and negative, increases steadily as x increases, equals unity when x is zero, and increases without limit as x increases.

A random variable X is said to have a *normal distribution*—or, its frequency function is said to have the normal form—if the frequency function can be expressed for all real values of x in the form

(5) $$f(x) = \frac{1}{\sigma\sqrt{(2\pi)}}\, e^{-\dfrac{(x-\alpha)^2}{2\sigma^2}} \equiv (2\pi\sigma^2)^{-1/2}\exp\left[-\frac{1}{2}\frac{(x-\alpha)^2}{\sigma^2}\right]$$

where α is a real number and σ is a positive number. We say that α and σ are the *parameters* of the normal curve. It can be shown that α is the mean and σ is the standard deviation. By a change of variable from X to Y, the form of the distribution can be simplified if we set

(6) $$Y = \frac{(X-\alpha)}{\sigma}.$$

Then the frequency function of Y can be written as

(7) $$g(y) = \frac{1}{\sqrt{2\pi}}\exp\left[-\frac{1}{2}y^2\right] \equiv (2\pi)^{-1/2}\exp\left[-\frac{1}{2}y^2\right].$$

Thus every normal frequency function can be reduced to a standard form (7) by a linear transformation (6). This transformation corresponds to a change of origin and scale, whereby the mean of the new curve is at the origin and the standard deviation has the value unity. Therefore, the properties of the normal curves can be studied by inspection of the standardized curve (7), which appears in Figure IV.1.

The following properties can be deduced from (5) or (7). Since the curve is always above the baseline, $g(x) > 0$ at every point. The area between the curve and the baseline is unity, and most of this area lies within a few units of the mean. Indeed, only some 0.3% of the area lies outside ± 3 units in the standard curve or ± 3 standard deviations in the general curve given by (5). The curve is closely applied to the baseline at a

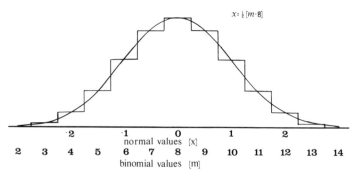

Figure IV.1. The approximation to the binomial, by the normal distribution.

distance more than, say, 3 standard deviations or units from the mean, and it is difficult to show graphically that the curve is distinct from the baseline at such distances from the mean. The curve is symmetrical and has a mode at the mean. Mean, median, and mode coincide. The curve extends to infinity in either direction. There is a point of *inflection* on either side of the mean at a distance of one standard deviation from the mean. Internal to these inflections, the curve is convex ·pward and external to them it is concave upward. At the points of *inflection*, there is no curvature—this is indeed the definition of inflection—and the tangent to the curve at the point of inflection follows the curve closely for some distance, crossing it at the point of inflection. If this straight line is produced, it cuts the baseline at a point 2 standard deviations from the origin. The area under the curve has been extensively tabulated, usually in a form that gives the total area under the curve outside specified points whose distance from the mean is expressed in standard deviations (s.d.). The quartiles are 0.67447 s.d. from the mean. In addition, 5 % of the area lies outside ±1.959964 s.d. (i.e., ca. 1.96 s.d. from the mean), 1 % of the area lies outsdie ±2.575829 s.d. from the mean, and 0.1 % of the area lies outside ±3.29053 s.d.

8. THE NORMAL APPROXIMATION TO THE BINOMIAL DISTRIBUTION

For the binomial variable X, let us write

(1) $$p_k \equiv \mathscr{P}(X = k) = {}^N C_k p^k q^{N-k}.$$

If we are testing the null hypothesis that p has a certain value, we shall need sums of the form

(2) $$P_j = \sum_{k=j}^{N} p_k$$

to be used as the test criterion of *significance*. If P_j is small, say less than α, the level of significance, an observation $X = j$ will be said to be *significant*. Since the computation of the sum in (2) may be lengthy, however, we would consult tables of the binomial distribution or use the *normal approximation* now to be explained.

If X has the distribution given by (1), then

(3) $$\mathscr{E}X = Np$$

where $\mathscr{E}X$ signifies the mean or expectation of X, and

(4) $$\text{var } X = Npq = \sigma^2, \text{ say.}$$

Suppose that neither Np nor Nq is small; neither is less than 5, say.

Suppose that rectangles of height p_k, are erected on the intervals $(k - \frac{1}{2}, k + \frac{1}{2})$ $k = 0, 1, \ldots, N$. Then the areas in these rectangles are approximated closely by the area under a normal curve having the same mean and standard deviation. It follows that the rectangle $(k - \frac{1}{2}, k + \frac{1}{2})$ is approximated closely by the area under a standard normal curve between the points $(k - Np - \frac{1}{2})/\sigma$ and $(k - Np + \frac{1}{2})/\sigma$. The sum in (2) is then approximated by the area under a number of such adjacent intervals beginning at $(j - Np - \frac{1}{2})/\sigma$ and ending at $(N - Np + \frac{1}{2})/\sigma$. However, there is little area under the normal curve beyond this point; thus we can equate the sum (2) to the area from $(j - Np - \frac{1}{2})/\sigma$ to infinity. We obtain

$$(5) \qquad P_j \cong \mathscr{P}\left[Y > \frac{(j - Np - \frac{1}{2})}{\sigma} \right],$$

where Y is standard normal and the probability can be obtained from the tables of the normal curve.

Example. Consider the binomial distribution with $N = 10$ and $p = \frac{1}{2} = q$. Then $\mathscr{E}X = Np = 5$, and the variance $\sigma^2 = (10 \times \frac{1}{2} \times \frac{1}{2})^{1/2} = \sqrt{2.5} = 1.581$. Then the exact binomial probabilities that X should be not less than 10, 9, 8, 7, and 6, computed by (1) and (2) are 0.001, 0.011, 0.057, 0.174, and 0.379, respectively. By the use of tables of the normal distribution, we find approximate values 0.002, 0.014, 0.057, 0.173, and 0.376. We show this excellent approximation graphically as Figure IV.1 where $p = \frac{1}{2}$, $N = 16$, $\sigma^2 = 16 \times \frac{1}{2} \times \frac{1}{2} = 4$, $\sigma = 2$.

EXERCISES

1. Assume $1! = 1$ and $(n + 1)! = (n + 1)n!$. Use this equation to verify that the factorials of 1, 2, ..., 10 are 1, 2, 6, 24, 120; 720, 5,040, 40,320, 362,880, 3,628,800.

2. In a tasting test of n solutions, it may be desirable to present the solutions to the taster in random order. There are $n!$ such orders, corresponding to the numbers of n permutations. Suppose that $n = 3$; then $^3P_3 = 6$, and the permutations are 123, 132, 213 231, 312, 321. Assign the numbers 0, 6, 12, ..., 90 to the first of these, 1, 7, 13, ..., 91 to the second; 2, 8, 14, ..., 10 to the third; ..., 5, 11, 17, ..., 95 to the sixth, and use a table of random sampling numbers to obtain a set of five permutations to be used in a tasting experiment.

3. Write down the 2-combinations of three objects A, B, and C. After each 2-combination, record the corresponding 2-permutations and verify that $r! \, ^nC_r = \, ^nP_r$ in this special case. For example, to the 2-combination AB, there correspond the permutations AB and BA.

4. Similarly, write down the 2-combinations of four objects A, B, C, and D and the corresponding 2-permutations and verify the formula, $12 = \, ^4P_2 = \, ^2P_2 \, ^4C_2 = 2.6 = 12$.

5. Compute the terms of $(\frac{3}{4}t + \frac{1}{4})^2$ and of $(\frac{1}{2}t + \frac{1}{2})^2$.

6. Compute the terms of $(pt + q)^2$, $(0.2t + 0.8)^2$, $(0.3t + 0.7)^2$, and $(0.4t + 0.6)^2$, respectively. Note that if p is a simple fraction, r/s say, it may be simpler to compute $s^{-2}(rt + s - r)^2$ than $[(r/s)t + (s - r)/s]^2$.

7. Write the general term of the binomial distribution as p_r. Then

$$p_0 + tp_1 + t^2p_2 + \cdots + t^np_n = (pt + q)^N$$

and

$$p_r = {}^NC_r p^r q^{N-r}.$$

Show that $p_{r+1}/p_r = (N - r)p/[(r + 1)q]$ and $p_{r+1} \geq p_r$ if $r \leq Np - q$. Two successive terms in the binomial expansion can be equal if $Np - q$ or $(N + 1)p - 1$ is an integer.

8. In a mating of the form $Aa \times Aa$, the possible genotypes are AA, Aa, and aa. It is assumed that the offspring obtains any particular allele from the first parent independently of the allele obtained from the second. Assuming that, of a pair of alleles at the locus, there is equal probability that either gene passes to the offspring, compute the probabilities of the various possibilities of the matings $AA \times AA$, $AA \times Aa$, $AA \times aa$, $Aa \times Aa$, $Aa \times aa$, $aa \times aa$.

9. A disease has a case fatality of q and the fatalities of the cases are mutually independent. Prove that the proportions of 0, 1, 2, ..., N deaths are given by the coefficients of the powers of t in the expansion of $(qt + p)^N$. Give numerical results for $q = \frac{1}{5}$, $N = 5$; $q = \frac{1}{10}$, $N = 10$; $q = \frac{1}{100}$, $N = 100$.

10. Draw a normal curve with the aid of statistical tables. Choose the ordinate scale so that one unit of height of the curve is represented by 10 in. and one unit of abscissa is represented by 2 in. By counting complete squares and adding $\frac{1}{2}$ for each incomplete square under the graph, estimate the total area, verifying that it is 20 in.^{2}. Estimate how much of the area lies beyond 0.67, 1, 2, 2.5, 3 s.d. distance from the origin.

NOTES

Permutations and combinations come within the branch of mathematics known as combinatorics or combinatorial mathematics. A classic in the field is Whitworth's (1901) *Choice and Chance*, in which little preliminary knowledge is assumed. The field has developed enormously in recent years. Riordan (1958) and Ryser (1963) are modern texts on the subject, which have surprisingly little overlap. Gregor Mendel's contribution to genetics was to introduce combinatorial ideas! His work has been translated as Mendel (1965). Many interesting combinatorial problems continue to arise in genetics and in the theory of the coding of the DNA molecule.

CHAPTER V

Medical Aspects of the Census and Official Statistics

1. INTRODUCTORY

The first English census was held in 1801, more than a century after William Petty in 1690 had written of the value of regular censuses. By 1841 the census in England had assumed a form not unlike that of modern times; it was based on a descriptive list, drawn up on uniform lines and collected in a uniform manner by paid enumerators, of all persons who slept in each house on a given night. Most censuses now follow the English census in recording residence on a *de facto* basis. Persons are recorded as being where they slept on the particular night chosen. In the *de jure* method, the residence is considered to be the usual place of residence. Usually a census is taken at a time when no great discrepancies are likely to occur between the *de facto* and *de jure* methods. In countries where the rate of literacy is high, the head of the household is responsible for filling in the schedule. The collector is responsible for checking that the forms have been completed properly. In countries in which the rate of literacy is lower, the schedules are completed by a canvasser or enumerator. The householder method has some advantages: the liability to err is diminished, since the householder has the responsibility to give the correct answer; errors due to haste are less likely to occur; the time of the enumerator is saved (thus effecting an economy in manpower); the labor of writing out the particulars is divided, resulting in fewer errors due to fatigue; the census can be made synchronous throughout the whole country. The householder method, however, requires a high level of general education and also the cooperation of the population. The system would clearly break down if the householders could not read and write.

At a meeting of the International Statistical Congress at St. Petersburg in 1872, a minimum list of questions was set out. These requirements were: (1) that the census be taken decennially and be completed within 24 hours, (2) that residence be recorded on a *de facto* basis, and (3) that information on individuals include name, age, sex, relationship to the head of the household, conjugal condition, occupation, religion, language, education, birthplace, nationality, and infirmities, such as deafness and blindness. Some countries have preferred to concentrate on a restricted number of topies in order to obtain accurate information on a few points rather than to risk exhausting the patience and dispersing the energy of the householder over too long a questionnaire.

Many countries now supplement the information obtained at the time of a census by sample surveys of the population, perhaps acquiring more detailed information than would be possible as a routine over the whole population. Moreover, in sample surveys, collectors specially versed in the field can secure comparative information that might never be elicited if different, untrained persons are answering questions that require judgment.

2. MEDICAL INFORMATION FROM THE CENSUS

Demographic, social and economic, ethnographic and statistical data from the censuses are often of medical interest.

(i) Total Population Numbers

The most obvious purpose of a census is to determine the total number of inhabitants of a community. The total population is used as the denominator in the computation of the crude death rates and crude birth rates.

Sometimes, as in comparing the population of a city or state over a number of years, care must be taken to verify that the definitions have not changed. For example, the boundaries of a city or country may change, and new classes of inhabitants (especially nomads) may be enumerated, or certain classes, such as the military, may not be enumerated.

(ii) The Population by Sex

Sex is an obvious criterion for classification. Migration and wars can bring about great changes in the proportion of the sexes. The influence of sex on certain forms of morbidity and mortality is obvious. For example, the rates of mortality from violent and accidental causes are higher in males than in females. However, it is not known why pertussis should cause higher infection rates and higher case fatality rates in females.

(iii) The Population by Age

Many diseases have a characteristic age distribution, and the numbers of the population by age and sex can be considered to be the most important medical data of a census, since they enable us to compute age- and sex-specific death rates. The influence of age is especially important in cancer incidence and mortality. Comparisons of the crude cancer death rates over a period of time in one country can be very misleading, since there may have been a considerable aging in the population over the span of years considered.

(iv)   Immigrant Population

Migrants may have special medical characteristics, such as a high incidence of tuberculosis, cancer, or previous experience of measles. Many authorities believe that migrants from the cities of Europe, particularly the United Kingdom, carry with them to the new lands an increased susceptibility to lung cancer (Dean, 1962).

(v)   Geographical Distribution

Malaria and other tropical diseases clearly have a geographical distribution, but so do many other diseases—skin cancer and rickets, for example. It is often desired to compare rates of mortality between different areas. Differences in mortality rates between country and city were known to the early observers, including John Graunt in the seventeenth century. Many of these urban–rural differences were due to the high incidence of infective diseases in the cities. With the recent amelioration of the conditions of life in the cities, these differences have tended to disappear. Geographical isolation due to the sea or impassable mountains greatly modifies the behavior of the epidemic diseases, and we return to this feature in Chapter XVI.

(vi)   Conjugal Conditions

It is necessary to know the conjugal condition and sometimes the parity of the females in order to calculate certain fertility indices, although this factor is of less medical interest than age or sex. The incidences of some cancers, notably of the breast, uterus, and prostate, are affected by the conjugal state. Cancer of the cervix is commoner in those who marry young.

(vii)   Ethnic Type

Information on ethnic type is available in the censuses of some countries. It is possible that there is a varying susceptibility to disease. Lack of skin pigment is an important predisposing factor to skin cancers in the lower latitudes. However, many of the supposed ethnic differences in mortality have been or probably can be explained by social and economic differences. The effects of race, economic status, history, geographical area, and social customs are confounded. Possibly the very high tuberculosis rates of races when they first become urbanized can be explained partly on genetic grounds, but social and other factors may also contribute to the explanations.

(viii)   Nationality

Customs within a federal community may vary between national groups, affecting both fertility and mortality. Such national differences may cause the formation of small enclaves of one nation within another. This has led on occasion to high rates of inbreeding in the smaller national groups and a high incidence of recessive defects from cousin marriages.

(ix)   Social Factors

Social factors are of special importance in the incidence of malnutrition and the infectious diseases. Halliday (1928) found a marked social gradient in the incidence of measles in infants and children in the cities of Scotland. Possibly the most important step in the establishment of effective hygiene in a community is the attainment of literacy. In a literate community, it is easy to direct campaigns against known bacterial hazards or to instruct mothers in child hygiene.

(x)   Occupation

By a complete enumeration of the population, it is possible to obtain, by age and sex, the numbers engaged in the various professions. In the past, many associations between disease and occupation have been established.

(xi)   Prevalence of Disease or Disability

Questions on deafness and blindness have often been asked in censuses. In recent times, there have been attempts to assess the prevalence of chronic diseases such as rheumatic disease, tuberculosis, or other chronic disabilities. The determination of disease prevalence at the censuses has usually had administrative and humanitarian motives. The incidence of deaf-mutism as described in Section I.1 seems to have been an isolated example of a finding of epidemiological importance. However, special *medical censuses*—that is, the enumeration and physical examination of all or a sample of the community—often have yielded information of epidemiological importance and interest.

3. OTHER OFFICIAL SOURCES OF MEDICAL STATISTICAL INFORMATION

A great amount of information on individuals is collected in a modern state—some by the state itself and some by other bodies. Much of it is stored in ordinary documentary form, but some of it is prepared for storage and retrieval by automatic methods in *data banks*. The ease with which such information can be transferred from one file to another has raised the question of the desirability of *data linkage*; that is, the supplementing of information collected from one source by information collected from a second source, or even a third source. This apparently attractive idea raises grave problems of *confidentiality*. For example, should information collected by one organization be made known to a second without the consent of the subject? Indeed, is such sharing *desirable* (since the quality of the answers to some inquiries will fall if there is a risk that the responses will be passed on to a second organization)? We first briefly list the sources of such data, making a few marginal comments, proceeding next to consider the methods of linkage and the problems raised by data linkage.

Data of possible interest to the vital statistician are collected under such headings as:

1. *Vital Events.* Data on births, deaths, and marriages are collected as a routine in all civilized countries, but access to them is frequently limited. Sensitive points include marriage certificates, legitimacy, and cause of death.

2. *Electoral Registers.* Voting rolls are usually published and present no difficulties of confidentiality.

3. *Telephone Directories.* Subscribers' names and addresses are usually published.

4. *Professional Directories.* If registration is a legal requirement, the directory is usually published or freely available. Sometimes, the professional union or learned society publishes the list of its members.

5. *Population Register.* Every state is entitled to know the existence and address of its citizens in order to remind them of their duties (e.g., payment of taxes, military service) or to confer on them the benefits of citizenship (e.g., to inoculate or educate their children or to provide old age or invalid pensions). It is a remarkable fact that some of the most advanced nations do not possess a population register.

6. *Social Insurance or Security.* Registers are kept of the employed and employees for purposes of workers' compensation, the collection of income tax, and so on.

7. *Income Tax.* Naturally a register is kept of persons once they have made their first return, but the department also has other sources of information.

8. *Health and Hospital Records and Statistics.* There is great variation in the thoroughness with which health and hospital statistics are collected and maintained.

9. *Educational Records.*

10. *Criminal Records.*

11. *Social Welfare Registers.* Private and public charitable and social welfare organizations make payments to individuals or to families. They may wish to avoid double payment or to determine areas of need.

12. *Property Registers.*

13. *Business Registers.*

Since there are so many sources of data on persons, it is sometimes asked whether the information should be pooled into a common *data bank*, from which the various bodies could draw the information they need.

The first simplification, already introduced in some countries, is to give every inhabitant a number that is to be used in every file. Since many surnames and even complete names (e.g., Fred Smith) correspond to different persons, it is helpful to identify the subject by his year of birth and by sex. If the same person can be identified in two files stored on magnetic tape in a data bank, it is a simple matter to form, by automatic processes, an entry that will contain the combined information on both files. It may be argued that such a consolidation is an advantage to all concerned, since it may result in less work for the subject. Moreover, in epidemiological research, we could check diagnoses from hospital records, and it is easy to imagine other situations in which such linkage of data would be valuable. However, already difficult problems have been introduced. Not everyone wishes to be identified by age and sex. Others will find it burdensome to carry the same name through life. For such reasons, even the construction of appropriately printed cards detailing the history of the subjects' vaccinations and inoculations throughout life has not become routine in many countries, although the convenience to attending physicians and the value to the patient are undoubted.

In the foregoing account, we have made use of Bachi and Baron (1969). The reader is referred to the other papers on the subject in Volumes 42 and 43 of the *Bulletin of the International Statistical Institute.*

4. MORBIDITY STATISTICS

In the past, mortality statistics have dominated the studies or views on health because the serious, disabling illnesses were often caused by the more lethal diseases and injuries. Here we think especially of tuberculosis, syphilis, the common infective diseases, and pneumonia, cancer, and violent and accidental causes. It was recognized that there were possibilities of controlling the infections, as well as violent and accidental causes, and attention was directed toward these ends by the public health workers. However, with the decline in frequency of some of these classical forms of death and disability, more emphasis came to be placed on the not-necessarily-fatal chronic diseases.

Morbidity can be defined as any departure, subjective or objective, from a state of physiological well-being, according to the World Health Organization (WHO) Expert Committee (1968). But this is rather too general a definition; usually a more operational definition is required by different governmental or other bodies—some prefer to make a definition incorporating a statement that the departure is such as to prevent the normal performance of the patient's usual occupation; others want to know whether the patient will need out-patient, in-patient, convalescent, home, or other treatment.

Morbidity data are collected from various sources as follows.

1. *Notification.* Notification is the traditional method of warning the health services that various diseases have occurred which will require specialized therapy and which may suggest special control methods. Notification was especially appropriate when exotic diseases were introduced or when isolation was indicated in endemic types of infections; however, food poisonings and accidents also were appropriately notifiable.

2. *Hospital In-Patient Statistics.* Since a large proportion of patients are treated in hospital, it seems reasonable to look at the total of diseases treated in such institutions. If the hospitals are all controlled by a central government, it may be quite easy to obtain statistics of the morbidity of serious diseases requiring hospitalization.

3. *Other Medical Care Statistics.* It is rather more difficult to secure good statistics on morbidity from convalescent homes, homes for the elderly, and the like, even though they are caring for serious chronic diseases. Possibly useful statistics can be obtained from the venereal disease clinics. General practitioners' records or experiences have also been analyzed. Sometimes it is possible to obtain these on a nationwide basis by means of a sample survey of the experiences of the general practitioners; but difficulties are encountered in that special types of practitioners will elect to enter the survey.

4. *Medical Insurance Schemes.* It is possible often to obtain the claims through medical insurance schemes and to make estimates of the various diseases from them.

5. *Social Security Data.* There is inevitably a wide overlap among medical insurance systems. In some countries, data from all the foregoing sources could be pooled by a linkage of records.

6. *Registers of Patients.* For some diseases (e.g., disseminate sclerosis), registers of patients may exist.

7. *Special Field Investigations.* The prevalence of particular diseases, such as malaria, trachoma, or diabetes, can sometimes be estimated by means of field surveys. In the case of diabetes, special care will be needed to differentiate the disease from hyperglycemia. Sometimes these surveys have been initiated by alert practitioners, noticing the effects of poisonings from industrial wastes or congenital malformations apparently attributable to thalidomide. Moreover, vigilant medical services can carry out special inquiries into the needs of sufferers from such diseases as rheumatoid arthritis, into the efficiency of therapy or control measures, and into the causation of chronic disease.

The *incidence rate* of a disease is the number of cases occurring per unit of time per person. One commonly used rate is the incidence per thousand per annum. The incidence rates can be calculated for the whole population or for age- or sex-specific subclasses of it. Usually incidence rates have been expressed as *notification rates.* Within recent years, incidence rates have been obtained by specially designed sample surveys, by records from hospitals, and from general practitioners' records. For acute infective diseases, incidence rates seem to be the appropriate rates to compute.

However, if the infective or other disability persists, a prevalence rate would appear to be more useful.

The *point prevalence rate* is defined as the number of illnesses existing at a specified point of time, divided by the number of persons exposed to risk at that time.

The *period prevalence rate* is an average of the point prevalence rate over an interval of time. It has come into use because some surveys on morbidity take the form of records kept over an interval of a week, a month, or another length of time. However, there are illnesses beginning before the interval and lasting right through the interval, those beginning before but ending during the interval, those beginning and ending in the interval, and finally those beginning in the interval and ending after it. The total of those in first class is multiplied by the number of days in the whole interval, and all the others are multiplied by the number of days in the fractional duration of the illness in the interval. The sum is to be divided by the *days at risk*, which is the total number of persons at risk multiplied by the number of days in the interval or, alternatively, by the sum of days at risk of each person.

Another index is the *average duration of the illness*, which is defined as the simple mean of the lengths of all illnesses recorded. As a rule, the mean of all illnesses observed on a particular day is greater than the mean of all the illnesses beginning on a given day or during a given interval of time.

NOTES

The *International Statistical Institute* was founded in 1885 (Nixon, 1960) to facilitate cooperation between the official statisticians of different countries. It remained the leading international statistical society until the formation of the League of Nations in 1920. Although many of its functions are now carried out by the agencies of the United Nations, the Institute remains an important forum for the discussion of problems in the collection, reporting, and analysis of official statistics. Furthermore, individuals at its Congresses can express opinions that might be thought quite inappropriate for publication in the journals of the United Nations or its agencies.

The Institute has done much to unify the procedures of collection and reporting of the results of the census and other official statistics. It has been closely associated with the International Commission for the Decennial Revision of the International List of the Causes of Death, which has met in Paris at the invitation of the French government.

The Institute publishes a regular journal, the *Review of the International Statistical Institute*, and its biennial meetings are published as the *Bulletin of the International Statistical Institute* by the host country. In recent years, the congresses and publications of the Institute have become increasingly concerned with distribution theory and with the theory of sampling surveys.

Of the agencies of the United Nations, the World Health Organization (WHO), the International Labor Organization (ILO), the Food and Agriculture Organization (FAO), and the United Nations Educational, Scientific, and Cultural Organization (UNESCO) all publish material that is relevant to medical statistics. For a general review of WHO, the reader can consult WHO Director-General (1970); for its publications, there are: WHO Bibliography (1958, 1964, 1969) and WHO Expert Committee (1969).

Of special interest to us here are *World Health Statistics Annual* (in three volumes): Vol. I, *Vital Statistics and Causes of Death*; Vol. II, *Infectious Diseases, Cases, Deaths and Vaccinations*; Vol. III, *Health, Personnel and Hospital Establishments; The Chronicle of the World Health Organization* and *Technical Report Series*. Under "WHO" in the bibliography, we have included a number of publications of WHO, which illustrate the sort of statistical work done by WHO.

The Population Division of the Department of Economic and Social Affairs of the United Nations publishes three series: *Population Bulletin of the United Nations, Population Studies*, and *Demographic Yearbook*, which have contained much material on mortality and other medical statistics.

We now briefly mention sources of primary data and vehicles of critical material on the official statistics of some countries, noting that there is a description of each of them in Koren (1918) and some further notes in H. Gille (1949).

Australia

The Bureau of Census and Statistics, Canberra, publishes a *Yearbook* that contains a good section on vital statistics and some bibliographical notes. The Bureau publishes extensive tables annually in *Demography* and *Causes of Death*. See also the bibliographies of Lancaster (1964*a*, 1973).

France

The Institut National de la Statistique et des Études Économiques publishes annually *l'Annuaire Statistique de la France* (formerly *Statistique Générale de la France*), and also *Bulletin de la Statistique Générale de la France*. The Institut National d'Études Démographiques publishes *Population*, and occasional publications *Cahiers de "Travaux et Documents."* The Societé Statistique de Paris publishes a journal, *Journal de la Société Statistique de Paris*.

Japan

The Bureau of Statistics was founded in 1871. The first census was held in 1920 [see a note in *Rev. Int. Statist. Inst.*, **36** (1968), 332–333]. There are extensive tables available in *Japan: Statistical Yearbook*.

New Zealand

The Department of Statistics publishes an annual, *Vital Statistics* (variously titled), and reports on the censuses, which have been held every five years since 1871 except in 1931, 1941, and 1946. The Department of Health has published *Report on the Medical Statistics of New Zealand* annually since 1948, as well as an annual report on mental health statistics for 1955–1963. An extensive bibliography of Donovan (1969) is available.

Norway

See notes on Sweden, also Koren (1918) and H. Gille (1949).

Sweden

It is difficult to consider the various Scandinavian countries separately because they have been combined politically or for statistical purposes at different times. The Central Bureau of Statistics, Statistisk Centralbyrån, publishes data on the censuses held in Sweden in years ending in 0 (i.e., 1970, 1960, ...), produces annual reports on the vital statistics, which are consolidated later into 10-year reports, produces every 10 years a life table, and gives an annual report on the causes of death. The National Board of Health publishes an annual report.

The Central Bureau publishes the *Statistisk Årsbok för Sverige*, *Statistisk Tidskrift, Statistiska Meddelanden,* and *Historisk Statistisk för Sverige* (respectively, the yearbook, review, reports, and historical statistics). The last-named volume is unique since it has vital statistics of interest from 1720 to 1950.

Skandinavisk Aktuarietidskrift is published by the Scandinavian actuaries from Stockholm. A number of the Scandinavian medical journals publish medical statistical or genetical monographs as supplements.

United Kingdom

Vital statistical information for Scotland and Northern Ireland is published by their respective Registrars-General. The publications for England and Wales includes *Registrar-General's Statistical Review of England and Wales— Part I, Medical; Part II, Civil; Part III, Commentaries, etc.* There are also various occasional publications of the Registrar-General; the most important for us are the Registrar-General's *Decennial Reports on the Census* and *Studies on Medical and Population Subjects.*

The Medical Research Council publishes a *Special Report Series*, which has contained many monographs of statistical interest. Much discussion of the official medical statistics has appeared in the *Journal of the Royal Statistical Society.* Among other journals worthy of mention here are: *Journal of Hygiene, Bulletin of Hygiene, British Journal of Preventive and Social Medicine, Journal of the Institute of Actuaries,* and *Transactions of the Faculty of Actuaries.*

United States

The U.S. Bureau of the Census was created in 1902 and is now responsible for the census, which has been held every ten years beginning in 1790. The Bureau publishes *The Statistical Abstract of the United States, Historical Statistics of the United States,* and various *Reports* on the Census.

The Journal of the American Statistical Association has made available much information of medical or vital statistical interest. The Population Association of America publishes *Demography.* Many reports are published by the U.S. Department of Health, Education and Welfare, including the *Public Health Reports* (U.S. Public Health Service).

Other journals published in the United States include *American Journal of Hygiene, American Journal of the Medical Sciences, Biometrics, Human Biology, The American Journal of Public Health, Milbank Memorial Fund Quarterly*, and *Population Index*.

Of international journals not already mentioned, *Acta Genetica et Statistica Medica, Metron, Genus, Biometrisches Zeitschrift, Biometrie-Praximetrie*, and *Sankhyā* (Series B) contain articles of medical statistical interest.

Some general discussion can also be found in the following:

Demography Texts

Barclay, 1958; Beaujeu-Garnier, 1956; Census Library Project, 1948; Chasteland, 1961; Eldridge, 1959; Koren, 1918; Landry, 1945; Milbank Memorial Fund, 1955; Naraghi, 1960; Sauvy, 1954a and 1969; Spiegelman, 1955; UN Population Studies nos. 4-7, 1949; no. 8, 1950; no. 9, 1951; nos. 17 and 18, 1953; no. 24, 1955; no. 25, 1956; Yates, 1960; Yntema, 1952.

Additional bibliography on the demography of various countries is given in the notes to Chapter VIII.

Census

Logan, 1951.

Demographic Analysis

UN Population Studies, no. 18, 1953.

Measurement of Health

WHO Study Group, 1957.

Morbidity

Hill, 1971; Rees, 1969; U.S. National Center for Health Statistics, 1965g, 1969, 1971; WHO Expert Committee, 1968; WHO (various authors), 1965.

Sampling Surveys

Dalenius, 1957, 1967, 1968; WHO Expert Committee, 1960.

Use of the Health Service

Ashford and Pearson, 1970.

Use of Records

Reid, 1957.

CHAPTER VI

Measurement of Mortality

1. INTRODUCTORY

Many interesting records of deaths have been handed down to us from times past. For example, S. Peller (1943, 1944, 1948) has analyzed the vital statistics of the German ruling classes, available from the genealogical records. Many important features emerge. Maternal death rates were high, and so were tuberculosis death rates in young adult life; violence and accidents caused a high mortality in young adult males. By its social isolation, the nobility was protected from the acute exanthemata and gastroenteritis in particular, and thus its infant mortality was low relative to that of the population as a whole; particularly was this true in the second half of the nineteenth century. It was also protected from famine, an important cause of death in Europe before 1750.

On a national basis, Sweden has records going back to 1721, because retrospective returns of the numbers of births and deaths from each diocese were required in 1736, for all the years since 1721. Age-specific death rates are available for Sweden from 1751 on, and Swedish statistics are particularly valuable for showing the predominance of the acute infections as causes of mortality.

In London, fear of the plague led Henry VIII to insist on adequate returns of the numbers of deaths from the plague, his aim being to take his court out of London whenever the weekly totals became high. The *Bills of Mortality*, begun in 1532, had become well established before John Graunt (1620–1674) made his famous *Observations* on them in 1662, in an attempt to determine the basic laws of human mortality, natality, and movement of population. Among other things, Graunt demonstrated:

1. The regularity of certain vital phenomena, such as births, deaths, and marriages.
2. The excess of male over female births and the approximately equal numbers of the sexes in the population.
3. The high rate of mortality in the earliest years of life.
4. An urban death rate that exceeded the rural death rate.

Graunt carefully examined the reliability of the data and inquired, for example, whether apparent changes over the years were due to transfer of cases of a disease to other rubrics. His work can still be read with interest because of the great insight he displayed in criticizing his sources and the caution with which he put forward new hypotheses.

Others have not always had the same insight; for example, William Heberden (1767–1845) noted the gradual decline of dysentery in the *Bills*, which he attributed to greater cleanliness, failing to recognize that "griping of the guts" was really infantile diarrhea and that there was a new tendency to transfer it to the rubric "convulsions" in later years. Graunt's contemporary and friend, William Petty (1623–1687), also made many observations on mortality and other vital statistical matters, proposing a system of censuses and registration that was far in advance of his time.

Although much good work was done by the demographers and actuaries in the study of mortality, the next great figure in the history of English vital statistics was William Farr (1807–1883), who entered the office of the Registrar-General in 1839 as compiler of extracts. He early urged the advantages of a uniform statistical nomenclature. At the "First Statistical Congress" in 1853, Dr. Farr and others were asked to prepare lists of diseases suitable for the classification of causes of death in the statistical offices. In 1893 Jacques Bertillon (1851–1922), following a classification of diseases based on anatomical sites after the manner of William Farr, presented a draft of a nomenclature, which was adopted by United States, Canada and Mexico. This *International List of the Causes of Death* was introduced in 1893 by the International Statistical Institute and was reviewed by it in 1899. In 1900, 1909, 1920, 1929, and 1938, the International Commission for the Decennial Revision of the International List of the Causes of Death, at the invitation of the French government, revised the *List*. These revisions were followed by the publication of manuals by various governmental agencies, notably the U.S. Bureau of the Census; not only did the manuals recommend assignments of single causes, they also contained instructions on priorities to be observed in making assignments when the certifier has given several possible distinct causes on the certificate of death.

In connection with the *International List of Causes of Death*, up to and including the fifth revision, three points are of great importance: (1) only the order, naming, and numbering of titles (or rubrics) are common among different countries; (2) there had been no international agreement on a list of assignments of individual diagnostic terms to the various titles or rubrics of the *International List*; (3) no guidance was laid down for selecting a single cause for tabulation from a statement of multiple causes.

Difficulties and differences caused by the first and second points just enumerated are relatively unimportant compared with those which arise under the third. The need to select a single cause for tabulation is dictated by the practical difficulties in the presentation of tabulations showing a classification by more than one cause of death. The selection of this single cause ("primary cause" or "underlying cause," as it is frequently termed) created a difficulty that has been met in different countries in various ways.

The sixth revision of the *International List* in 1948 introduced fundamentally new principles. The *List* was to be used for the classification both of causes of death and morbidity and of hospital admissions for diagnosis and childbirth. An attempt was to be made to cite the cause believed by the certifying physician to have initiated the chain of events leading to death. To mark this break, the *List* was superseded by the *International Classification of Causes of Death*, prepared by an Expert Committee of the World Health Organization and approved by an International Conference held by WHO in 1948. It was necessary to add new rubrics to the *Classification* in view of its stated aims. A seventh revision of the *International Classification* was made in 1955 and an eighth revision in 1965.

We believe that, notwithstanding the revisions of the *List* and the *Classification*, it is possible to obtain series of mortality rates for almost all causes of death important at ages under 50 years. However, such great changes have been made to the assignments to the classes of cardiovascular, nervous, and genitourinary diseases, and of senility, that it is impossible to follow them through separately. Nevertheless, the combined contribution of these four groups to mortality, as measured by the age-specific rates, has been rather stable. In making comparisons over the other classes of disease, the principal requirement is to transfer such infective causes as meningitis, gastroenteritis, and hydatid to the infective class for the deaths classified under the earlier revisions.

The death certificate is primarily a legal document. The state decides what are the most important facts to be brought out, and it assigns an order of priority to the causes of death. In general, preference in order is given to those forms of death which legislation and state action may be able to prevent; for example, first priority is given to violent and unnatural causes, such as war, homicide, suicide, legal executions, traffic accidents, poisonings, accidental drownings, deaths due to physical causes (e.g., cold and burns), attack by venomous animals, and therapeutic accidents. High priority is also accorded to infectious, especially the exotic infectious diseases, occupational diseases, diseases of pregnancy, childbirth, and the puerperal state, and diseases peculiar to the first year of life. For in all these causes, it is evident that state intervention may be required.

2. DEFINITIONS OF DEATH

As a rule, there is little doubt about the fact of death or its registration; but there are three instances in which some care must be taken in the making of international comparisons. First, there may be legal doubts regarding whether death has occurred as in certain cases of murder, civil war, and drownings at sea, when no body is recovered. In cases of violent and accidental deaths, the fact of death may even be unknown. From a numerical point of view, this class of death is usually unimportant. Second, deaths in war time may not be published in the official statistics for security reasons. Third, there have been varying definitions of "live birth" and "stillbirth" and, especially in making comparisons over the years before 1960, the following points have to be noted.

In some countries, including notably Belgium and the Netherlands, infants who died within the first three days before registration were registered as "presented dead." If a public holiday intervened, the period might be extended to six days. The statistics of the "presented dead" are given separately in these countries, and such births and deaths did not appear otherwise in the official statistics. In Italy, however, children who are born and die before registration are registered as "stillborn;" but for statistical purposes they are counted as "live births" and "infantile deaths." Signed articles on this topic and some of the implications of the divergences of practice appear in two issues of the *Epidemiological Reports of the World Health Organization* (Pascua, 1948; Stowman, 1949). Therefore, care must always be taken in interpreting international comparisons. Moreover, even within a given political entity, there may be provincial variations in registration practice.

Some attention has been given by some clinicians and epidemiologists to the legitimacy of the exclusion from the mortality statistics of the very immature foetuses delivered. The foetuses of small weight, say under 19 oz or 539 g, have very slender chances of survival under present conditions, yet the statistics treat them in the same tables as the usual run of infants born at term. This question is really full of difficulties. It is very hard to determine or define at what age the foetus becomes viable. The medico-legal textbooks are singularly uninformative on the question. It appears essential, if all abortions are not to be registrable (as they are in the State of New York), that there should be a lower limit to the length of gestation at which stillbirths are notifiable. It seems even more difficult to set the lower limit to the length of gestation of "live births" for registration purposes. Probably we shall not err if we continue to register all infants who show any signs of life as "live births," whatever their presumed length of gestation, for we can easily imagine advances in technique that would give any product of conception separated alive a good chance of survival. Fortunately, there is a period of pregnancy from the fourth to the seventh month when relatively few abortions or births occur.

It appears, then, that we must continue to register and to include in the statistics of infant births all live births, regardless of whether the foetuses are stated to be "nonviable" or previable." Any deaths in this class will then automatically come under the heading of "infantile death." Morevoer, it is important for the purpose of preventive medicine to be able to determine how many infant deaths are due to this excessive degree of immaturity— especially since the bulk of the infant deaths nowadays are ascribable to immaturity. One possible solution is to provide special forms for infant deaths on which some of the more relevant details could be supplied. Foremost among these details are age, parity and disease of the mother, weight of the infant, and plurality of birth. Finally, there should be a tabulation in addition to the usual infant mortality tables, showing the birth weight (where it appears on the certificate) of infants that die. It would be desirable to have the corresponding information for all confinements. Mortality by birth weight is becoming available in some countries, such as the United States and New Zealand.

Member states of the United Nations are going over to the standard definition of live birth, which in effect means that any product of conception that makes any movements after complete expulsion from its mother, will be classified as a live birth. Thus pulsation of the cord and movements of the voluntary muscle are evidence of life, as they should be. It is not held necessary for the child to aerate his lungs before being classified as alive. Aeration of the lungs as evidence of a live birth was a legal requirement for use in actions brought against women for concealment of birth and infanticide.

Model definitions run as follows:

1. *Live birth* is the complete expulsion or extraction from its mother of a product of conception, irrespective of the duration of pregnancy, which, after such separation, breathes or shows any other evidence of life, such as beating of the heart, pulsation of the umbilical cord, or definite movement of voluntary muscles, whether the umbilical cord has been cut or the placenta is attached; each product of such a birth is considered live born.

2. *Foetal death* is death prior to the complete expulsion or extraction from its mother of a product of conception irrespective of the duration of pregnancy; the death is indicated by the fact that after such separation the foetus does not breathe or show any other evidence of life, such as beating of the heart, pulsation of the umbilical cord, or definite movement of voluntary muscles.

3. *Stillbirth* is defined as synonymous with late foetal death; that is, a foetal death occurring after 28 or more completed weeks of gestation.

The first two resolutions above are given in the words of the recommendation of the Expert Committee (1950) "Improvement of Statistics on Foetal Mortality," *Chron. World Health Org.* **4**, 172–176. The third is consistent with their statement. See also Section VIII.2.

3. THE POPULATIONS AT RISK

The absolute number of deaths is not sufficient for comparisons. We need to reduce them to rates per thousand or per million per annum. The divisors are the *population at risk*. Estimates of the population at risk can be constructed as follows. For a single calendar year, the concept of the population at risk presents no difficulty; thus if the death rate for the whole population is to be computed for a certain year, we take the population at the midyear as the measure of the mean number of persons alive during the year and, thus, of the total number of years lived by persons at risk in the year.

If the deaths are being considered pooled over a number of calendar years, we calculate the number of person-years at risk (e.g., during a decade) in the following manner. In the first year there will be, say, P_1 persons alive at the midyear, in the second year there will be P_2 persons, and so on up to the tenth year, when there will be P_{10} persons alive at the midyear. Clearly, P_1 years of life have been experienced by the population during the first year, P_2 during the second year, and so on. Expressed differently, the total number of person-years, or simply years, experienced during the 10-year period is $(P_1 + P_2 + \cdots + P_{10})$. To obtain the mortality rate for the 10 years, the deaths during that decade are summed, and the sum so obtained is divided by the total numbers of years experienced during the corresponding period.

The populations for the first five years of life can be computed as follows. Approximately half the years lived at age under one year in 1961 will be lived by children born in 1961; half will be lived by those born in 1960. But of these, not all will live a complete year; therefore, a correction is made equal to half the mean of the deaths at ages under one year in 1960 and 1961. Similarly, the years of life lived by children aged one year in 1962 will be obtained as the mean of the births in 1960 and 1961, less the mean of the infant deaths in 1960 and 1961, and less half the mean of the deaths at the age of 1 year in 1961 and 1962. In effect, we are estimating the years lived in the various calendar years by a cohort or group of children born, on an average, at the beginning of 1961. By a repetition of this process, we can build up the estimates of the child populations at ages 0 to 4 and 5 to 9 years.

4.   THE AGE–SPECIFIC DEATH RATES

For any serious comparisons between populations, it is usually necessary to compare the death rates of classes that are similar with regard to age and sex, for populations can differ considerably in their distributions by age and sex. The terms "death rates" and "mortality rates" are used synonymously. Experience has shown that, for most purposes, the age groups are conveniently defined by ages in years at the last birthday as follows: 0, 1 to 4, 5 to 14, 15 to 24, ..., 65 to 74, 75 and over. There is some need to limit the number of operations to be performed, while retaining age groups that are comparable throughout a great range of actual populations. This is because wider age groups, say 15 to 44 years, are apt to give groups that may not be strictly comparable in age composition between, for example, a rapidly growing population and a declining population. Distortions introduced by such differences in age composition are not likely to be great in the 10 yearly age groups previously enumerated. Death rates can be made specific with respect not only to age and sex but also to disease, occupation, and geographical or economic, and other factors.

The *age-specific death rates* are obtained by dividing the number of deaths in a defined group of persons by the years of life experienced by the same group (i.e., the years at risk) in the same period. *We assume that all age-specific death rates are also sex-specific.* The death rates are usually given as deaths per annum per thousand, per million, or other power of 10. In other words, the death rates are decimals, and it is usually more advantageous to present them multiplied by a thousand or by a million, in order to obtain results in whole numbers. This practice, although uncommon is far more convenient from the point of view of the printer than giving precisely the same figures expressed as rates per annum per hundred thousand to one decimal place (Yule, 1934).

It may be noted that the infant and maternal mortality rates are not age-specific mortality rates as defined earlier.

5.   THE RELATION BETWEEN m_x AND q_x

For various reasons, the measurement of mortality has been discussed more frequently by actuaries than by medical or health workers. The actuary always has the concept of a life table before him, and he tends to describe mortality in terms of q_x, the probability of a person aged x years dying before he becomes aged $x + 1$ years; q_x and m_x are closely related. Let us drop the subscripts for the moment and consider l persons who have all attained a certain age. A proportion q of them will die before the end of the year—that is,

lq die. For the l persons, $l - lq$ have lived a whole year and lq have lived a fractional part of a year. We assume that the deaths are evenly spread over the year and that each person dying during the year thus has lived on an average a half-year. We thus have years at risk equal to $(l - lq) + \frac{1}{2}lq = l - \frac{1}{2}lq$. Since m, the mortality rate, is the number of deaths, divided by the years at risk, we have

(1)
$$m = \frac{lq}{l - \frac{1}{2}lq} = \frac{2q}{2 - q},$$

and consequently, after a rearrangement, we write

(2)
$$q = \frac{2m}{2 + m}.$$

If the age is specified as x, we have

(3)
$$m_x = \frac{2q_x}{2 - q_x}, \qquad q_x = \frac{2m_x}{2 + m_x}.$$

Examples. It is observed that m_x does not attain the value 0.05 until about age 70 in modern experience. Let us calculate q for specified values of m by (2). When $m = 0.001$, $q = 0.000999$, and other pairs of values are as follows: 0.002, 0.001998; 0.004, 0.003992; 0.01, 0.009950; 0.02, 0.019802; 0.04, 0.039216; 0.05, 0.048780.

The use of m_x in vital statistics has several advantages over the q_x. First, as a rule, the q_x require one more computation than the m_x. Second, the m_x are more readily partitioned into components due to individual causes of death. Third, in the age groups above 75 years, the q_x obtained from the life tables are often greatly affected by interpolation methods. On the other hand, the q_x are often available for comparison when the m_x are not for example, as in various census reports and in follow-up records in cancer or other clinics.

6. THE STANDARD ERROR OF m_x

The standard error of the probability of dying q, in a year, can be obtained by common statistical methods. If n persons begin the year and each has a probability of dying within the year, the deaths will follow the binomial distribution, and the expected number of deaths will be nq. The variance of the number of deaths is $nq(1 - q)$ or npq, where $p = 1 - q$; thus the standard error, or deviation, of the number of deaths is $\sqrt{(npq)}$ as we showed in Section IV.8. But q is usually quite small, and p is consequently close to unity. The standard error of the number of deaths is thus $\sqrt{(nq)}$ approximately.

The probability of death in the year is the number of deaths divided by n. Therefore, the standard error of the observed probability or proportion of death is $\sqrt{(nq)}/n$ or $\sqrt{(q/n)}$ and the standard error of q is the square root of the number of deaths divided by n.

If the proportion has been multiplied by a factor to obtain a rate, say per thousand, the standard error is $1000\sqrt{(qn)}/n$. This can also be written $1000q/\sqrt{(nq)}$, or the calculated death rate divided by the square root of the number of deaths. As q, the probability of dying within a year, and m, the death rate, approximate closely, we can assume that a good approximation to the standard error of a death rate m is the same death rate divided by the square root of the number of deaths. The standard error of the rate can be diminished by calculating the death rate from as many deaths as possible. The age group chosen should not be too narrow, and usually the experience of several years should be pooled.

7. THE ANALYSIS OF THE AGE–SPECIFIC DEATH RATES

Let us consider the statistics of a large country where the death rates have been calculated for each year of life for each calendar year over a long period, say from 1800 onward. We consider the rates for one sex only and form a table; down the first column are the calendar years, 1800, 1801, 1802, ..., and along the first row are the ages in years, 0, 1, 2, ... In the body of the table are written the death rates for the year 1800 and at ages, 0, 1, 2, ..., in the first row; for 1801, we have the death rates at ages 0, 1, 2, ..., in the second row, and then the rates for the succeeding years in the appropriate positions in the table.

Such a table can be read in several ways. First, the rates can be compared by rows for single calendar years—the so-called *calendar method*. The rates can be thought of in a graph as in Figure VII.1 or read off a table such as Table VI.1. Death rates from all causes can be considered. The graph begins at rather a high point, for at age 0 years, we are considering infant mortality. The curve falls throughout childhood, attaining a minimum at the age of 11 years. In both sexes, the graph rises throughout adolescence and also throughout most of adult life. Two exceptions could be made to these statements if we were to consider mortality rates for recent times as in Australia, 1961–1965; there has been a local maximum for the graph of the male death rates in early adult life, and the graph of the female death rates in adult life has had only a slight slope between ages 20 and 40 years.

It is convenient for many purposes to plot the rates on a semi-logarithmic grid; when this is done, the remarkable fact emerges that much of the graph can be represented by a straight line. This is the Gompertz law, as modified by Makeham. No information of any biological value seems ever to have arisen from the study of the constants in the Makeham-Gompertz formula (Greenwood, 1928); but in the past, the formula has been of assistance to the actuaries in their computations. The assumption that underlies the use of the Gompertz or related graduation formulas is that the constants measure a feature in the biological population which is increasing with age. This theory seems to be rather artificial when mortality is divided into its causes, and particularly when mortality from violence or the infections is being considered. Perhaps it is less artificial in the case of mortality from cancer, for in this case explanations might be achieved by way of suitable models of carcinogenesis, as by Armitage and Doll (1961) and Arley (1961), or from arteriosclerosis.

In the second system for using the age-specific death rates, the data are read down the columns of the table. Thus at age 0 year, the trend of the infant mortality can be followed or, the trend of mortality at ages 1 year, or 2 years, and so on, can be studied. In times of declining mortality, analyses by columns will show declines, more marked in the years of infancy and childhood than in later years of life.

In the third method, the mortality of a group born in a certain year is followed. Thus the top left square will have the death rates aged 0 year of those born about the beginning of 1800. In one year's time, this group or cohort will have grown one year older, and the death rate will be found in the second position along the diagonal. The rates along the diagonal will continue to belong to this same cohort. The death rates of other cohorts will be found along lines parallel to the diagonal. The fundamental importance of this cohort or generation method has been realized only in recent years. It has led to satisfying interpretations of the forms of the curves of the death rates from diseases of long standing, such as tuberculosis and lung cancer, which we discuss in greater detail in Sections VIII.7, VIII.8, and VI.11. We give as Table VI.1 the age-specific mortality rates for all American males, recorded at ten yearly intervals, as an example of modification of the methods necessary in the treatment of real data. The calendar method uses the rates in a row. The experience of the cohort of 1900 is given by the rates 1791, 205, 30, 48, 49, 59, 107, and 231. For some purposes, it might be appropriate to extrapolate for the higher ages using the rates 512, 1018, and 2119.

8. THE CRUDE DEATH RATE

The *crude death rate* is the ratio of deaths to the years at risk in the whole population, multiplied by a suitable factor, such as one thousand, to give a rate of deaths per thousand per annum. The use of the crude death rate has led to many fallacious conclusions, especially in the quantitative

Table VI.1

AGE-SPECIFIC MORTALITY RATES

(FOR ALL AMERICAN MALES. RATES PER TEN THOUSAND PER ANNUM)

	All Ages	Age Groups (years)										
		Under 1	1–4	5–14	15–24	25–34	35–44	45–54	55–64	65–74	75–84	85+
1900	179	1791	205	38	59	82	107	157	287	593	1283	2688
1910	156	1455	146	30	48	69	100	152	287	587	1274	2558
1920	134	1036	103	28	48	64	82	126	246	545	1221	2530
1930	123	770	60	19	35	49	75	136	266	558	1191	2367
1940	120	619	31	12	23	34	59	125	262	542	1215	2437
1950	111	373	15	7	17	22	43	107	240	493	1043	2164
1960	110	306	12	6	15	19	37	99	231	491	1018	2119
1966[a]	110	266	10	5	17	20	39	98	233	512	[b]	[b]

[a] WHO. *World Health Statistics Annual for 1966*
[b] Rates unavailable.

study of cancer. The crude death rate is very dependent on the age structure of the populations compared. Thus, if two populations have the same death rates from cancer at every age, the population having the greater proportion of persons at the high ages will exhibit the greater cancer death rates, since cancer is predominantly a disease of the aged. The crude death rate should not be used when more refined measures are available; however, in the analysis of the history of epidemic diseases (e.g., in the analysis of the evolution of mortality in such countries as Sweden over a long period of time), the use of the crude death rates may be inevitable.

9. STANDARDIZATION OF THE DEATH RATES: DIRECT METHOD

It may be desired to compare the mortality in one epoch from a set of diseases in one country with those in another country at the same epoch, or even those in the same country at a different epoch. As a rule, the age-specific death rates are calculated at ages 0 to 4, 5 to 14, 15 to 24, ..., 65 to 74, and 75 years and over. There are thus nine rates to be compared. It is often desirable to combine these rates to permit the use of a single measure for the comparison. One type of measure is obtained by multiplying each rate by an appropriate weight and summing; this is the *standardized death rate*.

As an example of the methods, we standardize the death rates from cancer of males in Australia in 1931 to 1940 onto the life-table population constructed from the Australian Census of 1933. The procedure is to specify the numbers by age of the standard population, which can be chosen with particular considerations in mind. The death rates in each age group in the actual population are then written down, as in Table VI.2. In the final column, the number of deaths to be expected in each age group in the standard population is calculated. For example, 24 deaths per million might be expected at ages, 0 to 14 years, since this is the rate in the actual population. But the standard population has only 221,691 persons at this age, so the expected number is worked out by proportions, namely, 24 × 221,691/1,000,000, or 5 deaths. Similarly, the expected deaths can be computed at ages 15 to 24 years, and so on. These expected deaths can then be summed to give the expected deaths per annum in the standard population of one million, 1825 in this example.

Another commonly used standard million, or million of standard population, is derived by taking a suitable proportion of the numbers enumerated by age and sex in the Census of 1901 in the United Kingdom.

A still simpler standard population consists of one-thirteenth of a million persons in each five-yearly age group, 0 to 4, 5 to 9, 10 to 15, ..., 60 to 64. This standardized rate, which is referred to as the *equivalent average death*

Table VI.2

THE PROCESS OF DIRECT STANDARDIZATION[a]

Age Groups (years)	Number of Males in the Life-Table Population	Death Rates for Males in the Actual Population (per million per annum)	Number of Deaths in the Standard Population	Number of Females in the Standard Population	Death Rates for Females in Actual Population (per million per annum)	Number of Deaths in the Standard Population
0–	221,691	24	5	211,607	21	4
15–	144,491	41	6	138,995	33	5
25–	141,010	98	14	135,816	130	18
35–	136,146	316	43	131,323	596	78
45–	127,312	1,106	141	124,446	1,614	201
55–	109,614	3,445	377	112,130	3,253	365
65–	78,255	8,374	655	88,050	6,072	535
75+	41,481	14,085	584	57,633	10,539	607
Total	1,000,000	1,123	1825	1,000,000	1,069	1813

[a] The standard populations have been computed from the life tables constructed from the data of the 1933 census in Australia. The members of the standard population have been imagined to be subjected at each age group to the same mortality rates from cancer as obtained in the actual population of Australia in the years 1931 to 1940.

rate, has been much used in occupational statistics since its introduction by Yule (1934). The computation of this rate is very simple, for it is the average of the rates for the thirteen 5-year age groups. If rates are only available for 10-year age groups, the rate in a 10-year age group is considered to be the average of the two 5-year age groups which it contains. The rates in childhood are reckoned from the experience of the children of those engaged in the occupation under scrutiny.

10. STANDARDIZATION OF THE DEATH RATES: THE INDIRECT METHOD

For completeness, although the method is not a true standardization, we now describe the *indirect method of standardization*. Suppose that the numbers of years at risk in the target population observed are T_1, T_2, T_3, ... and that a total of D deaths are observed. Let a standard population be chosen with t_1, t_2, t_3, ..., years at risk at the same ages and a schedule of death rates $q_1 = d_1/t_1$, $q_2 = d_2/t_2$, $q_3 = d_3/t_3$, ... The first step is to determine how many deaths, δ, would occur in the target population if it were submitted to the death rates of the standard population. We have then

(1) $$\delta = q_1 T_1 + q_2 T_2 + q_3 T_3 + \cdots.$$

We also know the death rate in the standard population, namely,

(2) $$r = \frac{d_1 + d_2 + \cdots}{t_1 + t_2 + \cdots}.$$

We now assume that the indirectly standardized death rate R for the target population bears the same ratio to r as do the deaths D in the target population to the expected deaths δ; thus we have

(3) $$\frac{R}{r} = \frac{D}{\delta},$$

or, after rearrangement,

(4) $$R = \frac{rD}{\delta}.$$

It may be noted that only D and not the individual numbers of deaths by the age groups in the target population is used in the computation. This is sometimes convenient in examining target subpopulations of, say, the counties of England and Wales, or the individual states of the United States, for deaths by age and cause may not be available for appropriate age groups in such smaller geographical areas of interest. It was the conclusion of Yule (1934) that the standard errors of the direct and indirect methods of standardization were of the same order. We give an example of the process in Table VI.3.

Table VI.3

THE PROCESS OF INDIRECT STANDARDIZATION[a]

Age Groups	Standard Population		Hewers		Solicitors	
	Numbers	Death Rates	Numbers	Expected Deaths	Numbers	Expected Deaths
20–24	1,381	3.52	1,589	5.59	99	0.35
25–34	2,591	3.99	3,249	12.96	1,581	6.31
35–44	2,499	6.39	2,577	16.47	2,645	16.90
45–54	2,151	11.56	1,809	20.91	2,839	32.82
55–64	1,378	25.72	776	19.96	2,836	72.94
	10,000	5.118	10,000	7.589×10	10,000	12.932×10
Death rates						
Observed		5.118		6.966		12.223
Standardized		5.118		4.698		4.838

[a] The figures in columns 5 and 7 are the rates (column 3) applied to the populations in columns 4 and 6, respectively, to give the number of expected deaths among hewers and solicitors. The observed death rates of hewers in column 5 is obtained by dividing the actual deaths [9,788] by the years at risk [1,405,182] and expressing the result as a rate per thousand. Similarly, $12.223 = 10^3 \times 513/41,970$. The standardized rates are obtained as explained in the text: $6.996 \times 5.118/7.589 = 4.698$. The data are from Yule (1934).

11. FORECASTING THE MORTALITY RATES

Forecast mortality rates serve in estimations of population numbers in future years and, more rarely, as a test of a particular hypothesis. Age- and sex-specific rates are used. The commonest technique is to fit a straight line to the rates or the logarithm of the rates for a given age and sex. Sometimes the fit of a straight line to the logarithm of the rates is good, and satisfactory results are obtained from the extrapolation. This is the method of extrapolating down a column of the rates as given in a table such as Table VI.1. An alternative method is to assume that the shape of the curve of the mortality rates for a cohort has a given form; then if the first few years of experience are known, the remainder can be forecast by taking simple proportions.

A more biological method is to consider for each age group the possible effects of projected public health measures or therapy on the mortality from individual diseases. Thus we might assume a negligible mortality from tuberculosis, no change from the mortality from cancers generally, but an increase in the mortality from lung cancer, and so on. These estimated rates can be summed to give the projected death rate.

EXERCISES

1. The registered deaths for white males in the United States in the three years, 1939 to 1941 are given in the following table, together with the estimated population at July 1, 1940. Consider the years at risk in each age group to be three times the population at the midpoint of three years and compute the age specific death rates from the following table.

Age Groups	Registered Deaths, 1939–1941	Estimated Population, 1/7/1940	Age Groups	Registered Deaths, 1939–1941	Estimated Population, 1/7/1940
0–4	186,541	4,697,251	50–54	142,217	3,461,903
5–9	16,716	4,736,987	55–59	173,192	2,808,550
10–14	17,062	5,234,717	60–64	201,341	2,238,579
15–19	28,507	5,511,945	65–69	229,887	1,749,889
20–24	35,522	5,131,965	70–74	235,612	1,190,567
25–29	37,146	4,905,853	75–79	208,875	683,763
30–34	42,405	4,588,155	80–84	157,479	342,554
35–39	53,285	4,253,778	85–89	76,515	114,282
40–44	72,956	4,021,881	90–94	23,084	25,165
45–49	105,256	3,841,840	95–99	4,396	4,292
			100+	626	573

Plot the age-specific death rates on a rectangular grid; plot them also on a semi-logarithmic grid. Comment on the shape of the curves and on the difficulty of bringing out mortality features at all ages on the rectangular grid.

2. Compute the equivalent average death rates from the rates computed in Exercise 1.

3. Condense the table of Exercise 1 to give deaths and midpoint populations at ages 0 to 4, 5 to 14, 15 to 24, ..., 55 to 64, and 65 and over. Compute the age-specific death rates for these age groups. Compute the deaths in a standard million (i.e., the standardized death rates) given by the following table:

Males (standard million) England and Wales, 1901		Females (standard million) England and Wales, 1901	
Age Groups	Population	Age Groups	Population
0–4	117,961	0–4	110,799
5–14	216,800	5–14	203,525
15–24	195,832	15–24	195,658
25–34	158,052	25–34	164,881
35–44	122,831	35–44	122,866
45–54	88,769	45–54	89,645
55–64	57,726	55–64	61,628
65–74	30,382	65–74	35,606
75+	11,647	75+	15,391
Total	1,000,000	Total	999,999

4. Compute the equivalent average death rate from the rates in Exercise 3, noting that the rates at ages 0 to 4 are counted once and that each of the other rates 5 to 14, ..., 55 to 64, is counted twice before dividing through by 13. Compare the answer with the rate computed in Exercise 2.

5. Between 1961 and 1965, the midyear populations of Australian males and the deaths were as follows:

Year	Midyear Population (thousands)	Deaths from All Causes
1961	5.312	50,248
1962	5,402	52,378
1963	5,506	53,212
1964	5,615	56,246
1965	5,728	55,170

Compute the crude death rates for Australian males for each year. Sum the populations to give the total years at risk and sum the deaths. Compute the crude death rate for 1961 to 1965 as the ratio of these two sums. (In such cases when the populations at risk are of the same order of magnitude, the mean of the ratios is approximately the ratio of the means.)

6. The numbers of females, aged 45 to 49 years, estimated for the midyear, and the number of deaths from various cancers in Australia and from all causes are given in the following table:

Year	Midyear Population	Deaths from Cancer	All Deaths
1961	335,890	676	1974
1962	334,810	774	2106
1963	331,267	823	2106
1964	328,073	739	2042
1965	329,732	741	1999

Compute the age-specific mortality rate from cancer at ages 45 to 49 years for females in Australia during 1961–1965. Compute also the age-specific mortality rate from all causes.

7. The births and deaths at ages under 5 years for white males in America have been given as follows [Greville (1946), p. 113]:

Year	Births	Deaths at Ages (years)				
		0	1	2	3	4
1934	975,804	60,319				
1935	969,916	56,424	7183			
1936	966,332	56,970	7491	3834		
1937	991,356	55,540	6781	3671	2461	
1938	1,030,398	54,121	6366	3255	2334	1729
1939	1,019,021	50,201	5292	2759	2012	1572
1940	1,064,067	51,477	4929	2592	1731	1432
1941	1,133,394	52,191	4717	2517	1756	1363

Compute the infant mortality rates (deaths per thousand births) for each calendar year. Compute the survivors of the cohort of the 975,804 births of 1934 to age 1, assuming that half the deaths at age 0 in 1934 and half the deaths at age 0 in 1935 have been of the group. Similarly, subtract half the deaths at age 1 in 1935 and half the deaths at age 1 in 1936 to obtain the survivors to age 2. Continue similarly and find the survivors to ages 3, 4, and 5 years.

8. Calculate q_x from (3) of Section VI.5 for $m_x = 0.001$, 0.005, 0.006, 0.007, 0.008, 0.009, 0.01, 0.02, 0.03, 0.04, 0.05, 0.10, 0.20, 0.30.

9. The standard error of a death rate has been computed on the assumption that the various events leading up to the deaths are independent. This independence breaks

down for the infective diseases. Comment on how the variance of the death rates would be affected by plane crashes or natural disasters. Comment also on the variance of death from rare causes, such as hemochromatosis.

10. Given the following data obtained at the Australian Census of 1947, work out the death rate standardized onto the life-table population. Also give the equivalent average death rate for males under 65 years of age.

Age Groups	Deaths in Australia of Males, 1947	Males Enumerated in Australia, 1947	Males in the Life-Table Population of Australia, 1933
0–4	3,578	388,301	74,896
5–14	512	579,458	146,795
15–24	933	607,014	144,491
25–34	1,093	595,028	141,010
35–44	1,822	543,317	136,146
45–54	4,017	443,896	127,312
55–64	7,768	358,085	109,614
65–74	9,565	193,430	78,255
75+	11,468	88,841	41,481

11. Calculate the crude death rate, the age-specific death rates, and the mortality rate from cancer, standardized onto the life-table population of Exercise 10, using the following data:

Age Groups	Deaths from Cancer, Males	Total Years of Life Experienced by Males in Australia, 1931–1940 (thousands)
0–14	218	9,060
15–24	250	6,163
25–34	538	5,484
35–44	1,475	4,674
45–54	4,413	3,991
55–64	9,105	2,643
65–74	13,704	1,637
75+	8,783	624
Total	38,486	34,276

CHAPTER VII

The Life Table

1. THE PURPOSES OF THE LIFE TABLE

For a biologist, the primary aim of a life table is to give a numerical description of the deaths and survivals in a group (or cohort) of animals which have been followed through their lives; for some populations, it is impossible to fulfil this aim. Instead, there is given a set or *schedule* of mortality rates, and it is required to estimate the survivors to each age of a group of animals passing through life exposed to this schedule. In the past, the schedule of mortality rates has been estimated for every age at the time of a census or for a span of years between censuses; an ideal population or *mathematical model* has then been set up and the members have been supposed to be submitted to the same schedule of rates observed in the actual population. However, the schedule of rates might equally well have been predicated on the basis of a hypothesis about possible changes in environmental or hygienic conditions and the consequences of these death rates worked out by means of the life table. First computed for human populations, life tables are now used in the study of natural or laboratory animal populations. It has been found convenient to empty the same methods for the study of plants, for determining the rates of wastage of equipment and the growth of families, and for many other purposes.

A direct observational method for the construction of life tables is practicable for short-lived animals such as flies or mice. We observe, say, a thousand mice from birth and count the survivors to age 1 day, 2 days, 3 days, until finally all are dead. This simple procedure, which would seem "natural" to a biologist, is usually not feasible in human populations, although it is practicable in, for example, follow-up studies of patients treated for cancer. The direct observational method is seldom used in the study of human populations, principally because of the administrative and technical difficulties in following a number of persons throughout their lives—

expense, migration, wars, resistance of persons to any form of continued observation, and the lack of continuity in a project of long duration, are among the obstacles to such an approach. Generation or cohort life tables, however, can supply information that is close to what would be yielded by the direct observational approach.

2. SELECT LIFE TABLES OR MORTALITY STUDIES

The life tables constructed by the official statisticians from the mortality experiences of various countries have been usually of the whole population; but studies on selected groups can also be of great interest. Thus William Farr could construct life tables for the "healthy" English counties and compare them with those of the "industrial" counties. Similarly, life tables for various American states have demonstrated considerable variation in mortality in the United States. It is always of interest to examine the most favorable tables that can be constructed for a given country, since they indicate that hygienic or social changes may make such favorable rates or tables possible over a much wider area.

One form of *select life tables* is constructed by the insurance companies from their experiences of insured lives; that is, of persons accepted as risks suitable for life insurance. Since these persons are "selected" by medical or other examination, the select life tables give the experience of a group of initially healthy persons. The tables are usually of doubtful comparative value, however, because it can never be known whether the criteria of selection have remained constant over a period of time. Another feature of this type of table is that among those treated as 24 years old, say, at entrance, are some whose age is 24 years—but others are included who are 23 years old and have been "weighted" one year by the company, or 22 years old, weighted two years, and so on. This practice greatly detracts from the value of the tables made by the life insurance companies.

Life tables of great historical interest have been constructed by Peller (1948), from records of the noble families of the old German and central European states, and by Russell (1948) from medieval English records. Such mortality inquiries are continuing in other countries, particularly France, using parish records and other old documents. The observer using the records of the noble families is in the same position as is the observer of a *Drosophila* colony, for he can count the number of persons entering the experience at birth, the number surviving to the first, second, ..., birthday; thus he is relieved of the necessity to compute the death rates first.

Life-table methods are useful in clinical studies and in follow-up studies of patients (e.g., in diabetes or cancer clinics).

3. THE FUNDAMENTAL ASSUMPTIONS OF THE LIFE TABLE

In modern language, the life table would be considered to be a mathematical model of the order of dying out of persons observed through their lives, the *Absterbeordnung* of German authors. In this model, it is assumed that the deaths are occurring according to some law. As an approximation, it usually suffices to assume that the deaths are uniformly distributed throughout the year, except at ages under 1. A further assumption that the death rates at a point of time could represent the death rates of a group passing through life is also made. The rates chosen in the mathematical model need not be those holding in some calendar year or epoch. They might be chosen as appropriate to a cohort, for example, of people born in France in 1872. They might be chosen as possible rates in a population after the mortality from certain groups of diseases had been eliminated. The rates might even be chosen according to hypotheses on the future progress of mortality.

4. THE LIFE–TABLE FUNCTIONS

In the life table, the values of the various functions computed are usually determined only for integer values of the age; that is, at ages 0, 1, 2, 3, ..., years, usually up to age 105 years.

(i) Survivors

The number of survivors from l_0 born into the life table to age x years is written l_x and is spoken of as the *survivors* to age x years. We can chose l_0 arbitrarily; usually it is put equal to unity or 100,000. With the second choice, decimals are avoided; but for theoretical work $l_0 = 1$ is often more convenient.

(ii) Probability of Survival for One Year

The probability of a person surviving from aged x years to aged $(x + 1)$ years is written p_x. The probability is to be read here as a proportion. The number who survive to $x + 1$ years is l_{x+1}; thus we have

(1) $$p_x = \frac{l_{x+1}}{l_x} \quad \text{and} \quad l_{x+1} = l_x p_x.$$

Therefore, given l_0 and $p_0, p_1, p_2, \ldots, l_1, l_2, l_3, \ldots$, can be computed in turn.

(iii) The Number of Deaths at Age x Years

The number of deaths between age x and age $x + 1$ years is written d_x. Since persons alive at age x must either die in the next year or survive to age $x + 1$, we can write

$$(2) \qquad\qquad l_x = d_x + l_{x+1}.$$

Thus the number of deaths at age x is simply the difference between those who reach x and those who reach $x + 1$ years.

$$(3) \qquad\qquad d_x = l_x - l_{x+1}.$$

$$(4) \qquad l_x = d_x + l_{x+1} = d_x + d_{x+1} + l_{x+2} = d_x + d_{x+1} + d_{x+2} + \cdots,$$

since (2) can be applied repeatedly with x replaced by $x + 1, x + 2, \ldots$.

(iv) The Probability of Death at Age x Years

The probability that a person who has reached x years will die before he attains the age $x + 1$ years is written q_x. Once again, the probability is to be interpreted as a proportion. It follows from the definition that

$$(5) \qquad\qquad q_x = \frac{d_x}{l_x} = \frac{l_x - l_{x+1}}{l_x}.$$

It is evident also from the definitions that

$$(6) \qquad\qquad q_x + p_x = 1, \qquad p_x = 1 - q_x.$$

(v) The Mortality Rate at Age x Years

The mortality rate in the life table at age x years is written m_x. Being a mortality rate, it is the ratio between the deaths at age x and the years at risk as measured by the number of years lived at age x in the life table. This number of years will be greater than l_{x+1}, which includes only the number of completed years. On the other hand, it will be less than l_x, which would represent the number of years that would be lived by the group if all the deaths took place at the end of the year. Evidently the number lies between l_{x+1} and l_x. Graphical considerations show that this number of years is close to the mean of l_x and l_{x+1}. Thus we know that number of years lived in the life table between ages x and $x + 1$ years is approximately $\frac{1}{2}(l_x + l_{x+1})$.

$$(7) \qquad\qquad m_x = \frac{d_x}{\frac{1}{2}(l_x + l_{x+1})}.$$

The figure given for the years at risk is equivalent to saying that everyone lives, on an average, half a year at the age at which he dies. Since this relationship is not very exact in the first year of life, other methods are used to obtain q_0. In practice, an estimate is made from the statistics of births and infant deaths of the number of survivors to age 1 year exactly.

(vi) The Expectation of Life

The complete expectation of life, usually called the *expectation of life*, is the average length of life that a person at age x years can be expected to live in the life table and is written $\mathring{e}_x$; this value is obtained by dividing the number of years lived above age x by l_x. The number of years will be complete if the person lives from x to $x + 1$, $x + 1$, to $x + 2$, and so on. The total of completed years is thus $l_{x+1} + l_{x+2} + l_{x+3} + \cdots$. The deaths can be assumed to be scattered throughout each year, making the total of the incomplete years approximately $\frac{1}{2}l_x$, since each person will live half a year, on an average, in the year he dies. The expectation of life can now be computed.

$$(8) \qquad \mathring{e}_x = \frac{\frac{1}{2}l_x + l_{x+1} + l_{x+2} + \cdots}{l_x}.$$

$\mathring{e}_0$ is the complete expectation of life at birth or average length of life. It is much used by popular writers on health and population affairs. The expectation of life at any age, which is an average, need not tell us anything precise about the mortality experience at higher ages.

(vii) The Force of Mortality

The force of mortality is the ratio of deaths from age x to age $x + \delta$ to the number of years lived in between the ages x to $x + \delta$ years, as δ is taken smaller and smaller. This limit would be given by

$$(9) \qquad -\mu_x = \lim_{\delta \to 0} \frac{l_{x+\delta} - l_x}{\delta l_x} = \frac{dl_x/dx}{l_x} = \frac{d}{dx} \log_e l_x$$

5. CONSTRUCTION OF THE LIFE TABLE

It is not intended to discuss here the technical details of life-table construction. It is sufficient to note in passing that usually a process of graduation is used and that a series of values for q_x and hence p_x is obtained. Every value of l_x is then computed. It is regrettable that the actuaries have concentrated far too much of their attention on such graduation procedures. Our account is very much like the procedures usually referred to as the *abridged method*. The first step is to equate the mortality rates in the life table to the corresponding rate in the actual population. The infant mortality rate can be obtained from the statistics of births and deaths. This is set equal to q_0. At other ages, m_x is given:

(1)
$$m_x = \frac{\text{number of deaths at age } x}{\text{number of years experienced at age } x}$$

$$= \frac{d_x}{\frac{1}{2}(l_x + l_{x+1})} = \frac{l_x q_x}{\frac{1}{2}(l_x + l_x - l_x q_x)}.$$

Or, dropping the subscripts for the time being, we can write

(2)
$$m = \frac{q}{\frac{1}{2}(2 - q)} = \frac{2q}{2 - q}.$$

After rearrangement, we have

(3)
$$q = \frac{2m}{2 + m} \quad \text{and} \quad q_x = \frac{2m_x}{2 + m_x}.$$

Note that m_x is usually quite small and that q_x is quite close to m_x throughout almost the whole life table.

The values of $p_x = 1 - q_x$ are next obtained, and we have $l_{x+1} = p_x l_x$, as in (1) of Section VII.4, which we apply for $x = 0, 1, 2, 3, \ldots$. We next obtain d_x by taking differences between the l_x, $d_x = l_x - l_{x+1}$, as in (3) of Section VII.4.

6. DESCRIPTION OF THE LIFE–TABLE FUNCTIONS

Strictly speaking, m_x is not a life-table function. The schedule of mortality rates $\{m_x\}$ has usually been observed in an actual population, but it may have been constructed on some hypothesis. The value of q_x is closely related to m_x and, for the x's for which m_x is small, q_x can be considered in place of m_x or μ_x. As we have seen, $q_x + p_x = 1$; thus we only need consider q_x, which we do. We consider the graphs of the functions as they would appear in the official statistics of any well-developed country, actually Australia in 1961. The q_0 is the infantile mortality, which means that the graph of q_x begins at a relatively high point in Figure VII.1. The graph falls throughout childhood, principally because the child is becoming immune to the childhood infections or better able to cope with any infections that occur. A minimum is reached at about age 11 years in both sexes, and the curves continue to rise throughout life, with the possible exception of a local maximum at young adult life for males, due to violent and accidental deaths.

The curve of l_x in Figure VII.2 begins at 100,000 and falls rapidly because

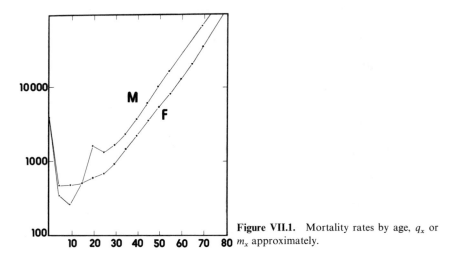

Figure VII.1. Mortality rates by age, q_x or m_x approximately.

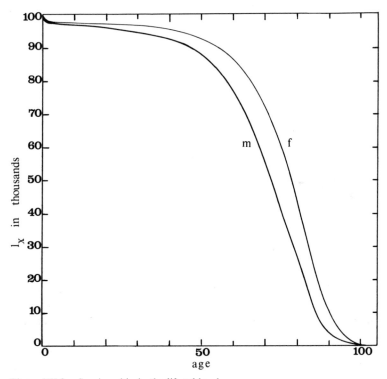

Figure VII.2. Survivorship in the life tables, l_x.

93

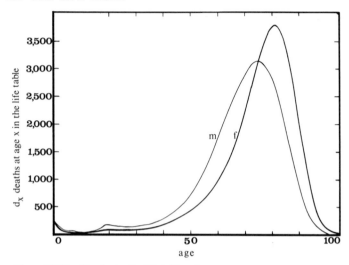

Figure VII.3.   Deaths in the life tables, d_x.

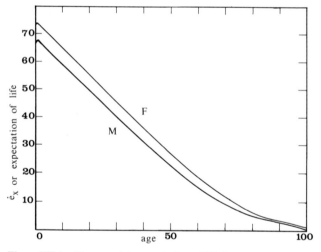

Figure VII.4.   The complete expectation of life $\mathring{e}_x$.

of the high infant mortality. The curve is then rather flat, although tending downward, from infancy until the middle fifties. It becomes increasingly steep, attaining maximum steepness at about ages 75 and 80 years for men and women, respectively.

The curve of d_x is approximately the curve of the slope of l_x by (3) of Section VII.4. It begins at a high level in infancy, falls to a minimum at age 11 years, rises slowly at first (possibly attaining a local maximum at age 21 years or nearby), rises to a maximum at ages 75 or 80 years, and falls steadily to zero (see Figure VII.3). The complete expectation of life $\overset{\circ}{e}_x$ begins at a high level but increases to a maximum at age 1 year and falls steadily throughout life, as in Figure VII.4. In countries having high infant mortality or high child mortality rates, $\overset{\circ}{e}_x$ has attained a maximum for $x = 7$. Before 1920 in most countries of the world, $\overset{\circ}{e}_5$ was greater than $\overset{\circ}{e}_0$. We state without proof that $\overset{\circ}{e}_x$ can be an increasing function of x whenever the force of mortality exceeds the reciprocal of the expectation of life. This is approximately equivalent to the condition that $m_x > 1/\overset{\circ}{e}_x$ or $q_x > 1/\overset{\circ}{e}_x$. It is seen in countries having high infant and child mortality rates.

EXERCISES

1. Normal mice were observed from their entry into certain cages (and not from birth, for there is cannibalism among mice in captivity). Mice were observed first at age about 100 days, or "cage age zero." At cage ages 0, 50, 100, 150, ..., 850 days, the numbers of mice alive were: 269; 269, 265, 263, 259, 258; 254, 249, 244, 237, 223; 193, 162, 140, 105, 76; 51, 22. The l_x are thus directly observed. Plot the values of l_x as a graph and compare it with the human life table. Compute the d_x for the 50-day intervals. Compute $\overset{\circ}{e}_x$, assuming that on an average a mouse lives 25 days in the interval in which it dies. [These data, due to A. B. Hill, were cited by Greenwood (1928).]

2. Mice were observed by Murray with a commencing point about 200 days after birth at cage ages (in days) of 0, 50, 100, ..., 650. The survivors were: 619; 553, 494, 421, 353, 308; 259, 213, 172, 133, 95; 62, 36, and 23. Calculate mortality rates at ages 0 to 49, 50 to 99, 100 to 149, ..., days, by assuming that each mouse lives 25 days in the period in which he dies. Compute $\overset{\circ}{e}_x$ for the beginning of each interval. Plot the graph of l_x. [Data, due to J. A. Murray, cited by Greenwood (1928).]

3. The number of *Drosophila* were observed at days 1, 7, 13, 19, 25; 31, 37, 43, 49, 55; 61, 67, and 73 to be as follows: 2822, 2781, 2753, 2693, 2522; 2337, 2109, 1763, 1436, 1070; 510, 272, and 111. Compute the life table functions l_x, q_x, m_x, d_x, $\overset{\circ}{e}_x$ at days 1, 7, 13, ... (Data of R. Pearl, cited by Greenwood, 1928.)

4. Give an account of how you would study the order of dying-out of either mice or men with complete observations extending over a period longer than the life span. Why is this method of observing the subjects over their life span seldom considered to be practical in man? Detail in general terms the procedure adopted by the statistician to form a life table, defining in turn m_x, the death rate in the population at age x years, and the life-table values q_x, p_x, and l_x.

5. In a certain follow-up of cancer cases after treatment, it was learned that 10 died in first year, 23 in second, 35 in third, 60 in fourth, 44 in fifth, 32 in sixth, 15 in seventh, and the remainder, 9, in the eighth. What was the expectation of life for these patients at the time of treatment?

6. The expectations of life for males for various countries are given in Table M of Greville (1946) as follows:

Age (years)	Australia 1932–1934	Belgium, 1918–1932	England and Wales, 1930–1932	Mexico, 1930	United States (whites), 1939–1941
0	63.48	56.02	58.74	32.44	62.81
1	65.49	61.25	62.25	40.64	64.98
5	62.57	59.21	60.11	44.97	61.68
10	58.02	54.88	55.79	44.57	57.03
15	53.36	50.29	51.19	40.80	52.33

Comment on these expectations of life, especially noting that $\overset{\circ}{e}_0$ is in no table the greatest of the $\overset{\circ}{e}_x$'s. Compare these figures with the table of Exercise 13.

7. The following is a table of l_x for total males in the United States for the years 1959 to 1961.

x	l_x	x	l_x	x	l_x	x	l_x
0	100,000	25	94,631	50	86,199	75	38,950
1	97,087	26	94,466	51	85,325	76	36,210
2	96,911	27	94,306	52	84,369	77	33,468
3	96,800	28	94,148	53	83,333	78	30,732
4	96,714	29	93,990	54	82,222	79	28,006
5	96,643	30	93,826	55	81,039	80	25,300
6	96,580	31	93,656	56	79,783	81	22,619
7	96,522	32	93,479	57	78,451	82	19,983
8	96,469	33	93,293	58	77.032	83	17,439
9	96,420	34	93,097	59	75,513	84	15,045
10	96,375	35	92,889	60	73,887	85	12,845
11	96,333	36	92,666	61	72,151	86	10,819
12	96,290	37	92,426	62	70,308	87	8,980
13	96,242	38	92,166	63	68,361	88	7,333
14	96,182	39	91,883	64	66,316	89	5,876
15	96,107	40	91,572	65	64,177	90	4,609
16	96,014	41	91,230	66	61,947	91	3,534
17	95,905	42	90,854	67	59,631	92	2,648
18	95,779	43	90,441	68	57,235	93	1,939
19	95,641	44	89,988	69	54,770	94	1,387
20	95,491	45	89,492	70	52,244	95	970
21	95,330	46	88,950	71	49,665	96	665
22	95,158	47	88,359	72	47,040	97	446
23	94,981	48	87,709	73	44,375	98	293
24	94,803	49	86,992	74	41,676	99	187

The material for Exercises 7 to 14 has been taken from *United States Life Tables*: *1959–1961, Life-Tables: 1956–1961*, Vol. 1, No. 1. U.S. Department Health, Education and Welfare, 1964.

8. Compute q_x from the l_x of Exercise 7 for $x = 0, 1, 2, 3, 4, 5, 10, 15, 20, \ldots, 90$, and plot the graph of q_x against the age.

9. Calculate q_x from the l_x of Exercise 7 for $x = 8, 9, 10, 11, 12, 13$, and $x = 20, 21, 22, 23, 24, 25, 26, 27, 28, 29$, and hence determine the minimum of q_x and the corresponding x in childhood, the relative maximum of q_x in early adult life, and the relative minimum in the late twenties. Give an explanation for these minima and the relative maximum.

10. Compute $\overset{\circ}{e}_x$ by (8) of Section VII.5, for $x = 90, 85, 80, \ldots, 5, 0$, cumulating the sums, $l_{100} + l_{99} + \cdots + l_{96}$, $l_{100} + l_{99} + \cdots + l_{91}$, $l_{100} + l_{99} + \cdots + l_{86}, \ldots$, and then using the formula, assuming that a person lives an average of a half year in the year in which he dies.

11. Compute $\overset{\circ}{e}_x$ by a modification of (8) of Section VII.4, for $x = 90, 85, \ldots, 5, 0$, by cumulating the sums l_{100}, $l_{100} + l_{95}$, $l_{100} + l_{95} + l_{90}$, $l_{100} + \cdots + l_{85}, \ldots$, $l_{100} + \cdots + l_5 + l_0$.

The completed five-year stretches will be the sums just given; $\overset{\circ}{e}_{40}$, for example, will be given by

$$\overset{\circ}{e}_{40} = 2.5 + \frac{5(l_{100} + l_{95} + \cdots + l_{50} + l_{45})}{l_{40}}.$$

Compare these approximate results with those of the previous exercise.

12. The q_x for certain ages for white males in the United States are given in the *United States Life Tables 1959–1961* as follows:

x				q_x			
	1959–1961	1949–1951	1939–1941	1929–1931	1919–1921	1909–1911	1900–1902
45	0.00558	0.00637	0.00766	0.00929	0.00926	0.01264	0.01263
50	0.00955	0.01012	0.01155	0.01278	0.01174	0.01553	0.01537
55	0.01475	0.01587	0.01737	0.01819	0.01653	0.02150	0.02118
60	0.02271	0.02381	0.02548	0.02644	0.02462	0.03075	0.02859
65	0.03389	0.03445	0.03685	0.03865	0.03499	0.04379	0.04166
70	0.04871	0.05027	0.05454	0.05796	0.05463	0.06214	0.05894
75	0.07066	0.07499	0.08313	0.08526	0.08191	0.09253	0.08843

Draw a graph of these rates and comment on them.

13. The following table presents the average remaining life time or expectation of life, $\overset{\circ}{e}_x$, for males in the United States for various ages and epochs:

$\overset{\circ}{e}_x$						
x	1959–1961	1949–1951	1939–1941	1929–1931	1919–1921	1909–1911	1900–1902
---	---	---	---	---	---	---	---
0	67.55	66.31	62.81	59.12	56.34	50.23	48.23
5	64.61	63.77	61.68	59.38	58.31	55.37	54.43
10	59.78	58.98	57.03	54.96	54.15	51.32	50.59
50	23.22	22.83	21.96	21.51	22.22	20.39	20.76
60	16.01	15.76	15.05	14.72	15.25	13.98	14.35
65	12.97	12.75	12.07	11.77	12.21	11.25	11.51

Use these figures to criticize the following statement: "there is a larger proportion of elderly persons in the American population in 1961 than in 1901 because persons are living to a higher age," and the common notion that $\overset{\circ}{e}_0$ has increased because of improvements in mortality at the high ages.

14. In the tables for 1900–1902 and 1909–1911, data for the life tables were collected from the death-registration states, 10 states plus the District of Columbia; 24 more states were added for 1919–1921. For 1929–1931, 1939–1941, and 1949–1951, the whole of the continental United States was included. In 1959–1961, Alaska and Hawaii were added. Speculate how this changing area might have affected the mortality rates for the total population.

15. The death rates by age groups for white males in the United States, the populations by age for white males in the United States and in some individual states, and the crude death rates for 1960 are given in the following table. (Data from Grove and Hetzel, 1968.)

Age Groups	Deaths/ million per Annum for Entire United States	Population of Entire United States (thousands)	Population of Arkansas	Population of California	Population of Massachusetts
Under 1 year	23,577	1,784	13,800	161,859	54,617
1–4	952	7,065	55,477	637,883	215,918
5–14	439	15,658	140,457	1,400,311	462,973
15–24	991	10,483	98,286	984,278	313,111
25–34	1,236	9,940	75,257	971,908	301,624
35–44	2,604	10,564	83,991	1,040,095	328,513
45–54	6,923	9,114	83,475	830,441	285,166
55–64	16,328	6,850	64,546	588,862	226,960
65–74	37,398	4,702	50,051	393,599	160,067
75–84	88,272	1,874	21,542	157,101	63,232
85+	203,545	330	3,880	26,757	11,766

Calculate the expected death rates in Arkansas, California, and Massachusetts by applying the U.S. rates at each age to the state population. The observed death rates in the three states were 9.7, 10.0, and 12.0. Standardize these rates onto the population of the United States by multiplying the state observed rate by the U.S. rate divided by the state expected rate. These three numbers are the rates indirectly standardized onto the U.S. population.

16. Use the result of Exercise 7 of Chapter VI to determine l_1, l_2, ..., l_5, by following the experience of the birth cohort of 1934.

NOTES

Texts: Coale and Demeny, 1966; Dublin, Lotka, and Spiegelman, 1949; Greenwood, 1922; Greville, 1946; Pearl, 1940; Spiegelman, 1955.

Graunt's Table; Glass, 1950, 1963, 1964.

Halley's Table: Greenwood, 1942; Halley, 1693.

Australian Life Tables: Lancaster, 1951c, 1964a.

English Life Tables: Registrar-General's Decennial Supplement, 1957.

American Life Tables: Greville, 1946; Grove and Hetzel, 1968; Smith, 1948.

CHAPTER VIII

Mortality in Human Populations

1. INTRODUCTORY

A detailed and fully documented account of the progress of mortality throughout the countries of the world would require more space than is available in this text. We would have to compare the mortality rates by country, age, sex, and cause, and by social and economic conditions. These comparisons would require numerous tables and graphs. However, certain aspects of these comparisons seldom receive adequate treatment in texts of statistics or epidemiology.

There is now available much commentary on the mortality of individual countries, not only in the yearbooks and other official publications but also in journal articles and the discussions of learned societies. At the end of the chapter we furnish bibliographical references that may assist the student wishing either to trace the progress of mortality in one country or to make international comparisons. Much commentary on mortality can now be found in Australia, England and Wales, France, New Zealand, Sweden, and the United States. Also there are good official statistics available from Canada and Japan.

2. INFANT MORTALITY

The *infant mortality* is usually computed by dividing the deaths of infants under 1 year in a given calendar year by the number of live births in the given year; of course, the calendar year might be replaced by any other convenient unit of time. A preferable rate is obtained by considering the deaths of infants under 1 year related back to the births of a given year or other period. In normal times, when the birth and infantile death rates are not in a state of rapid change, the two rates give almost identical results, especially in countries having a low rate, when most of the infantile deaths occur in the first week of life (*UN Population Studies*, No. 13, I and II, 1954). In making international comparisons, it is as well to note the varying definitions of live birth and stillbirth (Pascua, 1948); fortunately, under the influence of the World Health Organization, definitions are tending to become uniform throughout the world.

The WHO Expert Committee (1970) recommends that fetal deaths be classified as *early fetal deaths* up to and including 500 g, as *intermediate fetal deaths* over 500 g up to and including 1000 g, and as *late fetal deaths* over 1000 g, noting that the weights of 500 and 1000 g correspond approximately to the gestational ages of 20 and 28 weeks. The Committee suggests that the *perinatal mortality ratio* be defined as "late fetal and early neonatal deaths weighing over 1000 g at birth expressed as a ratio per thousand live births weighing over 1000 g at birth." The Committee also proposes that birth registration be as complete as possible and that, as soon as is practicable, birth weight be added to the official birth certificate used in each country; furthermore that the birth weights should be classified in 500 g weight groups. Consistent with these definitions the *infant mortality rate* is the proportion of deaths among live births of weight over 1000 g, conveniently expressed as a ratio per thousand, deaths and births being observed over the same time and area. The Committee favored 500 g as the weight below which products of conception could be considered to be "nonviable," unless the infant survived some specified length of time. Such "nonviable" products would not be counted in the statistics of births and infant deaths.

Infant mortality can be considered for the *neonatal period* of 28 days and for the rest of the first year. In the neonatal period, much of the mortality is due to congenital defects (about 4 deaths per thousand infants), to the trauma of birth, and to respiratory difficulties. *Prematurity* is often a result of the first class of deaths and a cause of the second and third classes of deaths. In earlier times, there would have been more neglected or abandoned children dying in the neonatal period. In developing countries now, malnutrition and severe anemia are major factors leading to a high neonatal mortality. The prenatal health of the mother is of great importance. Peller (1948) emphasized this point in his studies on the German noble families, for their infants suffered only very low neonatal mortality rates and, indeed, remarkably low infantile mortality rates.

In the industrialized nations at the beginning of this century, deaths in the remaining 11 months of the first year of infant life were due almost entirely to respiratory infections, meningococcal and tubercular meningitis, gastro-enteritis, and the diseases "peculiar to the first year of life," many of these being partly due to the infections already mentioned. In recent years in the industrialized nations, the death rates in these 11 months have fallen greatly. In the developing countries, however the infections, together with malnutrition and anemia, still cause very high infant death rates.

Considering the whole first year of life, we can summarize the experience of the industrialized nations by saying that the infant mortality rates were in excess of 120 deaths per thousand births in the years before 1900 and that they have fallen to levels in the neighborhood of 20 deaths per 1000 births. Table VIII.1 presents rates for a few countries. The rates for males have always been higher than those for females, and high masculinity of the infantile mortality rates has become more pronounced as the rates have fallen.

Table VIII.1

Infant Mortality

(rates are per thousand live births)

Year	United[a] States	England and Wales[b]	Denmark[c]	Australia[d]
1903	132·6[e]	151·4	115·9	111·4
1908	133·2[e]	129·0	123·2	77·8
1913	114·8[e]	121·4	93·5	72·2
1918	100·9	100·6	74·2	58·6
1923	77·1	85·6	82·9	60·5
1928	68·7	76·6	80·8	53·0
1933	58·1	71·8	67·6	39·5
1938	51·0	59.5	58·7	38·3
1943	40·4	54·4	44·8	36·3
1948	32·0	38·7	35·3	27·8
1953	27·8	29·8	27·2	23·3
1958	27·1	25·3	22·4	20·5
1963[f]	25·2	23·7	19·1	19·6
1968[g]	21·8	18·3	14·8	17·8

[a] From Table 38, Grove and Hetzel (1968).
[b,c] U.S. National Center for Health Statistics (1968c), (1967c).
[d] Demography, Canberra, Australia.
[e] As deaths per thousand infant years of life.
[f,g] UN Demographic Yearbooks (1964, 1969).

3. THE MORTALITY OF CHILDHOOD

Up to the end of World War II, the mortality of childhood had been due almost entirely to the infections, such as gastroenteritis, meningococcal and tubercular meningitis, scarlatina, measles, diphtheria, whooping cough, and infective diseases of the respiratory system, and to accidental and violent causes. The mortality from the diseases mentioned had been falling in the developed countries since the later part of the nineteenth century, and thus childhood mortality rates in the 1960s were very low compared with the rates at the beginning of this century. Most of these declines had occurred in the absence of any effective specific therapy. However, the introduction of the chemotherapeutic and antibiotic drugs accelerated the general decline. It appears that the improvements in the death rates from the infections had been due to a diversity of changes in hygienic and social conditions, which tended to prevent or lower the probability of the passage of organisms from person to person, to raise the age at infection, and to favor the patient who had acquired the infection. It is possible that only a small portion of the declines in mortality can be attributed to changes in therapy and that planned public health activities were assisted by changes in social conditions. However, in the years since 1945, effective antibacterial agents have resulted in a more rapid fall in the rates from some of the infections. There have also been improvements in the mortality from violent and accidental causes, although these deaths now account for higher proportions of deaths during childhood than formerly.

4. THE MORTALITY OF YOUNG ADULT LIFE

Now let us consider the mortality of young adults; that is, people between the ages of 15 and 24 years. The classic causes of mortality at these ages were: in both sexes, tuberculosis; in males, violent and accidental causes; and in females, accidents and diseases associated with childbearing. The rates from tuberculosis tended to be higher in females than in males, but the rates in either sex at these ages had already declined to low levels by 1940. Violence and accidental causes have always been important in males at these ages. There have been great declines in the peace-time mortality rates, notwithstanding a slight increase recently due to the growing number of deaths from automobile accidents. However, deaths in war tend to be excluded from the deaths used to calculate death rates in modern times, whereas they are naturally included in such historical surveys as Peller (1947). It might be said that deaths from warfare were like deaths from an endemic disease in the period 1300–1600, say, whereas in this century they have been epidemic.

As a rule, deaths at ages 15 to 24 are high under pioneering conditions. At these ages, we find an interesting exception to the rule that the mortality rates increase steadily from age 11 years. In many modern experiences there is now a local maximum at about the age of 21 years in males (see Figure VII.1). This relative maximum is almost entirely due to violent and accidental causes (see Lancaster, 1960).

5.   THE MORTALITY OF ADULT LIFE

As we pass from the mortality of young adults to that of old age, a larger proportion of the causes cited by the certifying physician become unsatisfactory. However, even at ages 55 to 64 years, most diagnoses are satisfactory and only a few come from the cardiovascular–renal–neurological–indefinite class. However, at most ages over 65 years, diagnoses tend inevitably to become more difficult, since often the patient has been failing from old age or from a combination of diseases, perhaps even from diseases in different anatomical systems. In such cases, the certifying physician must try to give a diagnosis that will convey this idea and yet be acceptable to the official statisticians.

There have been overall declines in mortality, as we saw in Table VI.1. In the early decades of the century, about 5% of deaths at ages 55 to 64 years were due to infective causes other than tuberculosis, syphilis, and the respiratory diseases.

Tuberculosis death rates had fallen considerably before 1950, but the declines were accelerated by the widespread adoption of efficient chemotherapy. For syphilis, chiefly *locomotor ataxia* and *general paralysis of the insane*, the decline in the male rates came later than one might have expected from the known value both of the organic arsenicals in the early stages of the disease and of shock treatments in the later stages.

The death rates from *cancer* and other tumors reveals a slight but definite downward trend for the females, but the rates have remained almost stationary for males. These have been substantial decreases in the death rates from cancer of the mouth and of the liver, very slight declines in those of the stomach, an increase in those of the pancreas and of the prostate. The death rates from cancer of the lung at ages 55 to 69 has markedly increased.

No satisfactory secular comparisons can be made for mortality rates from causes included in the *nervous, cardiovascular, genitourinary,* and *ill-defined diseases* classes of the *International Statistical Classification.* This is because there have been changes in assignment according to the rules of the *Internation Statistical Classification* which make it very difficult to compare different periods; in addition, changes in diagnosis have occurred in certain disease systems—ill-defined diseases, indeed, are almost entirely "senility."

6.   THE MORTALITY OF OLD AGE

Findings and discussion similar to the material of the previous section apply to mortality at ages over 65 years. However, the difficulties are greater in tracing the real cause of death. Many deaths at these ages were recorded in the earlier decades as due to senility, although in later decades the same conditions would have been referred to the classes of diseases of the cardiovascular, genitourinary, or nervous systems. Once again, the death rates consisting of the totals of *cardiovascular, nervous, genitourinary,* and *all other* diseases, have shown an increase for males and a moderate decrease for females.

7. MORTALITY FROM TUBERCULOSIS

Andvord (1921) can be given the credit for realizing that tuberculosis mortality should be considered on a cohort or generation basis. He believed that the experience of a cohort was largely determined by the infection rates in childhood. Later workers have shown that this hypothesis explains adequately the changes in the form of the curve of the death rates from tuberculosis. The following discussion taken from Lancaster (1950a) applies particularly to the Australian experience of tuberculosis mortality but, as our quotations from Frost (1939) indicate, it applies also to the American experience and generally to that of the developed countries.

For any period (e.g., 1911–1920), the rates from Table VIII.2 or Figure VIII.1 begin at a high level because of the existence of childhood forms of tuberculosis, particularly tuberculous meningitis; rates decline to a minimum in the ages 5 to 14 years, rise to a high value in adult life, and decline again in old age. For a more recent period (e.g., 1941–1950), the high rates in infancy and early childhood have disappeared, and there is a gradual increase in the rates with age until late adult life, followed by a decrease in old age.

The form of this maximum in the rates in late adult life in recent times is often misinterpreted as being due to a delay of the time of first infection into adult life, whereby the tubercle bacillus is infecting adult persons who have had no experience of the bacillus in their childhood. But the men aged 55 to 64 years in 1941 to 1950 did not enjoy the low rates of infection of 1941 to 1950 when they were aged, 5 to 14 years. They had been aged 5 to 14 years a half-century earlier (i.e., 1891–1900) and had been exposed to very high risks of infection. It is evident from Table VIII.2 that the greater part of the mortality from tuberculosis had disappeared before the advent of the modern chemotherapeutic and antibiotic agencies, such as isoniazide and streptomycin.

Important factors may have been the prevention of infections in childhood by improved home conditions, whereby fewer children were exposed to high dosages of bacilli from "open" cases, often within the family. Other factors such as nutrition and social conditions are no doubt important but there is great difficulty in assessing their importance. Nor can the role of genetic

Table VIII.2

Tuberculosis Mortality in Australia by Cohorts Age-Specific Mortality Rate[a]

Age Group	Years Stated						Years Stated					
	1866	1876	1886	1896	1906	1916	1866	1876	1886	1896	1906	1916
5-	—	—	173	157	108	67	—	—	161	172	128	76
15-	—	904	582	529	373	197	—	864	934	762	642	373
25-	1903	1150	1104	844	447	230	1755	1384	1074	866	607	344
35-	1548	1365	1056	707	435	84	1215	935	667	469	311	67
45-	1587	1336	982	774	209	64	745	562	338	242	65	26
55-	1318	1225	1095	441	151		488	372	242	70	31	
65-	1089	1314	666	338			390	333	114	52		
75+	898	727	578				296	164	93			

[a] The rates for 1961–70 have been assumed to be close to those for 1961–1967, which are given above on the lowest diagonals. The rates are given in "calendar" form in Lancaster (1950a)

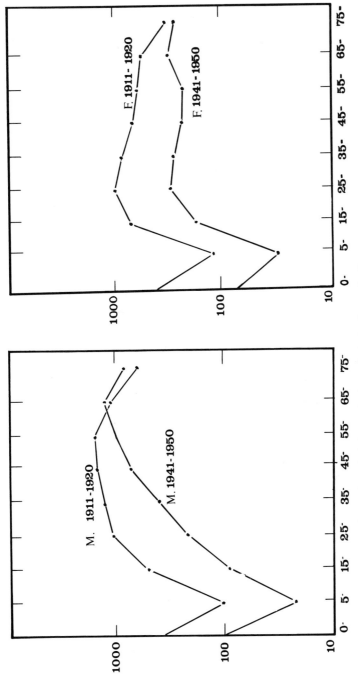

Figure VIII.1. Mortality rates from tuberculosis by age in Australia (calendar method).

MALES

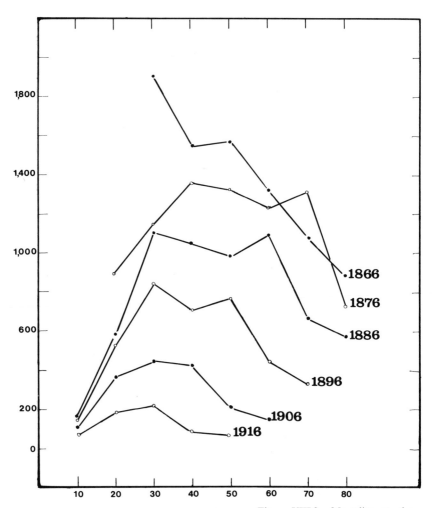

Figure. VIII.2. Mortality rates from

FEMALES

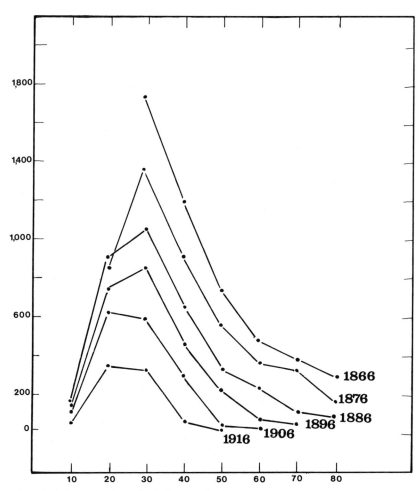

tuberculosis by age in Australia (cohort method).

changes in the human population be lightly dismissed, although possibly its importance has been exaggerated by some writers—as we pointed out in Section V.2 in the comparisons made to test genetic differences, genetic or ethnic differences have usually been confounded with social and economic conditions.

Figure VIII.2 plots the death rates from tuberculosis, appropriate to certain cohorts. There is a maximum for the tuberculosis mortality rates for each of the first four cohorts in the age group 25 to 34 years, but in the cohort of 1906 it appears that the maximum is in the age group 15 to 24 years. Given a finer dissection of the rates with unit of time for the age groups of five years, we should expect to find the maximum mortality rate in any case close to the age of 25 years. The maximum as observed in the cohorts is sharper than that of the rates in the calendar period method outlined previously. The results of the application of the cohort method to the rates of mortality are less definite for the males than for the females, although it appears in Figure VIII.2 that there is usually a maximum in the age group 25 to 35 years. In any case, the maximum in the later age groups, observed in a single period by the first or calendar method, is not observed for the cohorts.

There has been a disturbing factor in the case of the male rates, due either to (a) the war and the consequent increased radiographic diagnosis of tuberculosis in recruits to the armed forces, or (b) the increase in awareness of the disease in the susceptible occupations. It may be suggested that there is a maximum in the male rates at the age of approximately 35 years for each cohort.

Such also has been the experience in other countries exhibiting a declining death rate from tuberculosis, as can be illustrated by the conclusions of W. H. Frost (1939) on the tuberculosis mortality in Massachusetts. Frost found that at every age the mortality is lower in the later period but that the general form of the graphs of the rates is similar in the two periods, even though the age of the highest rate of mortality comes at the age of 50 to 60 years in 1930, whereas formerly it was at the age of 20 to 40.

These conclusions would fit the data of Figures VIII.1 and VIII.2. Frost says that he once believed that the change in age of the highest rate was due to a loss of the immunizing infections of childhood; but examination of the rates by the generation method had shown that this conclusion was fallacious. Persons aged, say, 50 years in 1935, have passed through greater mortality risks in the past, as indicated by the very high rate for children aged 10 years of a period 40 years earlier—that is, 1895.

The cohort or generation method reveals that the age distribution of the rates observed for a cohort can be very different from the age distribution presumed from an inspection of the rates at any given time, such as 1931 to 1940 or 1941 to 1950. The age distribution in the cohorts has been uniform—that is, the maximum occurs at approximately the same age in each cohort. We can conclude with Frost (1939) that the constancy of age selection (relative mortality at successive ages) in successive cohorts suggests rather constant physiological changes in resistance (with age) as the controlling factor and that, although both frequency and extent of exposure to infection in early life have decreased progressively decade by decade, there is no indication that this amelioration has had the effect of exaggerating the risk of death in adult life due to lack of opportunity to acquire specific immunity in childhood. The present-day "peak" of mortality does not represent postponement of maximum risk to a later period; rather, it seems to indicate that the present high rates in old age are the residuals of higher rates in earlier life.

We find little to add to Frost's conclusions on the Massachusetts data. The contrary conclusion that the protection of the young endangers their life at a later period of life appears to be founded on an analogy with the doctrine of the "survival of the fittest." Frost rejected the survival-of-the-fittest notion, concluding instead that if the rates are high in childhood, the survivors are so badly damaged that they will have a higher mortality rate than would have been the case, had there been lighter rates of infection in childhood. The statistics, then, do not controvert the thesis that it is good to avoid infection with the tubercle bacillus in childhood.

There was certainly no effective antibacterial agent before 1948, and such measures as collapse therapy probably played only a very small role in reducing mortality. The only therapy known was comprised of such nonspecific measures as rest, sunshine, and attention to diet. Effective chemotherapeutic and antibiotic agents (including streptomycin, paraaminosalicyclic acid, and isoniazide) have hastened the decline of tuberculosis as a cause of death in recent years. The decline in the death rates has been accompanied by lowered morbidity rates, indicating that the declines in death rates have not kept alive a number of persons in a state of invalidity. Public health measures against infection with tuberculosis from milk have been important in reducing bone and meningeal disease; case finding and other measures including Bacille Calmette-Guérin (BCG) vaccination are also important in reducing the number of cases suffering at an early age from infections by the human tubercle bacillus.

8. MORTALITY FROM LUNG CANCER

It has long been suspected that cigarette smoking caused clinical syndromes, such as cancer of the lung, emphysema, and arterial disease; however, sound epidemiological evidence was lacking prior to the clinical surveys of

Doll and Hill (1950), Müller (1939), and Wynder and Graham (1950).

It was known in the early postwar years that cases of lung cancer were appearing with increasing frequency and that the age-specific death rates from cancer of the lung were climbing, especially in men. Although other observers had produced evidence in favor of the hypothesis that cigarette smoking was the principal cause of the increase, none had been so careful in comparing their cases with controls, rigidly defined, as were Doll and Hill (1950). After reading their evidence, it was difficult for many not to believe that cigarette smoking had been the principal cause. However, numerous critics assailed the hypothesis, especially attacking the information on inhalation. It has since become evident that the definition of degrees of inhalation are too difficult to establish for such clinical surveys. Many clinical surveys have confirmed the main observations. However, once the *prima facie* case had been made against cigarette smoking, the hypothesis could be tested in a prospective survey, as by Hammond and Horn (1958) and Doll and Hill (1964). Their results have confirmed that the cancer risk increases with the acquisition of the cigarette smoking habit and with the amount smoked.

The industrial cancers of the lung of the miners in uranium in St. Joachimsthal and Schneeberg are well-known (Lorenz, 1944) and are of interest because they were an early indication that environmental factors could cause cancer.

A statistical point of interest arose in the study of lung cancer. The age-specific mortality rate increases steadily with age in almost every other cancer; however, there was a maximum at ages about 60 years for the lung cancers. Kennaway and Waller (1953) demonstrated that this was a generation effect and that the graph of every birth cohort had the same approximate form, although later cohorts had graphs elevated above earlier cohorts. The result is that the apparent maximum at a point of time is displaced toward the younger ages. This is the reverse of what happened to the maximum from tuberculosis, a disease with rates declining with time.

The increase in the lung cancer rates has resulted in a net increase in age-specific cancer death rates in most countries.

9. MORTALITY FROM OTHER CANCERS

We can consider the statistics of deaths from all forms of cancer, in the sense of malignant neoplasm, to constitute an example of the difficulties of making comparisons of the rates over a long period of time. Cancer has always had a high priority under the rules for classifying deaths of the statistical offices. Even in the most recent revisions, which no longer feature rigid rules for classification, there is a tendency to favor cancer as a cause of death, especially if it appears that other causes mentioned are terminal or complicating features of the cancer.

Over most of the period for which statistics are available, the appearance of the word "cancer" on a death certificate ensured that the death would be assigned to a cancer rubric by the statisticians. Cancer was preferred to almost any disease other than the rarer infective diseases, or violence. There has been, perhaps, only a small loss because of deliberate failure of the certifying physician to diagnose cancer on social grounds. More serious losses have occurred in the past, particularly at the high ages, through the common use of vague terms such as "senility." Between 1911 and 1920, for example,* the death rates of males from senility at ages over 65 years were some 22 per thousand per annum. There were also deaths of cancer patients transferred to other rubrics when the patient died suddenly or was found dead; for in such circumstances the coroner gave a verdict of "death due to natural causes" if he had no suspicion of foul play, and he made no effort to obtain a medical certificate rendering a more precise diagnosis.

It is difficult also to assign any numerical value to the effect of improved diagnosis in recent years, because of the greatly increased use of the clinical techniques of biopsy and endoscopy, and because of the availability of laboratory aids from radiology and pathology. Moreover, there has been a greater interest recently in malignant disease, since now surgical treatment can be attempted in a far greater range of cases than was possible in earlier years. In addition, the frequency of autopsy is higher than it was previously, and the possibility that a patient with a cancer will be given that diagnosis, either clinically or at autopsy is greater now than formerly.

Studies on certification that have been made by various authors writing on cancer, as on other diseases, have probably overemphasized the difficulties of certification, particularly at the younger ages. It is difficult otherwise to explain the continuity of the cancer mortality statistics over many years in various countries—that is, these authors fail to account for our ability to construct series going back a hundred years for cancer deaths as a whole or for, say, deaths from cancer of the breast. In other words, if the rules for assigning deaths, or even the fashion of diagnosing the conditions, varied too greatly over the years, we should expect discontinuities between epochs in the death rates from, say, cancer of the breast.

If we examine the cancer statistics for a given country at a point of time, we see that the rates are rather low in childhood and youth, increasing steadily and markedly with age. This feature has led to many incorrect conclusions about the increasing incidence of cancer as a whole,

* in Australia

when the crude death rates from cancer have been used as the basis of comparison.

The cancer death rates also vary with sex, being higher for males, except between the ages of 25 and 55 years. Some of these differences have an explanation that can be related directly to organs of sex. Cancers of the uterus and then cancers of the female breast cause mortality at an earlier stage in life than many of the other major cancers, whereas cancer of the prostate tends to occur at higher ages. However, differences in the rates between the sexes also occur in the cancers of organs, where sex might not be thought to be relevant. Cancers of the buccal cavity, stomach, rectum, and skin are commoner in males, cancers of the intestine and liver appear more often in females.

There has been a tendency, more evident in the females, for the death rates from cancer to fall at the different ages. The tendency has been counterbalanced in the males by the great increase in the lung cancer death rates. Let us mention some individual sites. Cancer of the stomach has declined in importance in many countries, but few would point to surgery as the cause of these declines. The rates from cancer of the breast have remained remarkably stable over the last century—a feature that has occasioned frequent comment. The death rates from cancer of the cervix have declined. For the comparisons of the death rates from cancers over time, we refer the reader to the works of Clemmesen (1965), Gordon, Crittenden, and Haenszel (1961), and Lancaster (1964a).

10. MORTALITY FROM VIOLENT AND ACCIDENTAL CAUSES

Violent and accidental causes—more briefly, violence—account for about 5% of the total mortality in the developed countries. They are important because they form the only large class of causes, other than the infections, that can be or have been controlled under present conditions. At some ages, the violent deaths form a considerable proportion of all deaths. Thus in males at ages 15 to 24, and 25 to 34 years, violent deaths constituted 71% and 56%, respectively, of all deaths. Violent causes include drownings, falls, suffocation, accidental poisoning, homicide, judicial executions, civil strife, and war. The war deaths are often excluded from the official statistics. In the developed countries, there have been considerable declines in the mortality rates from violence. The reasons for these declines include control of the causes (as in accidents to children and in industrial accidents) and improvements in surgical techniques. As we mentioned in Section VIII.4, deaths from violence have often been the cause of a relative maximum in the age-specific death rates in early adult life. It should be mentioned that the mortality rates from road accidents for those over 65 years now exceed the rates at ages 15 to 24 years—the elderly dying as pedestrians rather than as passengers or drivers.

In the notes to this chapter we furnish references to problems of accidents and also to the special problem of catastrophes, such as earthquakes, tidal waves, cyclones, and other natural events.

11. CAUSES OF THE DECLINES IN MORTALITY

A general discussion of the causes of the declines in the mortality rates has been published by Lancaster (1967), and we give a shorter version of that account.

(i) Isolation

Isolation, which can be defined here as any condition that leads to a diminished contact between persons, takes many different forms. Isolation may result from distance; in this sense, Australia, Iceland, and the many island groups throughout the world are isolated. High mountain ranges can also produce isolation. Arid regions may support only small groups of persons. Such separation into small groups occurs throughout the marginal lands of the world—for example, the low-rainfall areas of Australia and the ice-bound areas of northern Europe.

However, mere distance is not the only cause of geographical isolation. Isolation was a marked feature of the New Guinea populations before the arrival of Europeans, for there was little contact among warring groups. Often infants and small children are effectively isolated because their only contact with the community is apt to be through their parents. This form of isolation has led frequently to great "social gradients" in the mortality of infants. Isolation may have a political and social basis; differences in religion, language, or social standing may produce great differences between groups living in the same area, which are reflected in their fertility and mortality. Examples of such social isolation come readily to mind in Europe and in India. Besides these natural and social forms of isolation, there are the quarantine measures and the deliberate isolation in hospitals of persons suffering from certain infections.

The effect of isolation is particularly enhanced if the isolated unit of population is small, for then any infective disease will die out if the carrier state does not occur and if the incubation and infective periods are not overly long.

The effect of the formal isolation of affected persons within a country is not always clear. Isolation from other members of the family will be valuable in cases of leprosy and tuberculosis. Children are particularly susceptible to these diseases, and they must not be submitted to the risk of exposure to massive doses of bacilli. In other diseases, the effect of isolation on epidemic spread may be less than is popularly supposed, especially in epidemic diseases in which the ratio of cases to carriers is low. Thus, although it may be true that the isolation of poliomyelitis patients does not greatly influence the course of the epidemic, prophylactic isolation can be defended on the grounds that it reduces the possibility of large infective doses being given to other members of the patient's family. The isolation of pneumonia patients has rarely been attempted. Isolation of diphtheria patients can be justified, particularly if there are other members of the same family or group at school who might be expected to be exposed to a high risk of infection and a high initial dose. In some epidemic diseases, such as meningitis and scarlet fever, the carrier rate is possibly so high that it would be impracticable to isolate all patients and carriers.

(ii) Surgery

Surgery has been particularly valuable against the results of violent and accidental causes. Surgery is efficacious in the treatment of burns, scalds, fractures, and injuries arising from road or other accidents. First let us note that measures such as aseptic surgery, the correct treatment of shock (including blood transfusion), modern anesthetic methods, and the formation of hospitals or of teams within general hospitals devoted to the treatment of accident victims, have all helped to render the treatment of accident patients more efficient than ever before. Accident patients can now be brought by modern transport immediately after the accident, into special accident wards, where standard resuscitative methods can be immediately applied by specially trained staff. Such therapy, including aseptic and antiseptic therapy and measures against shock and operative techniques, has certainly been of great importance. The recent rise in mortality rates from automobiles may be said to be small compared with the declines previously achieved.

The surgical treatment of infections of the bone and of the skin and subcutaneous tissues has been of value, but the number of deaths from these causes was never large. The surgical treatment of hernia and intussusceptions has been successful, but these conditions have not been numerically important from the broader view of total mortality. Similar remarks could be made about the closure of patent *ductus arteriosus* and cardiac surgery generally.

When we leave the treatment of injuries due to accidental causes and the small group of diseases just mentioned, we find that surgery must be valued as palliative rather than curative. Cancers of the lip, like other cancers of the skin, are now treated by radiotherapy and other local agents. Here education and improved hospital outpatient attention have also been important, early treatment being possible. Cancer of the cervix has yielded to surgery and/or radiotherapy, and perhaps also to hygienic changes, including smaller families and changes in social customs (e.g., the practice of circumcision).

The record for the other major cancers is less clear. Cancer of the lung usually seems to be beyond effective treatment when first diagnosed or, perhaps, when first capable of diagnosis. Few surgeons are happy with the results of treatment of cancer of the prostate, breast, stomach, intestines, or rectum—the sites of most of the common major cancers. Little progress has been made in the treatment of leukemia, Hodgkin's disease, and melanoma.

(iii) Drugs and Antibiotics

Effective remedies against the cause of disease—as opposed to remedies to alleviate symptoms or to counteract physiological disturbances resulting from the disease process, have been available only in recent years. Mercury had been used against syphilis in European medicine since about 1500, and quinine against malaria since 1630. Digitalis has been used to control certain defects of cardiac rhythm, but it has been correctly used only since about 1900. Aside from these few drugs, the remainder of the drugs in the pharmacopoeia in use before the twentieth century were either inert or efficacious only in controlling disease symptoms. The effect of these drugs on the important group of acute infective diseases and the respiratory diseases had been negligible. Near the beginning of the century, the disinfectants, such as the phenol derivatives, were widely used to protect wounds against infections, in accordance with the teaching of Lister.

Later, under the influence of Lister and the bacteriologists, a rational antiseptic and aseptic surgical technique was developed. Up to 1900, however, no drug had been discovered that could destroy bacteria in wounds or in the tissues, without undue damage to the host. Paul Ehrlich began in 1904 his sytematic search for the *magna therapia sterilans*, the drug capable of killing the infecting organism within the tissues without damaging the host. Salvarsan, the first of the organic arsenicals, the the first drug to approach Ehrlich's ideals, was effective against the spirochete of syphilis.

The pharmacologists in the first quarter of this century had found many new drugs active against the infections usually associated with tropical medicine. However, it was only after the development of the sulfonamides and the report of Domagk, in 1935, that chemical agents became available against the common infections of the temperate zone, such as pneumonia and the streptococcal infections. There has followed an intensified search for other chemotherapeutic agents.

(iv) Immunological Methods

Vaccination has been effective in controlling smallpox, and prophylactic immunization has successfully combated diphtheria and tetanus. Serum therapy against these two diseases has not been equally important, and we can assert that serum therapy generally has been of little value in reducing mortality.

(v) Other Factors

Additional causes of the decline in mortality can be listed briefly as follows:

1. *Endocrine Therapy.* Little effect on mortality has been produced by endocrine therapy.

2. *Vitamins and Nutrition.* Nutrition is obviously of major importance on a worldwide basis. But in the developed countries, starvation has ceased to be a cause of mortality except under the stress of war. Nevertheless, improvements in nutrition have been significant in the advanced nations, particularly in infancy and childhood. At higher ages, the consumption of abundant food is often considered to be a leading cause of cardiovascular disease and diabetes.

3. *Municipal Services.* Improved water supply, sewerage, and adequate garbage disposal have all been valuable in reducing the mortality from bowel infections.

4. *Insect Vectors of Disease.* The control of insect vectors of diseases, such as malaria-carrying mosquitos, has been important.

5. *Radiotherapy.* Although radiotherapy has been of value in the control of skin cancer, it cannot be said to have greatly reduced the mortality from the major cancers.

6. *Social Factors.* A certain amount of importance must be attached to social factors.

7. *Genetical Control of Diseases.* The application of genetical theory to the control of disease has had no impact on mortality.

EXERCISES

1. (a) Plot the mortality rates from all causes against the age on an arithmetic grid and on a semilogarithmic grid, using the data of Table VIII.3.

Table VIII.3

DEATHS PER MILLION PER ANNUM FROM CERTAIN SELECTED CAUSES IN THE UNITED STATES IN 1960, BY AGE AND SEX[a]

Causes	Sex	All Ages	Ages Groups (years)										
			Under 1	1–4	5–14	15–24	25–34	35–44	45–54	55–64	65–74	75–84	85+
All causes	M	11,045	30,593	1,195	557	1,521	1,879	3,728	9,922	23,095	49,144	101,784	211,863
All causes	F	8,092	23,213	984	373	613	1,066	2,294	5,267	11,964	28,718	76,331	190,084
Tuberculosis (001–019)	M	89	9	6	1	5	23	62	144	266	393	522	649
	F	33	9	6	1	7	24	42	45	51	91	178	235
Syphilis and its sequelae (020–029)	M	24	10	—	0	1	2	6	27	86	152	131	127
	F	9	4	—	—	0	1	3	11	28	38	52	74
Malignant neoplasms (140–205)	M	1,625	77	124	76	102	188	489	1,708	4,599	8,905	13,894	17,412
	F	1,364	68	93	60	65	201	700	1,830	3,377	5,602	9,241	12,639
Diabetes (260)	M	138	5	3	3	8	27	51	121	319	761	1,446	1,706
	F	196	3	3	5	10	20	40	121	437	1,084	1,785	1,887
Major cardio-vascular-renal diseases (330–334, 400–468, 592–594)	M	5,917	145	28	28	90	303	1,406	5,018	13,068	30,306	69,212	154,912
	F	4,539	97	21	25	79	214	629	1,926	6,034	18,023	55,050	145,962
Rheumatic fever and chronic rheumatic heart disease (400–402, 410–416)	M	99	0	2	7	19	47	105	199	290	310	352	461
	F	106	1	2	7	21	48	99	195	284	312	379	580

(continued)

Table VIII.3—(Continued)

Causes[a]	Sex	All Ages	Age Groups (years)										
			Under 1	1-4	5-14	15-24	25-34	35-44	45-54	55-64	65-74	75-84	85+
Influenza and pneumonia (except of newborn) (480–493)	M	432	2,677	168	27	34	51	115	268	602	1,547	4,220	12,700
	F	315	2,094	156	25	27	45	71	127	272	751	2,774	10,350
Ulcer of stomach and duodenum (540, 541)	M	96	27	1	0	2	11	39	116	265	494	850	1,143
	F	31	10	1	1	1	4	12	32	56	129	293	547
Appendicitis (550–553)	M	13	3	4	4	4	3	6	15	32	55	98	116
	F	8	3	3	4	2	2	4	5	13	27	51	88
Hernia and intestinal obstruction (560, 561, 570)	M	51	259	6	1	2	5	13	35	93	224	513	1,049
	F	51	188	3	1	2	5	14	35	75	181	487	1,122
Cirrhosis of liver (581)	M	153	8	2	1	2	31	144	368	485	574	451	400
	F	75	9	1	2	3	27	93	186	179	201	220	217

Hyperplasia of prostate (610)	M	50	—	—	—	—	0	1	5	42	243	923	2,642
Congenital malformations (750–759)	M	135	4,070	129	38	32	22	25	30	30	37	30	55
	F	109	3,404	129	35	22	19	19	24	28	19	26	18
Certain diseases of early infancy (760–776)	M	443	18,705	1	0	—	—	—	—	—	—	—	—
	F	308	13,839	1	0	0	—	—	—	—	—	—	—
Ill-defined conditions (780–795)	M	136	677	32	6	15	29	57	139	253	462	1,066	3,254
	F	92	545	24	4	10	22	36	63	111	220	622	2,990
Motor vehicle accidents (E810–E835)	M	318	86	115	104	612	401	299	316	356	458	660	627
	F	110	75	84	54	151	92	91	116	152	190	230	220
Other accidents (E800–E802, E840–E962)	M	411	944	243	163	317	319	359	461	526	740	1,703	5,192
	F	213	755	187	63	46	59	80	112	163	416	1,745	6,300

a This table has been abstracted from Table I. M, *Vital Statistics of the United States, 1960*, Vol. II, *Mortality Part A*, Govt. Printing Office, Washington, D.C. 1963. The numbers in parentheses in the first column refer to the rubrics of the seventh revision of the *International Statistical Classification*, WHO manual (1957).

(b) Give possible explanations for the high masculinity at the higher ages of tuberculosis, syphilis, malignant neoplasma, major cardiovascular-renal diseases, influenza and pneumonia, ulcers of the stomach and duodenum, and cirrhosis of the liver to be observed in Table VIII.3.

2. Since the infective diseases tend to have a higher case fatality and more serious symptoms at the younger ages, improvements in hygiene lead to less morbidity and mortality from them. There are exceptions, however. Name the exceptions among tuberculosis, syphilis, diphtheria, measles,rubella, scarlatina, mumps, smallpox, poliomyelitis.

3. Which of the following diseases should be studied with the aid of generation death rates techniques: tuberculosis, syphilis, diphtheria, measles, acute rheumatic fever and its sequelae, cancer of the cervix, cancer of the stomach, and respiratory cancer?

4. It is of some interest to obtain the probability of conversion from the tuberculin-negative to the tuberculin-positive state at various ages. A survey is carried out at a single point of time, and the tuberculin-positive rates, r_x say, are known for $x = 0, 1, 2, \ldots$. Is $r_x - r_{x-1}$ a reliable estimate of the conversion rates at age x?

5. How would you measure the mortality from tuberculosis in a country? What vital statistical rates would you use: (a) to study the evolution of tuberculosis in a country, and (b) to compare the mortality in two different countries? Your answer should make clear the concepts of the age-specific mortality rates, the generation death rates, and the standardization.

6. Why is the infant mortality rate not an age-specific death rate?

7. Determine any diseases in the list of Exercise 1 which have a marked departure from equality of the rates in the two sexes and, where possible, explain the departures.

8. Use the official statistics of the United States or of Australia to test the hypothesis that sunlight may be effective in producing melanoma (see also Dorn and Cutler, 1954).

NOTES

The following bibliography of articles and books on mortality and related topics may assist the reader in obtaining data or in making the necessary comparisons on mortality.

Measurement of Mortality

Grove and Hetzel, 1968; Lancaster, 1951b, 1964a; Lancaster and Donovan, 1966; Lancaster and Willcocks, 1950; Larsson, 1965; Linder and Grove, 1943; UN Population Studies No. 18, 1953; UN/WHO Joint Committee, 1970.

Nomenclature, Classification of Diseases, and Related Topics

Logie, 1933; *Manual of the International Classification*, 1949; Thompson and Hayden, 1961; U. S. Bureau of the Census, 1911, 1924, 1931, 1940; WHO Manual, 1967.

International

Benjamin, 1966; Brockington, 1967; Milbank Memorial Fund, 1956; Powell, 1947; Secretary General to the UN, 1961; Stolnitz, 1955, 1957; Stowman, 1949 (see also, WHO and UN references); UN/WHO Joint Committee, 1970.

Mortality, General

Spiegelman, 1956; Stocks, 1950; Sutter and Tabah, 1952; UN/WHO Joint Committee, 1970.

Disappearance of Causes

Schwartz and Lazar, 1961.

Geographical Comparisons

Africa. Brass et al., 1968; Kuczynski, 1948–1953; Scott, 1965.
America, Latin. Centro-Americano de Bioestadistica, 1955; Ferrero, 1965.
Asia. Bose and Dey (Eds.), 1964; Fredericksen, 1961; *Symposium,* 1961.
Australia. Lancaster, 1964*a*; Pedersen and Moodie, 1966; Wickens, 1930.
Canada. Urquhart and Buckley, 1965.
Chile. U.S. National Center for Health Statistics, 1964*b*.
Czechoslovakia. U.S. National Center for Health Statistics, 1969.
Denmark. Mathiessen, 1965.
England and Wales. Carr-Saunders, Caradog Jones, and Moser, 1958. E. Grebenik, in Hauser and Duncan, 1959; Greenwood, 1924, 1936. Hamer, 1934; Humphreys, 1883; Logan, 1950; McKenzie, Case, and Pearson, 1957; McKeown and Record, 1962; Martin, 1960; Parsons, 1899–1900; Pike, 1966; Royal Commission on Population, 1949, 1950; Rudd, 1962; Russell, 1937; Sainsbury, 1955; Studies in Official Statistics No. 4, 1959; Taylor, 1951; U.S. National Center for Health Statistics, 1965*f*.
France. Institut national d'études démographiques, 1952, 1956; Reinhard, 1961; Sauvy, 1954*b*: Sauvy in Duncan and Hauser, 1959. Toutain, 1963.
Germany. Schubnell, in Duncan and Hauser, 1959.
Greenland. Fog-Poulsen, 1957.
Iceland. Jonsson, 1844; Schleisner, 1851; Sigurdsson and Tomasson, 1968.

India. C. Chandrasekaran, in Hauser and Duncan, 1959; Learmonth, 1965.

Ireland. Honohan, 1960.

Italy. A. Costanzo, in Hauser and Duncan 1959.

Japan. *Japan Yearbook*, annually; U.S. National Center for Health Statistics, 1968*a*.

New Zealand. Donovan, *passim*, in *New Zealand Medical Journal*; Donovan, 1969; Lancaster and Donovan, 1966.

Norway. Backer, 1961; Backer and Aagenaus, 1966; Central Bureau, 1952; Selmer, 1967.

Oceania. Audy, 1964; McArthur, 1967; Norman-Taylor, 1964; *Symposium* 1961; I. E. Taeuber, in Hauser and Duncan, 1959; Thompson, 1959.

Scotland. Harley and Hytten, 1966; Stark, 1851; U.S. National Center for Health Statistics, 1966*b*.

Sweden. Arosenius, 1925, 1927, 1930, 1933; Cramér and Wold, 1935; Greenwood, 1924; Heckscher, 1949; Hendriks, 1862; *Historisk Statistik för Sverige*, 1955; Larsson, 1965; Ryder, 1955; Sundbärg, 1906, etc.; Thomas, 1941.

Undeveloped Countries. Audy, 1964: Béhar, 1964; Bose and Dey (Ed.), 1964; Coale and Demeny, 1966; Edge, 1932; Johnson, 1964; Mackintosh, 1964; Stolnitz, 1956*a*, 1956*b*; Taylor and Hall, 1967; WHO Expert Committee, 1967.

United States. Ashburn, 1947; Blake, 1959; U.S., Bureau of Census, 1960; Dublin, 1948; Fitzpatrick 1957*a*, 1957*b*, 1958; Grove and Hetzel, 1968; Hermalin, 1966; Lerner and Anderson, 1963; Linder, 1958, 1962; Rosenberg, 1962; Shapiro, Schlesinger, and Nesbitt, 1968; Sydenstricker, Dublin, and Lotka, 1934; Taeuber, Haenszel, and Sirken, 1961; Taeuber and Taeuber, 1958; Twaddle, 1968; U.S. National Center for Health Statistics, 1965*b*, 1968*a*, 1970*c*; U.S. National Health Survey, 1958*a*, 1958*b*, 1959*a*, 1959*b*; R. B. Vance, in Hauser and Duncan, 1959; Whelpton, 1947; Wright and Hunt, 1900.

Mortality by Cause*

000   **Cholera.** Pollitzer, 1959; Rosenberg, 1962.

020   **Plague.** Baltazard, 1960; Creighton, 1894; Hirsch, 1883; Hirst, 1953; Mullett, 1956; Pollitzer, 1954; Rowntree, 1901; Shrewsbury, 1970.

040–046   **Poliomyelitis and Related Diseases.** Paul, 1955.

010–019   **Tuberculosis.** Andvord, 1921; Doege, 1965; Frost, 1939; Haybittle, 1963; Lancaster, 1950*a*; Springett, 1950.

---

* The rubric numbers according to the eighth revision of the *International Statistical Classification* are given to the left of the "cause."

080   **Typhus.** Zinsser, 1935.

050–079   **Viruses.** Conference, 1968; Fenner, 1968; Fenner and White, 1970; Stocks, 1942; see also, Notes to Chapter XVI.

140–239   **Cancers.** Case, 1966; Chaklin, 1962; Clayson, 1962; Clemmesen, 1965; Cutler and Latourette, 1959; Dorn and Cutler, 1954; Gagnon, 1950; Gordon, Crittenden, and Haenszel, 1961; Greenwood, 1926; Haybittle, 1963; Hueper, 1950, 1961, 1962, 1966; Kennaway and Waller, 1953; Lorenz, 1944; McKenzie, Case, and Pearson, 1957; Robertson, 1968; Roe and M. C. Lancaster, 1964; Stewart and Herrold, 1961; Stocks, 1953; Thompson and Slaughter, 1957; U.S. Public Health Service Publication, 1960; WHO Bibliography on Cancer, 1970; WHO Committee on Health Statistics, 1959; WHO Study Group, 1960; Wynder and Graham, 1950.

Carcinogensis. Clayson, 1962; Hueper, 1961, 1962.

Virus. Bryan, 1961.

Radiation. Robertson, 1968; Urbach, 1968.

Lung Cancer. Clemmesen, 1965; Doll and Hill, 1950, 1964; Hammond and Horn, 1958; Hueper, 1966; James and Rosenthal, 1962; Kennaway and Waller, 1953; Lorenz, 1944; Mueller, 1939; U.S. Public Health Service, 1971; Wynder and Graham, 1950.

Melanoma. Mackie and McGovern, 1958; McGovern, 1952; McGovern and Lane, 1969, Lancaster and Nelson, 1957.

250   **Diabetes.** Renold and Cahill, 1960; Stocks, 1944.

290–299   **Psychiatry.** Moran, 1969.

390–458   **Circulatory.** de Haas and Rusbach, 1964; Epstein, 1965; Robb-Smith, 1967; Sackett and Winkelstein, 1965; Schuman, 1965; Stallones, 1965; Standing Committee, 1971; WHO Study Group, 1957.

460   **Respiratory**

Asthma. Speizer, Doll, and Heaf, 1968.

Bronchitis. Smart, 1961.

712   **Rheumatic Arthritis.** Scotch and Geiger, 1962.

740   **Congenital Neurological Defects.** WHO Scientific Group 1970.

760   **Maternal.** Willcocks and Lancaster, 1951; Tandy, 1935.

E990–999   **War.** Greenwood, 1942; Hauser, 1942; Willcox, 1923; Urlanis, 1960.

E800–999   **Accidents, Disasters.** Adams, 1969; Ayers, 1969; Black, 1969; Blake, 1969; Dainty, 1969; Hewitt, 1957; Irwin, 1964; Latter, 1969; Norman, 1962; Robens of Woldingham, 1969; Rudd, 1962.

Accident Proneness. Cresswell and Froggatt, 1963.

Aircraft Accidents. Stevens, 1970.

E950–959   **Suicide.** Daric, 1955; Sainsbury, 1955.

Sudden Death. Kuller, 1967.

Generation Death Rates. Case, 1956; Kennaway and Waller, 1953; Kermack, McKendrick, and McKinlay, 1934; Jacobson, 1964; Lancaster, 1950a, 1957; McKendrick, 1926; Springett, 1950.

Zoonoses and Animal Diseases. Goret, 1966; Fenner and Ratcliffe, 1965; Hull (Ed.), 1963.

Mortality by Age

Infants. Butler and Bonham, 1963; Feld, 1923; Heady and Heasman, 1959; Henderson, 1968; Henry, 1968; Mathiessen, 1965; Pascua, 1948; Populations Studies, No. 13, 1954; Reports on Public Health and Medical Subjects, No. 94, 1949; Shapiro and Moriyama, 1963; Shapiro, Schlesinger, and Nesbitt, 1968; Solomons, 1958; *Symposium*, 1961; Studies I and II, 1954; Tabah and Sutter, 1948; WHO Expert Committee, 1970; U.S. National Center for Health Statistics, 1965a, 1965c, 1965d, 1965e, 1966a, 1967, 1968c.

Childhood. Apley, 1964; Béhar, 1964; Bose and Dey, 1964; Gordon, Wyon, and Ascoli, 1967; Henderson, 1968; Kendall, 1958; Rouquette and Corone, 1965; UN Population Studies No. 13, 1954; WHO Epidemiological Report, 1964.

Young Adults. Lancaster, 1960.

Adult Life. Office of Health Economics, 1966.

Longevity, Aging, and Senescence. Comfort, 1956; Forbes, 1967; McMullan, 1963.

Various Factors

Ancient Times. Egerton, 1968.

Historical. Blake, 1969; Henry, 1956; Peller, 1943, 1944, 1947, 1948; UN/WHO (Joint Committee) 1970; WHO (various authors), 1965.

Medical Students. Simon, 1968.

Meteorology. Tromp, 1963.

Navy. Lloyd and Coulter, 1961, 1963.

Nutrition. Drummond and Wilbraham, 1939; Salaman, 1949.

Occupation. Daric, 1949; Moriyama and Guralnik, 1956; Registrar-General, 1959; Reid, 1957; Stocks, 1938.

Peerage and Noble Families. Hollingsworth, 1957, 1965; Peller 1943, 1944, 1948. Young and Russell, 1927.

Remote Areas. Westergaard, 1880.

Sex. Vance and Madigan, 1956; UN Population Studies, No. 22, 1955; Valaoras, 1956.

Social Class. Antonovsky, 1967; Moriyama and Guralnik, 1956; Rountree, 1901; Stevenson, 1921, 1928.

Urban–Rural. Johnson, 1964; Mackintosh, 1964; Parsons, 1899–1900; Pickles, 1939; UN Population Studies, No. 8, 1950.

Working Life. Studies in official statistics No. 4, 1959; Wolfbein, 1949.

Population

Glass and Eversley, 1965; Lorimer, 1959; Pascua, 1952; Peller, 1943, 1944; Russell, 1937, 1941, 1945, 1948; Slicher van Bath, 1963; Underwood (Ed.) 1953.

CHAPTER IX

Fertility and Population Dynamics

1. DEFINITIONS AND INTRODUCTORY

In demography, the term *fertility* is used in the sense of offspring borne, whereas *fecundity* is used to refer to the potential for bearing offspring. It is possible for fecund women not to be fertile. There has often been confusion in the literature with respect to these two words, but "fertility" is now universally used in the sense of actual production or bearing of offspring and "fecundity" in the sense of the corresponding potential.

We now consider the measurement of fertility, noting that the interaction between mortality, fertility, and migration determines the age distribution of the population, which has many medical implications. In some countries, migration has been of minor importance in changing the age distribution of the population. However, fertility can fall rapidly, as it did in the years around 1930 in western Europe, and in Japan after World War II, causing great changes in the age structure of the population.

The *numbers of births* in each year or even in each month are available for many countries and often can be obtained for small geographical units. Some countries publish the births by age of mother.

If fertility is to be compared between countries or over different epochs in the same country, it is necessary to reduce the numbers of births to a ratio or rate. This is analogous to the reduction of the deaths to death rates. The *crude birth rate* is defined as the ratio of the total number of births in a year to the mean population at risk during the year, usually estimated by the mid-year population, both births and population number being measured for the same population. The crude birth rate is usually expressed as so many births per thousand of total population per annum, by multiplying the ratio obtained in the following equation by 1000:

$$(1) \quad \text{crude birth rate} = \frac{\text{number of births in the population in a year}}{\text{mean population for the year}}.$$

Example i. There were 239,986 births in Australia in 1961. The population at the midyear was 10,508,186. The crude birth rate was thus 1,000

$\times$ 239,986/10,508,186 = 22.84 per thousand per annum. The definition of (1) can be modified if we consider the crude birth rate for a portion of a year or for a number of years by the formula

$$(2) \qquad\qquad \text{crude birth rate} = \frac{B}{Y},$$

where B is the number of births in the population and Y is the number of years of life experienced by that population over the same interval of time. For example, if the interval were 0.5 year, we would multiply the mean population over that time by one-half to obtain the estimate of Y. On the other hand, if the interval of time were 5 years we would: (a) add the mean populations of the years to obtain $Y = P_1 + P_2 + P_3 + P_4 + P_5$ or (b) make an estimation that would give an approximate estimate, such as $5P_3$.

Example   ii. The births in Australia in 1960 were 230,326, and the midyear population was 10,275,020. For the two years 1960 and 1961 combined, the births were 470,312 and the years lived were 20,783,206. The crude birth rate for the period was thus 1,000 $\times$ 470,312/20,783,206 = 22.63 births per thousand per annum.

Example   iii. There were 61,214 births in Australia in the second quarter of 1961. The population at the midpoint of this period was $\frac{1}{2}$(10,454,495 + 10,508,186); that is, half the sum of the values at March 31 and June 30. The years lived in this quarter was one-quarter of the population at the midpoint of the period; thus the crude birth rate is

$$\frac{1,000 \times 61,214}{\{\frac{1}{8}(20,962,681)\}} = 23.36.$$

The crude birth rates shares some unsatisfactory features with the crude death rate, since births obviously depend on the age and sex distribution of the population.

There are several advantages in relating the births to the female population; for example, since the mother can almost always be identified, an accurate age distribution of mothers at the time of confinement can be obtained. We can define the *age-specific fertility rate* as the ratio of the number of children born to women of a given age group to the number of women years at risk in the age group. If the observations are over a calendar year, the midyear population will be appropriate; for other periods of time, the appropriate denominator will be calculated as explained for the crude birth rate. The age groups usually chosen are 15 to 19, 20 to 24, ..., 40 to 44 years, on the last birthday. Sometimes this rate is defined using only female births.

Another informative rate is the ratio of the births in a year to the midyear population of women of ages 15 to 44 years. Rather less useful is a calculation

of the same rate, married women replacing the total female population at ages
15 to 44 years. This rate tends to be deceptive because the conceptions of many
first births occur before marriage, thus producing a spuriously high fertility of
young married women.

The age-specific fertility rates presented in Table IX.1 (next section) and in
Figure IX.1 for Australia, 1961, can be taken as representative of an

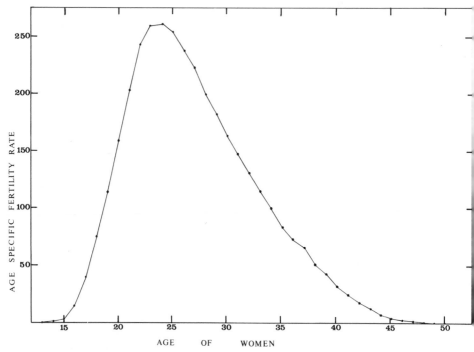

Figure IX.1.   Fertility rates by age in Australia, 1961 (data from Table IX.1).

industrialized society. The rates are negligible before the age of 15 years,
rapidly increasing between the ages of 17 and 22 years, attaining a mode at
ages 23 and 24 years and then declining, but rather more slowly than they have
risen. The graph of the fertility rates can be approximated by a normal curve,
a property to be used in a later section. It does not seem appropriate here to
discuss the causes of the fertility, but we remark that although the upper and
lower ages of fecundity (and thus of fertility) are fixed by physiological causes,
the fertility rates are determined by economic, religious, and social causes.
Here we are interested in the rates because they affect the total numbers and
age distribution of the population (i.e. the population dynamics) for which we
will set up models.

It greatly simplifies the analysis in the mathematical model if the population treated is of one sex. The female sex is usually chosen, since in actual populations data on births by age of mother are often available and need no further adjustment to ensure the counting of illegitimate births; thus appropriate parameters are more readily estimated. Furthermore, the female part of the population is less directly affected than the male part by war and migration. The analysis in the model is simplified if the fertility rates depend only on the age of the parent and not on numbers or proportions of the population by age and sex.

The general results of the theory of population dynamics can be stated. In a mathematical model, if the members of the population are imagined to be submitted to fertility and mortality rates at every age according to a fixed schedule of fertility and mortality rates, the population ultimately attains a fixed age distribution—*the stable age distribution*—and it increases or decreases at a fixed ratio between any two points of time, separated by a given interval.

2. GROSS AND NET REPRODUCTION RATES

The long-term implications of a given schedule of mortality and fertility rates are often sought. Will succeeding generations be increasing or decreasing? A partial answer to such a question is afforded by the *gross reproduction rate* (GRR), which is defined as the average number of female offspring born to women in a mathematical model in which there is no mortality and in which the fertility rates at every age are the same as those in the actual population observed. The gross reproduction is evidently the sum of all the fertility rates, multiplied by a factor f, the proportion of female births, which we can assume for this purpose to be substantially constant with the age of mother. Thus we have

$$(1) \qquad \mathrm{GRR} = f \sum_{x=0}^{\infty} f_x,$$

where f_x is the fertility rate at age x.

Example. The midyear population of women in Australia is given by single years of age in Table IX.1, together with the number of births to mothers of the respective ages. The fertility rates have been computed for each age and summed to give, after a multiplication by f, the GRR.

It may be that the fertility rates are given only for five-year age groups 15 to 19, 20 to 24, ..., years, respectively $f_{15}^*, f_{20}^*, \ldots$, say. A good approximation to the GRR is then expressed by

$$(2) \qquad \mathrm{GRR} = 5f(f_{15}^* + f_{20}^* + f_{25}^* + \cdots),$$

Table IX.1

Age of Women	Number of Women	Births	Age-Specific Fertility Rate
13	97,015	4	0.0000
14	104,268	66	0.0006
15	84,613	288	0.0034
16	84,207	1,281	0.0152
17	80,278	3,181	0.0396
18	72,165	5,463	0.0757
19	72,856	8,388	0.1151
20	69,158	11,047	0.1597
21	67,872	13,854	0.2041
22	67,136	16,384	0.2440
23	65,990	17,178	0.2603
24	65,768	17,193	0.2614
25	64,330	16,388	0.2548
26	62,691	14,915	0.2380
27	61,090	13,692	0.2241
28	62,784	12,573	0.2003
29	62,716	11,471	0.1829
30	70,834	11,543	0.1630
31	68,360	10.117	0.1480
32	70,030	9,157	0.1308
33	71,297	8,180	0.1147
34	71,304	7,191	0.1009
35	75,040	6,228	0.0830
36	75,400	5,507	0.0730
37	72,463	4,781	0.0660
38	75,895	3,877	0.0511
39	73,839	3,170	0.0429
40	77,997	2,490	0.0319
41	65,140	1,626	0.0250
42	64,917	1,115	0.0172
43	63,453	741	0.0117
44	63,087	441	0.0070
45	65,379	245	0.0037
46	66,820	125	0.0019
47	65,468	62	0.0009
48	64,110	17	0.0003
49	60,123	4	0.0001
50	63,642	3	0.0000
Total		239,986	3.5523

where $f^*_{15} =$ (births)/(midyear population), and the midyear population is the population at the central point of the year of observation of the births. We have computed the GRR in Table IX.2 by the second method, and no appreciable error seems to have been introduced thereby. In the event of the sex ratio of the births being unknown, f can be taken to be the factor 0.487, or even 0.5, without great error.

The GRR takes no account of mortality, nor does it allow for the generation effect. The mortality can be handled by calculating the net reproduction rate soon to be described, but the generation effect enters into the interpretation of either index. To see the difficulty clearly, we consider only first births and note that we must reject any calculation that raises the average number of first births to women above unity.

For the rates in our mathematical model, we choose a country that has been in a state of war, which has had the effect of delaying all marriages for a number of years; at the conclusion of the war, marriages are undertaken and some women bear their first children. Under such circumstances, the sum of the age-specific fertility rates for first births might exceed unity in the mathematical model. For example, it would not be unreasonable to imagine the first-born fertility rates at ages 18, 19, 20, 21, and 22 years to be 0.15, 0.20, 0.25, 0.25, and 0.25; these rates alone give a sum of 1.10, which indicates that the average number of first born would exceed 1.10 and, thus, unity, the maximum acceptable (since a woman can bear only one first child). Although the example is extreme, it shows that we cannot always interpret the experience of women in a particular year as equivalent to the experience of a woman passing through life. The same objection would hold for the projection of the marriage rates as estimates of marriage rates for the future. We have discussed generation effects in the study of tuberculosis mortality rates in Section VIII.7 and in the forecasts of Section VI.11.

We now wish to combine schedules of mortality rates and fertility rates. It simplifies the notation if we set l_0 equal to 1 in the life tables of Chapter VII. In the mathematical model, we now assume sets of mortality rates $\{m_x\}$ and fertility rates $\{f_x\}$. The set $\{m_x\}$ enables us to calculate $\{l_x\}$, which, we can assume, has been done. Of females commencing life in the mathematical model, a proportion l_x reach age x years, and of these $l_x f_x$ bear a child; the contribution of children at age x is thus $l_x f_x$, on an average. For the whole life, the average contribution of children is the sum of the $l_x f_x$ at every age or $\sum l_x f_x$. The contribution of female children will be the latter sum multiplied by the female proportion of the births; thus we have $f \sum l_x f_x$. Therefore, we define the *net reproduction rate* (NRR) by the equation

$$(3) \qquad\qquad NRR = f \sum f_x l_x.$$

However, a simplification of the computations is possible. Most of the births occur at ages 15 to 35 years; over this span of years, there is little change in l_x; in fact, l_{15} is about 0.97 and l_{35} is about 0.96 in modern life tables. Thus it is easily shown that little inaccuracy is introduced by multiplying every f_x by l_{25}, a central value. An approximate and easily calculated formula is

$$(4) \qquad \text{NRR} = l_{25}\, f \sum f_x = l_{25} \times \text{GRR}.$$

The gross and net reproduction rates can be computed for cohorts from the official statistics by the use of $\{m_x\}$ and $\{f_x\}$ schedules appropriate to the cohort. The computations of the gross and net reproduction rates appear in Tables IX.1 and IX.2. We have taken l_{25} to be 0.96984. By the longer method we find that the GRR is 1.73 and the NRR is 1.68, whereas by the shorter method the GRR is 1.72 and the NRR is 1.67. We have taken f to be 0.487.

Table IX.2

AGE-SPECIFIC FERTILITY OF WOMEN IN AUSTRALIA, 1961
(ABBREVIATED METHOD)

Age Group (women)	Number of Women	Births	Age-Specific Fertility Rates
13–14	201,283	70	0.0003
15–19	394,119	18,601	0.0472
20–24	335,924	75,656	0.2252
25–29	313,611	69,039	0.2201
30–34	351,825	46,188	0.1313
35–39	372,637	23,563	0.0632
40–44	334,594	6,413	0.0192
45–49	321,900	453	0.0014
50+	63,642	3	0.0000
		239,986	0.7079
		Total	3.5395

Note that $5 \times 0.7079 = 3.5395$.

*3. THE INTEGRAL EQUATION OF POPULATION GROWTH

Many important political, social, and medical problems arise from the relation of the population to its physical resources. We now set forth a general theory of the growth of populations, taking account of the fertility and mortality at every age. Naïve theory, which hopes to understand and forecast population changes by a study of the crude birth and death rates, is quite inadequate. However, we cannot presume to present a rigorous solution of the integral equation of population growth; we can only sketch briefly some aspects of it which appear relevant. It is supposed that schedules of rates of fertility $\{f_x\}$ and of mortality $\{m_x\}$ are given for each value of x. From $\{m_x\}$ a life table can be constructed in the usual manner, as explained in Chapter VII, and a schedule of values of the survivorship to age x years $\{l_x\}$ can be computed. It simplifies the notation if l_0 is set equal to unity, so that l_x becomes the proportion of persons entering the life table at age zero surviving to age x years.

A first approximation to the final theory is the use of matrix algebra, whereby the time and age variables t and x are considered as discrete variables, taking values 0, 1, 2, 3, ... This algebraic approach is equivalent to the following procedure. At time 0, we record the population, *taken simply to be the female population*, as the first row of a table, P_{00}, at age 0, P_{01} at age 1 year, P_{02} at age 2 years. By hypothesis, we are given the values of $\{m_x\}$ and hence of $\{l_x\}$; hence at time t, the members aged x in this initial population are age $t + x$. We then have that at time t, the population $P_{t,\,t+x}$ at age, $t + x$, are the survivors from P_{0x} at age x at time 0. But the proportion who survive from aged x years to aged $x + t$ years is the ratio l_{x+t}/l_x. We can then write

$$(1) \qquad P_{t,\,x+t} = \frac{P_{0x}\,l_{x+t}}{l_x},$$

or more generally, for the relation between the populations at times, t and t', where $t' < t$, we have

$$(2) \qquad P_{t,\,x+t-t'} = \frac{P_{t'x}\,l_{x+t-t'}}{l_x}.$$

Furthermore,

$$(3) \qquad P_{t,\,t-t'} = P_{t'0}\,l_{t-t'},$$

since $l_0 = 1$.

We show the populations by calendar year (time) and age in Table IX.3, in which we have indicated by arrows the progress of the cohorts, aged 0 at time 0, and age 0 at time t. We have hypothesized that the fertility rates are f_x; thus we have births equal to $f_0 P_{00} + f_1 P_{01} + f_2 P_{02} + \cdots$, who are those aged 0 at time 1.

$$(4) \qquad P_{10} = \sum f_x P_{0x},$$

Table IX.3

THE POPULATION BY AGE

Time			Age		
(epoch)	0	1	2	3	4
0	P_{00}	P_{01}	P_{02}	P_{03}	P_{04} ⋯
1	P_{10}	P_{11}	P_{12}	P_{13}	P_{14}
2	P_{20}	P_{21}	P_{22}	P_{23}	P_{24}
3	P_{30}	P_{31}	P_{32}	P_{33}	P_{34}
4	P_{40}	P_{41}	P_{42}	P_{43}	P_{44}

and more generally

$$(5) \qquad P_{t+1,\,0} = \sum f_x P_{tx}.$$

This procedure is readily formalized in the notation of matrix algebra, and results can be obtained on the ultimate rate of growth and age distribution. However, in some ways it is preferable to consider these variables as continuous, such that the number of the births at time t is derived from its values at times prior to t by an integration, whereas when discrete variables are used, the set of values of the population at the different age groups is derived from the values at the preceding instant of time by a matrix transformation. Let us now suppose that $B(t)\,dt$ births of females occur during the epoch, t to $t + dt$, dt being an infinitesimal, in the mathematical model. The births at different epochs can be related by the equation

$$(6) \qquad B(t) = \int f_x l_x B(t - x)\,dx,$$

where the limits of integration are zero and the greatest value of x, for which $f_x > 0$. Equation 6 assumes that the number of births to females at age x to $x + dx$ at time t is obtained by multiplying the fertility rate over this small interval by the number of survivors to ages in this small interval. The number of survivors in this small interval of age is very close to $B(t - x)l_x$ and could be written as $B(t - x)l_x$. The summation of all these contributions $f_x B(t - x)l_x$ is simply the integral as given in (6).

Let there now be defined

$$(7) \qquad R_0 = \int f_x l_x\,dx,$$

$$(8) \qquad R_1 = \int x f_x l_x \, dx,$$

and

$$(9) \qquad R_2 = \int x^2 f_x l_x \, dx.$$

The R_0 can be interpreted as the expected number of female births to a female entering the mathematical model and corresponds to the net reproduction rate of actual populations calculated by the cohort method. We can also interpret R_0 as the ratio between the numbers of two successive generations. Let $g(x)$ be defined by

$$(10) \qquad g(x) = \frac{f_x l_x}{R_0} \qquad \text{for} \quad x > 0$$

and

$$g(x) = 0 \qquad \text{for} \quad x < 0.$$

Now $g(x)$ satisfies the conditions $g(x) \geq 0$ and $\int g(x) \, dx = 1$, where integration is over the whole line, and the term can therefore be regarded as the density function of a statistical distribution. Now we can interpret $m = R_1/R_0$ as the mean and $v = (R_2/R_0 - R_1{}^2/R_0{}^2)$ as the variance of the distribution of the ages of females giving birth to female offspring.

Nothing yet has been said of the form of the function $g(x)$ of (10) if realistic hypotheses are made about human fertility, for example. It is found that the graph of $g(x)$ can be satisfactorily approximated by a normal curve with the same mean and variance, as is illustrated in Figure IX.1. It can be assumed that

$$(11) \qquad g(x) = (2\pi v)^{-1/2} \exp \frac{-\frac{1}{2}(x - m)^2}{v},$$

to a good order of approximation. By a well-known integration, the Laplace transform of $g(x)$ is given by

$$(12) \qquad G(t) = \int \exp(tx) g(x) \, dx = \exp(mt + \tfrac{1}{2}vt^2).$$

The general theory now suggests that we should attempt to obtain special solutions of (6). It is assumed that t is large so that special initial features of the population are no longer operative. A solution that gives a constant rate of increase can be considered, namely, such that we have

$$(13) \qquad \frac{1}{B(t)} \frac{dB(t)}{dt} = \frac{d}{dt} \log B(t) = \rho,$$

which corresponds to

(14) $$B(t) = A \exp(\rho t),$$

where A is a constant; consequently we can write

(15) $$B(t - x) = B(t)\exp(-\rho x).$$

The substitution of (14) into (6) yields

(16) $$B(t) = \int f_x l_x B(t - x)\, dx$$

$$= R_0 B(t) \int g(x)\exp(-\rho x)\, dx,$$

from the definition of $g(x)$. But (16) can be simplified by the use of (12) to

(17) $$1 = R_0 \int g(x)\exp(-\rho x)\, dx = R_0 G(-\rho)$$

$$= R_0 \exp(-m\rho + \tfrac{1}{2}v\rho^2).$$

It follows that

(18) $$0 = \log_e R_0 - m\rho + \tfrac{1}{2}v\rho^2,$$

and if ρ is small, an approximate solution is

(19) $$\rho = \frac{\log_e R_0}{m}.$$

This means that the instantaneous rate of increase is equal to the logarithm of the ratio between numbers in successive generations divided by the length of a generation. The exact solution of (18) is

(20) $$\rho = \frac{m}{v} - \sqrt{(m^2 - 2v \log_e R_0)/v}.$$

From either (19) or (20) we can put

(21)
$$\begin{aligned}
\rho > 0 \quad &\text{if} \quad R_0 > 1; \\
\rho = 0 \quad &\text{if} \quad R_0 = 1; \\
\rho < 0 \quad &\text{if} \quad R_0 < 1.
\end{aligned}$$

This can be paraphrased. In the mathematical model, the population ultimately becomes increasing, stationary, or decreasing, according to whether the net reproduction rate is greater than, equal to, or less than unity. The theory of integral equations shows that there is only one real root for (16) and that of all such roots, the real one has largest absolute value. The complex roots contribute periodic components that become negligible after a long lapse of time. Furthermore it can be demonstrated that the foregoing solution is a satisfactory approximation.

The general solution of (6) is obtained as a linear combination of the solutions of the form (14) where ρ is replaced by complex numbers

$$(22) \qquad \rho_j = a_j + ib_j, \qquad j = 1, 2, 3, \ldots; \qquad i = \sqrt{-1}$$

and where $\rho - a_j > 0$.
We then obtain

$$(23) \qquad B(t) = A \exp(\rho t) + \sum_{j=1}^{\infty} A_j \exp(\rho_j t).$$

However, from (23) we have

$$(24) \qquad B(t)\exp(-\rho t) = A + \sum_{j=1}^{\infty} A_j \exp(ib_j t)\exp([a_j - \rho]t).$$

Thus since $t \to \infty$, all terms on the right of (23) other than A can be neglected, and the (asymptotic) solution for large t is

$$(25) \qquad B(t) = A \exp(\rho t).$$

Now the element of population at age x at time t, is

$$(26) \qquad B(t - x)l_x = B(t)\exp(-\rho x)l_x,$$

which means that the element of population at age x at time t is proportional to $\exp(-\rho x)l_x$. The age distribution can then be written

$$(27) \qquad h(x; \rho) = \frac{\exp(-\rho x)l_x}{\int_0^{\infty} \exp(-\rho x)l_x \, dx}$$

and $h(x; \rho)$ is independent of t but evidently depends on ρ.

Further, as t becomes large, the age distribution in the mathematical model is constant; thus the population ultimately acquires a *stable* form, the form of the *stable life-table population*. If $\rho = 0$, the population form is stable and the total size is fixed. This is the *stationary life-table population*, often used in demography to calculate standardized death rates, as in Chapter VI.

Small changes in ρ can have a great effect on the age distribution. Thus values of ρ of 0.01 and -0.01 correspond to ratios of 1.28 and 0.78, respectively, between a generation and its predecessor. Such NRR or

implied "intrinsic rates of increase" have been attained by actual popula-
models are illustrated in Figure IX.2, in which one population is increasing
tions. The great changes that are brought about in the mathematical
at the rate of 1% per annum and the other decreasing by 1% per annum.

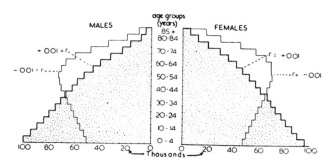

Figure IX.2. Population pyramids of increasing and decreasing populations (stable form).
Reproduced from *Med. J. Austl.*, **2**, (1954), 550.

The mode in the age distribution of the stable population occurs when
$h(x; \rho)$, which is proportional to $l_x \exp(-\rho x)$, is a maximum. We require
the maximum of

(28) $$\log[l_x \exp(-\rho x)] = \log l_x - \rho x.$$

Differentiating the expression on the right and setting the result equal to
zero in the usual manner, we obtain

(29) $$-\mu_{x'} = \rho,$$

where $\mu_{x'}$ is the force of mortality or $-$logarithmic differential of l_x when
$\rho < 0$; when $\rho \geq 0$, the maximum occurs at age 0, since both l_x and
$\exp(-\rho x)$ are decreasing throughout life. If $\rho < 0$, the value of the density
function for the population by age is the product of a constant times
$l_x \exp(-\rho x)$. At earlier ages, $-\rho x \equiv \log \exp(-\rho x)$ is increasing faster than
$\log l_x$ is decreasing, but at the higher ages $\log l_x$ is decreasing faster; thus the
expression $l_x \exp(-\rho x)$ attains a maximum when ρ is negative, and for a fixed
schedule $\{l_x\}$ the mode occurs higher as the absolute value of ρ increases.

Example.   As a modern example of the effect of a change in fertility
rates on the age distribution of a population, we reproduce the age-specific
fertility rates from the *Japan Statistical Yearbook* of 1967 as Table IX.4.
The effects of these changes are shown graphically as Figure IX.3, in
which the age distributions of the two sexes are shown as histograms,

rotated so as to give ages vertically and population numbers horizontally, males on the left, females on the right. The shape here, as usual, resembles that of a pyramid.

This pyramid is of interest because the official statistician has shown the year of birth against the appropriate population, permitting demographic history to be read from the pyramid. The population had been rapidly

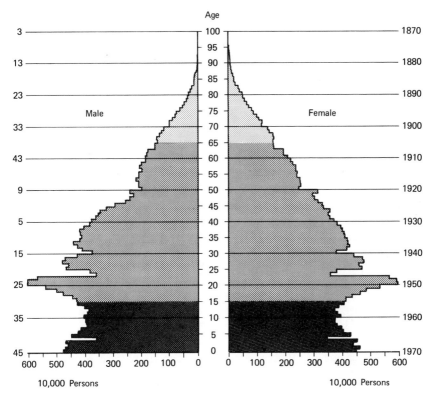

Figure IX.3. Population pyramid of japan, 1970. Reproduced from the *Japan Statistical Yearbook for 1971.*

expanding due to a high fertility rate. Births were low relative to neighboring years in 1919, 1939, 1946, and 1947, and 1958 and 1966. After 1950 there is an "undermining" of the pyramid, the survivors from the births of 1958 being the local minimum; measurements of the width of the graph or reference to the original tables reveal a marked preponderance of females over males at the higher ages, due to the effects of war and to more favorable rates of mortality in adult life.

Table IX.4

AGE-SPECIFIC FERTILITY RATES IN JAPAN[a]

Age Groups	Births/1000 Women per Annum							
	1925	1930	1937	1947	1950	1955	1960	1965
15–19	43	32	19	15	13	6	4	3
20–24	228	201	177	167	161	112	107	112
25–29	260	249	244	269	236	181	181	203
30–34	229	217	207	234	175	112	80	86
35–39	174	163	152	157	104	49	24	19
40–44	75	72	66	57	36	13	5	3
45–49	10	8	8	5	2	1	0	0
Total	1019	942	873	902	727	473	401	428
GRR	2510	2300	2130	2200	1760	1150	970	1040
NRR	1560	1520	1490	1670	1530	1050	920	1000
Ratio, NRR/GRR	.622	.661	.700	.759	.869	.913	.948	.962

[a] From Table 18 *Japan Statistical Yearbook* (1967, p. 40).

4. MORTALITY AND POPULATION INCREASE

It was formerly believed that in the absence of migration, population changes could be adequately measured by the difference between births and deaths. This view is reflected in the preoccupation of Pearl (1927) over many years with the study of the logistic curve of the total population and with the "vital index." However, changes in age distribution are also of importance, for fertility depends on age. Thus it is now well known that a population may be increasing in numbers at a time when its pattern of fertility and mortality imply its ultimate extinction. For example, England and Wales had such low fertility rates before World War II that, if the same rates had continued indefinitely, they would have led to a decline of about 20% per generation; yet the total actual population was increasing.

Measures such as R_0, the *net reproduction rate* (Boeckh, 1886; Kuczynski, 1928) and ρ, the *intrinsic rate of natural increase* of Lotka (1925) and Fisher (1930), which were discussed in Section IX.2, give the long-term implications of schedules of fertility and mortality rates. In so doing, they may be in contradiction with common-sense measures such as the "vital index" of Pearl. Thus in the 1930s the fertility rates and mortality rates of many European countries implied that these rates would ultimately decline and become extinct if they were to hold for an indefinite length of time; yet the population of no European nation actually declined (although the phenomenon of aging was apparent).

The declines in the mortality rates have naturally led to an increase in population. Some declines have occurred at the higher ages, resulting in more persons surviving under modern conditions from, say, 50 years to 70 years, than would have survived under conditions of mortality of the nineteenth century. However, the great contribution to total size has come from changes in mortality at the lower ages, for a person whose life was saved at birth, say, from infectious disease, may expect to live a further 70 years, on an average; thus he will have a greater effect on total population size than a life saved at, say, 65 years of age. The change in mortality at the lower ages has also contributed to population increase, in that the proportion of children who later enter the reproduction ages is higher now than formerly. This is true because, as we saw in Section IX.2, the NRR is approximately equal to the GRR multiplied by l_{25}. In the last century, l_{25} would have been of the order of 0.75, whereas now it is greater than 0.95.

If other conditions such as fertility remain constant, then, we can say that in recent experience, about 20% more persons out of every cohort commencing life are available as parents for the next generation than in the nineteenth century. If a balance had been present before these changes, the rates of increase would be more than 20% per generation after the change. For several generations, the death rates have been improving, hence contributing to an increase in the ratio between succeeding generations. Possibly, however, the changes are even more fundamental than these remarks would suggest. Young persons are entering adult life free of a succession of infections in childhood and free of chronic tuberculous infections—in better health than ever before—and this may mean that fecundity (i.e., ability to bear children) is higher than ever before. All observers, incidentally, agree that improvements in the death rates have been an important factor in the general increase of population in the countries of the world.

5. AGING OF THE POPULATIONS

During the 1930s the average age of persons in the western European nations, the United States, Australia, and New Zealand rose, as did the proportions of persons older than 65 years. Such changes are collectively known as *aging of the population*. Although it is common to ascribe all these changes to changes in mortality, our analysis in the preceding sections should lead to doubt this conclusion. The study of the life-table populations suggests that changes in the birth rate might well be more powerful than changes in mortality; indeed, this was known to William Farr (1885). Furthermore, it was noted in the years about 1935 that there were fewer children at ages 0 to four years than at ages 5 to 9 years. This circumstance cannot be explained by changes in mortality, but it is readily accounted for by changes in the birth rate. Moreover, the critical observation is that changes in mortality have occurred chiefly at the younger ages and have had the effect of retarding the aging—in fact, they have acted like an increase in the birth rate.

Let us imagine the population pyramid for a country in, say, 1947, reconstructed to allow only as many in the different age groups as would have survived had the mortality rates of, say, 1900 persisted. Since reductions in mortality have occurred chiefly at the younger ages, only the younger age groups, up to, say, the age of 50 years in 1947, would be affected. There would be fewer survivors in each age-group than were actually enumerated in 1947. The reconstructed population would exhibit definite undermining, expecially for the age groups up to age 35 years in 1947. Such an analysis would clearly reveal that mortality changes in the past have had the effect of delaying the aging of the population.

The problem of aging has been extensively studied in the European populations such as in Sweden, the United Kingdom, and France, in which countries migration does not confuse the picture as it does in Australia and the United States. In Figure IX.4 we present the population pyramids for Sweden for the years 1900, 1920, 1940, and 1960, illustrating the effects of the fall in fertility on the age distribution of Sweden in the early 1930s. There seems to be general agreement among demographers that the decreased fertility has been the cause of the aging and that, up to the present, the aging process had actually beeen delayed because the changes in mortality occurred principally at the younger ages (Kuczynski, 1928; Royal Commission on Population, 1949; Notestein, 1942; Coale, 1956; Sauvy, 1954a, 1954b). The Royal Commission (1949) believed that in the absence of catastrophic changes in the birth or death rates, the proportion of persons in the population at ages 15 to 64 years would remain at the 62 to 66% level for any projection forward of the fertility and death rates of England and Wales into the next hundred years or so. It is clear that the improvement in the mortality rates does not impose an impossible burden on the state, which will be expected to be responsible for the care of the aged and will have to help by pensions, hospital care, or other means.

It is possible that many of the more pessimistic views on the social problems associated with aging emanate from those working in teaching hospitals. Sheldon (1948), investigating a random sample in Wolverhampton, England, noted the importance of taking a true random sample of the population. Otherwise, he stated, biased views might result, for "the degree

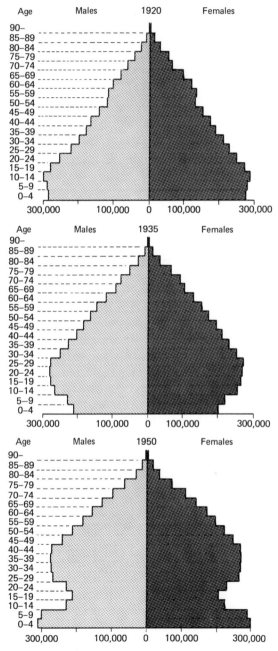

Figure IX.4. Population Pyramids for Sweden. From *Historisk Statistik for Sverige, Befolkning, 1720–1950.*

of self-selection imposed by the population on itself in regard to its approach to doctors inevitably gives anything other than a random sample a considerable bias."

Economic aspects of the problem are beyond the scope of this book. We may note that the actuarial problems of having each generation provide for its old age would be fairly easy to solve if it were not for the inflationary effects of wars, which have the effect of destroying savings and which are financed partly by devaluation of the currency. Economic depressions would have less importance than wars.

6. OTHER SOCIAL ASPECTS OF THE DECLINES OF MORTALITY

Certain social consequences of the declines of mortality possess some statistical interest, and we select a few of these for discussion now.

(i) Orphanhood

In distinguishing among *paternal, maternal,* and *complete orphanhood,* it is convenient to follow the method of Lotka (1931) and of Dublin, Lotka, and Spiegelman (1949) for estimating the orphanhood in a population. Lotka's method consists of noting that we can, without great error, consider all children as having been born of fathers of the one fixed age and of mothers of the one fixed age. Of course, owing to the increase in mortality rates with age, a child born to an old father will be more likely to become an orphan than a child born to a young father; but Lotka showed that the chances average out in such a way that their mean can be computed as if the age of the parents were fixed. The mean parental age at the time of conception can be taken to be 30 years for the father and 27 years for the mother. From the appropriate life table, the probability that the father will die before the birth of the child, before its first birthday, and so on, can be computed. Similar computations can be carried out for maternal orphanhood. For Australian experience, of children born between 1891 and 1900, about 1% would be born paternal orphans, about 10% would be so at their tenth birthday, and about 20% at their eighteenth birthday. According to the 1947 experience, only about 0.25% would be paternal orphans at their birth, about 2.6% at 10 years, and 7% at 18 years, which represents a great improvement. The experience of other countries, such as the United States or Sweden, would be similar.

(ii) Widowhood

At every age, the widows form a larger proportion of the female population than do the widowers of the male population. This is chiefly because bridegrooms tend to be about five years older than the brides, and because the rates of mortality of the females are more favorable. The two world wars have added, but not greatly, to this disparity. The declines of the mortality at ages 20 to 50 years have greatly lessened the social and economic problems of marriages broken by death and the care of orphaned children. Recent changes in the employment of women have further reduced the importance of such problems of widowhood.

(iii) Invalid Dependency

It is sometimes stated that modern advances in medicine may be increasing the rate of invalid dependency. This fear arises from a misconception of how and at what ages the improvements have occurred. It cannot be overstressed that almost all the improvements have taken place at the younger ages. In the past, much was made of the effect of a high infant and child mortality in weeding out the unfit. But this line of argument can be pushed too far; for example, the change of the age distribution of tuberculosis was formerly ascribed to loss of immunizing infections in childhood, as we noted in Section VIII.7. However, analysis by the generation method now seems to indicate that a favorable mortality experience in youth is followed by a favorable experience throughout life. There appears to be good reason for believing that the fall in tuberculosis death rates is being accompanied by a fall in morbidity and invalidity rates.

There seems to be good reason for also believing that the great changes in the incidence of the infective diseases of childhood will lead to lessened morbidity and invalidity; thus there will be less bronchiectasis due to measles and whooping cough and less chronic bronchitis; there will be less nephritis following scarlatina. With the great fall in incidence of the bowel diseases, children may be expected to grow up less susceptible to other infections. Modern treatment of syphilis and gonorrhea also should lessen invalidity. In Australia there is little need to reckon on unfavorable effects on morbidity at higher ages from treatment at younger ages for such diseases as malaria or schistosomiasis. These examples are mentioned merely to suggest that it is by no means axiomatic that successful therapy results in an invalid population, as is so often maintained. Other gains results from the improved treatment of accidents—(burns, scalds, etc.), as well as the special accidents and diseases of childbearing.

When we come to diseases of old age, it is well known that modern therapy has had little effect, with the notable exceptions of diabetes and pernicious anemia. It is possible that effective therapy for these two diseases increases the active period of life and decreases the period of invalidity once so inevitable as the illness progressed.

EXERCISES

1. The age-specific fertility rates, total births per thousand per annum, in 1960 are given by Grove and Hetzel (1968) as follows:

Age	Entire United States	Alabama	California	Massachusetts
All ages	23.7	24.7	23.7	22.4
15–44	118.0	120.9	115.9	113.4
10–14	0.8	1.8	0.6	0.2
15–19	89.1	108.9	102.8	50.6
20–24	258.1	251.9	267.3	230.7
25–29	197.4	179.9	189.1	220.7
30–34	112.7	107.8	103.4	133.5
35–39	56.2	56.8	48.3	65.7
40–44	15.5	17.8	13.0	17.2
45–49	0.9	1.2	0.7	0.7

Calculate the gross and net reproduction rates for the United States and for each of the three states in the tabulation. Use $f = 0.488$ for the ratio of female to all live births, and 0.964 for l_{25}. Compare the orders assigned to the United States and in the three states by the GRR and the NRR.

2. Grove and Hetzel (1968) give the fertility per 1000 women aged 15 to 44 years in the same areas as follows:

Year	United States	Alabama	California	Massachusetts
1940	79.9	106.1	69.3	63.1
1950	106.2	121.6	102.5	91.4
1960	118.0	120.9	115.9	113.5

Compare these figures with the results of Exercise 1. Comment on the development of these rates with time.

3. Calculate the ratio f of female live births to all live births for the various age groups and for the whole population, from the following data from the *Report of the Registrar-General for England and Wales, 1939.*

Age of Mother (years)	Total Live Births	Total Female Live Births
Under 20	28,513	13,827
20	140,239	67,976
25	200,348	97,868
30	144,103	70,188
35	77,431	38,066
40	23,618	11,661
45+	2,155	1,104
Total	616,407	300,690

NOTES

Population Texts

Hauser and Duncan, 1959; Keyfitz and Flieger, 1968; Mudd, 1964; Reinhard, 1949; (France): Reinhard and Armengaud, 1961; Royal Commission on Population, 1949; UN Statistical Papers, 1954; UN Population Studies No. 17, 1953; UN Population Studies No. 25, 1956; Wolfenden, 1954.

Aging

Bourlière, 1970; Kuczynski, 1928; Lancaster, 1965; McMullen, 1963; Sauvy, 1954b; Sheldon, 1948, 1960; Taylor, 1961; Twaddle, 1968; UN Population Studies No. 22, 1955; UN Population Studies No. 26, 1956.

Migration

UN Population Studies No. 24, 1955.

Population and Economic and Social Factors

Dorn, 1962; McKeown 1961, 1966; Sheps and Ridley (Eds.), 1966; Taylor and Hall, 1967; UN Population Studies No. 20, 1954; U.S. National Center for Health Statistics, 1970a; WHO Expert Committee, 1967.

Population of Eurasia

Usher, 1930.

Population Growth, Mathematical

Feller, 1939, 1940, and 1941.

World Population and Birth Control

Hartmann et al., 1951.

Fecundity and Fertility

Boeckh, 1890; Henry, 1961; James, 1963; Kuczynski, 1928; Milbank Memorial Fund, 1959; Pollard and Pollard, 1966; Registrar-General, 1959; Royal Commission, 1949; Ryder, 1955; Sheps and Ridley (Eds.), 1966; Sydenstricker and Notestein, 1930; UN Population Studies No. 6, 1949; U.S. National Center for Health Statistics, 1967a, 1968a, 1970a, 1970b.

Length of Pregnancy

Hotelling and Hotelling, 1932; Sutton, 1945.

Hour of Birth

Charles, 1953; Sutton, 1945.

CHAPTER X

Statistical Aspects of Human Genetics

1. GENETIC MODELS

It is well known that certain characters or characteristics are passed from parent to child. These characters are determined by the *genes*, which are arranged linearly on the *chromosomes*. In the human species, there are 22 pairs of *autosomes* and one pair of *sex chromosomes*. The sex chromosomes are referred to as the X- and Y-chromosomes. In the human species, the sexes are distinguished by the fact that the females carry two X-chromosomes and the males an X- and a Y-chromosome.

Cell division is of two types. In ordinary cell division, the chromosomes are duplicated, and after division both daughter cells possess copies of the 23 chromosome pairs; this is the process of *mitosis*. A new individual, the *zygote*, is formed at fertilization by the union of the *spermatozoon* (*male gamete*) and the ovum (*female gamete*). In the zygote, one member of each chromosome pair has come from each parent by way of the gamete. It is evident that there is some process by which only one member of each chromosome pair passes to the gamete. This is the special reducing subdivision, *meiosis*, of the chromosomes.

Reasons of symmetry suggest to us that a chromosome of any pair has probability equal to its fellow and, thus, a probability of $\frac{1}{2}$ of passing into the gamete. In its effect, the process of meiosis is analogous to the tossing of a coin. For a mathematical model of inheritance, the foregoing summary of biological theory can be formalized in a set of postulates.

Postulate i. The hereditary characters are transmitted by *genes* occurring at fixed positions, the *loci*, along the chromosomes. In each autosomal pair, genes for the determination of the same character appear in corresponding positions on the two members of the pair.

Postulate   ii. At a given locus, the gene can possess one of a set of alternative forms, the *alleles*. The particular form or allele remains fixed throughout life.

Postulate   iii. The two alleles appearing at a locus in an autosomal pair may be identical or distinct.

Postulate   iv. At meiosis, one allele from the pair at any locus passes to the gamete with probability equal to $\frac{1}{2}$.

Postulate   v. The passage of a particular allele at one meiosis to the gamete is statistically independent of the passage of the allele at the same locus at any other meiosis, or of the passage of any allele in any other parent.

Postulate   vi. At a given meiosis, the probability of an allele at one locus passing to the gamete is independent of an allele at any locus on another chromosome passing to the gamete.

Postulate   vii. The passage of the alleles at loci on a single chromosome are not mutually independent.

Postulate   viii. The gametes combine during fertilization to form a zygote, which then develops toward the adult form.

In the simplest case, there are two alleles to be considered, called *dominant* and *recessive*. Some authors use these terms even when the heterozygote can be distinguished from both homozygotes. In typical cases, the individuals possessing two dominant alleles cannot be readily distinguished from individuals possessing only one dominant. The class of individuals with a given genetic constitution is called a *genotype*, whereas the class of individuals with a given observable set of characters is called a *phenotype*. The phenomenon of dominance indicates that different genotypes may have the same phenotype.

For definiteness, we consider alleles A_1 and A_2 possessed by the male, and A_3 and A_4 possessed by the female parents. Alleles A_1, A_2, A_3, and A_4 may or may not be distinct. At meiosis A_1 goes to the *male gamete* with probability $\frac{1}{2}$, A_2 going with complementary probability, $\frac{1}{2}$; similarly, the *female gamete* contains A_3 with probability $\frac{1}{2}$ and A_4 with probability $\frac{1}{2}$. The mating, written $A_1 A_2 \times A_3 A_4$, can result in four mutually exclusive and exhaustive events at the locus: namely, the appearance of one of the pairs—$A_1 A_3$, $A_1 A_4$, $A_2 A_3$, and $A_2 A_4$. Graphically, we have

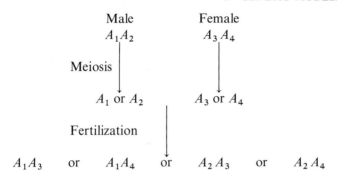

Example i. $A_1 = A_2 = D, A_3 = A_4 = D$. All four possibilities reduce to DD.

Example ii. $A_1 = A_2 = D$. $A_3 = D$. $A_4 = r$. $A_1 A_3 = DD$, $A_1 A_4 = Dr$, $A_2 A_3 = DD$, $A_2 A_4 = Dr$. In this case, DD occurs in two ways and Dr in two ways; DD occurs with probability $\frac{1}{2}$. We call DD and rr *homozygotes* and Dr *heterozygotes*.

Example iii. $A_1 = A_2 = D, A_3 = A_4 = r$. The possibilities now become Dr in each case. All offspring are heterozygotes.

Example iv. $A_1 = D, A_2 = r, A_3 = D, A_4 = r$. The four possibilities are now DD, Dr, rD, and rr; DD occurs with probability $\frac{1}{4}$, rr with probability $\frac{1}{4}$ and the heterozygote written Dr without respect to order occurs with probability $\frac{1}{2}$.

Example v. $A_1 = D$, $A_2 = r$, $A_3 = A_4 = r$. The four possibilities are Dr, Dr, rr, and rr; Dr occurs with probability $\frac{1}{2}$, as does rr.

Example vi. $A_1 = A_2 = r$, $A_3 = A_4 = r$. The only possibility is rr.

Although it is possible to write D and r in place of A_1, A_2, A_3, and A_4 in $2^4 = 16$ ways, all matings can be reduced to one of the six types given previously as examples by adopting the conventions that D is written before r in either pair A_1, A_2 or A_3, A_4 and that the pair with the greater number of D's is written first (e.g., r, D and D, r are combined and written as Dr as in Example iv). These results are summarized in Table X.1. Since A_1, A_2, A_3, and A_4 can each take the values a or A, we find that there are nine different forms of mating as given in Table X.1. The convention given for the D-r system would identify the matings—2 with 4, 3 with 7, and 6 with 8.

Table X.1

THE POSSIBILITIES OF MATING PAIRS AND OFFSPRING

Genotypes of Parents		Probabilities of Zygote		
F	M	Homozygous Dominant, AA	Heterozygous, Aa	Homozygous Recessive, aa
1. AA	AA	1	0	0
2. AA	Aa	$\frac{1}{2}$	$\frac{1}{2}$	0
3. AA	aa	0	1	0
4. Aa	AA	$\frac{1}{2}$	$\frac{1}{2}$	0
5. Aa	Aa	$\frac{1}{4}$	$\frac{1}{2}$	$\frac{1}{4}$
6. Aa	aa	0	$\frac{1}{2}$	$\frac{1}{2}$
7. aa	AA	0	1	0
8. aa	Aa	0	$\frac{1}{2}$	$\frac{1}{2}$
9. aa	aa	0	0	1

2. COMMENTARY ON THE MODELS

The postulates in Section X.1 constitute an abstraction from the theory of geneticists beginning with Gregor Mendel (1822–1884), whose principal works have been translated and commented upon by J. H. Bennett, R. A. Fisher, and W. Bateson in Mendel (1965). We now comment on the postulates and give some simple statistical tests of their adequacy in representing experimental findings.

Mendel's aims, which we write in modern language, were as follows:

1. To determine the number of different genotypes that could arise under various matings.

2. To arrange these forms according to the generations in which they appear.

5. To ascertain the statistical relations between the numbers of the different genotypes.

It is evident that the first two aims have a combinatorial aspect and that the third is thoroughly statistical.

Mendel began his experiments on pure lines with respect to a given character or characters. A *pure line* is a group of individuals so constituted that any mating among them will result in other individuals having the same form of the character. In terms of the model in Section X.1, every individual in a pure line must have a pair of identical alleles at the particular locus defining the character, and this pair is repeated in every individual in the given pure line. A pure line thus has genotype DD or rr. All matings in a dominant pure line are of the form $DD \times DD$, and these must result in DD offspring. Similarly, matings in the recessive pure line must be of the form $rr \times rr$, resulting in rr offspring. We suppose that the dominant phenotype cannot readily be separated into the class DD and Dr. A dominant pure line cannot contain Dr individuals, since this would lead to the possibility of the mating $Dr \times Dr$, yielding rr individuals.

From the two pure lines, matings of the form $DD \times rr$ can only yield Dr individuals by Postulate iv of Section X.1. Mendel called this the "hybrid" generation, but it now is usual to call it F_1. Matings can now be made between members of the F_1 generation, which are all of the form, $Dr \times Dr$. Postulates iv and v enable the genotypes and their relative proportions in the ensuing F_2 generation to be computed as in Example iv of Section X.1. The dominant phenotype occurs with probability 0.75 and the recessive phenotype with probability 0.25. There thus tends to be observed a $3:1$ ratio between the numbers of dominant and recessive phenotypes.

Example i. Mendel fertilized 253 F_1 plants with pollen from other F_1 plants and obtained 7324 seeds yielding 5474 dominants and 1850 recessives; thus the ratio was $2.96:1$. This result can be tested. The number of recessive phenotypes is a random binomial variable with index 7324 and probability $\frac{1}{4}$. The expected number is $7324 \times \frac{1}{4} = 1831$, and the variance is $7324 \times \frac{3}{4} \times \frac{1}{4} = 1373.25$. We also have $\sqrt{1373.25} = 37.06$, $1850 - 1831 = 19$, and $19/37.06 = 0.51$. Using the normal approximation, the observed value differs by only 0.51 of its standard deviation, and Mendel's observations agree well with theory.

Example ii. Mendel made two matings, which we could write $Aa\,Bb \times Aa\,Bb$, to obtain 315 AB phenotypes, 108 Ab phenotypes, 101 aB phenotypes, and 32 ab phenotypes. The results can be tabulated as follows:

	B-Dominant	B-Recessive	Totals
A-Dominant	315 (312.75)	108 (104.25)	423 (417)
A-Recessive	101 (104.25)	32 (34.75)	133 (139)
Totals	416 (417)	140 (139)	556 (556)

The expected numbers of A-dominants is $\frac{3}{4} \times 556 = 417$, and the variance is $556 \times \frac{3}{4} \times \frac{1}{4} = 104.25$. The difference, observed-expected, is $423 - 417 = 6$. The difference is thus only 0.59 of its standard error, since $\sqrt{104.25} = 10.21$ and $6/10.21 = 0.59$. Similarly, the difference of the number of B-dominants divided by its standard error is $(416 - 417)/10.21 = -0.098$.

Both these differences are well in accord with theory as expressed in Postulates iv and v of the preceding section.

However, we can test a further hypothesis. If the events at the A- and B-loci are mutually independent, the proportion of A-dominants should be the same for the B-dominants and B-recessives. The proportions observed are 315/416 and 108/140. The difference between these proportions is -0.0167, which has a standard error of 0.0423. The difference is thus 0.37 times its standard error.

It may be remarked that a combined test of the Postulates iv, v, and vi is the χ^2-test of Pearson (explained in Chapter XII), by which we take the sum of the quantities (observed $-$ expected)^2/(expected) in the four cells of the table, so that $\chi^2 = (315 - 312.75)^2/312.75 + (108 - 104.25)^2/104.25 + (101 - 104.25)^2/104.25 + (32 - 34.75)^2/34.75 = 0.470$, and this sum would have to be greater than 7.815 to be significant at the 5% level.

Postulate vi is usually referred to as the law of *independent segregation of the genes.*

Roberts, Dawson, and Madden (1939) reported an extensive set of experiments for testing the independent segregation of the genes in mice and rats. One set of results of a mating of the form *Aa Bb Dd* × *aa bb dd* can be written

	$A^- B^-$	$A^- B^+$	$A^+ B^-$	$A^+ B^+$	Totals
D^-	427	440	509	460	1836
D^+	494	467	462	475	1898
Totals	921	907	971	935	3734

The expected number in any cell in this table is $\frac{1}{2} \times \frac{1}{2} \times \frac{1}{2} \times 3734 = 466.75$. The variance of each entry is $3734 \times \frac{1}{8} \times \frac{7}{8} = 408.412$. The standard error is then 20.2. We should expect numbers in the range 466.75 ± 40.4 (i.e., in the range 426–507), and this is confirmed by the data. The table is good evidence in favor of independent segregation.

3. EQUILIBRIUM OF THE GENOTYPES IN A POPULATION

Elementary computations are sufficient to establish an important law named after G. H. Hardy and W. Weinberg. *Panmixia* is said to exist if every possible mating pair has equal probability of occurring. We suppose that the distributions of the genotypes *AA*, *Aa*, and *aa* are the same in the two sexes, and we write the proportions as *P*, *R*, and *Q*. Thus

(1) $P + Q + R = 1.$

The *gene frequency* of A in the population is the proportion, p, of A alleles at the locus; similarly, the gene frequency of a, q, is the proportion of a alleles at the same locus: $p + q = 1$. Furthermore, we can write

(2) $p = P + \frac{1}{2}R, \qquad q = Q + \frac{1}{2}R.$

One method of proving (2) is to observe that if there were a large number of individuals, N say, there would be $2N$ alleles at the locus, the NP homozygotes providing $2NP$ A-alleles and the NR heterozygotes providing NR A-alleles. The proportion, p, of A-alleles would be $(2NP + NR)/2N$ and so $P + \frac{1}{2}R$. Now we have $p = P + \frac{1}{2}R$. Similarly, $q = Q + \frac{1}{2}R$.

Let us consider a mating chosen at random. Since in either sex the probability of an allele A passing to the gamete is p, the contributions from this sex are A with probability p and a (or not-A) with probability q. The probabilities from the other sex are the same. The assumption of panmixia is that these events are independent; therefore, the offspring receives 2 A's, 1 A, or no A with probabilities p^2, $2pq$, and q^2, the coefficients of t^2, t, and 1 in $(pt + q)^2$. The gene frequencies are again p and q. A second set of matings under panmixia will result in the same frequencies and the same proportions. Thus *the stable distribution of the genotypes is attained in one generation under the condition of panmixia.* This is the famous Hardy-Weinberg law.

The foregoing proof can be given in an expanded form. Let us first consider the "stable" form of the population and possible matings. We are given $P = p^2$ dominant homozygotes, $Q = q^2$ recessive homozygotes, and $R = 2pq$ heterozygotes in the two sexes. The matings and their relative frequencies appears in Table X.2. It is evident that the genotypes of the offspring remain in the same ratios—namely, $p^2 : 2pq : q^2$—as the parent, and thus the term "stable" is justified.

Let us suppose now that P, Q, and R take any arbitrary values compatible with $P + Q + R = 1$. We can construct a mating table under panmixia as Table X.3, in which the matings are listed in the same order as in the Examples of Section X.1, A replacing D and a replacing r. Matings 2, 3, and 5 appear with a multiplier 2, since $AA \times Aa$ can occur in two ways (because AA can be the male or the female contribution).

Of course, this law relates to what happens in the mathematical model. Panmixia may occur rarely, but actual populations existing for many generations without migration often have genotype ratios that approximate to the stable condition.

The proportions of AA, Aa, and aa genotypes, P, R, and Q, can be represented on a trilinear graph as the distances from a point within an

Table X.2

MATINGS AND OFFSPRING UNDER HYPOTHESIS OF
PANMIXIA IN A STABLE POPULATION

Type of Mating	Frequency of Mating	Frequency of Offspring		
		AA	Aa	aa
$AA \times AA$	p^4	p^4	0	0
$AA \times Aa$	$4p^3q$	$2p^3q$	$2p^3q$	0
$AA \times aa$	$2p^2q^2$	0	$2p^2q^2$	0
$Aa \times Aa$	$4p^2q^2$	p^2q^2	$2p^2q^2$	p^2q^2
$Aa \times aa$	$4pq^3$	0	$2pq^3$	$2pq^3$
$aa \times aa$	q^4	0	0	q^4
Total	1.00	p^2	$2pq$	q^2

Table X.3

THE ATTAINMENT OF THE STABLE FORM UNDER PANMIXIA

Type of Mating	Frequency of Mating	Frequency of Offspring		
		AA	Aa	aa
1. $AA \times AA$	P^2	P^2	0	0
2. $AA \times Aa$	$2PR$	PR	PR	0
3. $AA \times aa$	$2PQ$	0	$2PQ$	0
4. $Aa \times Aa$	R^2	$\frac{1}{4}R^2$	$\frac{1}{2}R^2$	$\frac{1}{4}R^2$
5. $Aa \times aa$	$2RQ$	0	RQ	RQ
6. $aa \times aa$	Q^2	0	0	Q^2
Total	$\begin{array}{c}1\\ \equiv (P+Q+R)^2\end{array}$	$\begin{array}{c}(P+\frac{1}{2}R)^2\\ \equiv p^2\end{array}$	$\begin{array}{c}2(P+\frac{1}{2}R)(Q+\frac{1}{2}R)\\ \equiv 2pq\end{array}$	$\begin{array}{c}(Q+\frac{1}{2}R)^2\\ \equiv q^2\end{array}$

equilateral triangle to the sides. We show such a representation in Figure X.1, where a general point G appears at a distance R from the base XY, P from YZ, and Q from ZX. The perpendicular from G to the base divides it in the ratio $p : q$. In the equilibrium population, $R \leq \frac{1}{2}$. The points representing an equilibrium population all lie on the parabola shown.

In human populations, much interest is centered on diseases caused by a single dominant gene. Usually there is a selective advantage against such a gene, and it tends to die out. The gene frequency p is small, possibly of the

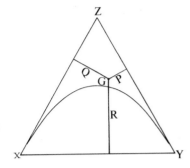

Figure X.1. Gene ratios in population (trilinear grid); P dominant and Q recessive homozygote ratios; R heterozygote ratio; G is a general point. The curved line includes all the equilibrium points under panmixia.

order (of size) of $1/10,000$ or 1 in 10^4. The dominant homozygote occurs with frequency $P = p^2$, which is of the order of 1 in 10^8; the heterozygote has probability $R = 2pq$, and has a frequency of the order of 1 in 10^4. In constructing genealogies or pedigrees of a dominant defect or disease, it is usually justified to assume that all marriages outside the family are with the recessive genotype. Similarly, if the deleterious gene is a recessive and the frequency is q, the corresponding defect will appear with probability $Q = q^2$. If q is small, Q will be small with respect to $R = 2pq$, and the proportion of carriers of a single gene will be high relative to the proportion of the defective. Furthermore, if q is small and an individual possesses the recessive, the proportion of carriers in that individual's relatives will be much higher than in the general population. Recessive defects, therefore, tend to show up in the offspring of consanguineous marriages (i.e., unions between individuals with a common ancestor).

4. PEDIGREES AND GENEALOGICAL RECORDS

The notion of a family tree or *pedigree* is familiar in history and in animal breeding. In genetical studies on man, pedigrees are essential in determining whether a given character is inherited and in ascertaining its mode of transmission. Some conventions in the description of pedigrees have become generally accepted. In British custom, a male is denoted by a circle with spear (of Mars) ♂, and a female by a mirror (of Venus) ♀; persons of sex unknown are recorded as circles ○. Affected persons are denoted by the same symbols with the circles "filled in."

In American custom, males are represented by squares and females by circles. Matings are represented either by horizontal lines □—┬—○ or

angled joins □⌐○, the male being written on the left, as a rule. This convention cannot be carried through if one of the pair has two mates; we can then write ▢ ⚲ ▢, showing that the female has

been mated to two males or ⚲ ▢ ⚲, where the male has been mated

with two females. The symbol └──┘ denotes marriage or mating as between I.1 and I.2 in Fig. X.2. The members of a sibship are joined by a horizontal bar. The line joining a parent to a child is to be interpreted in the same way, whether it be a simple straight line as between II.5 and III.8 in Fig. X.3 or a zig-zag line as between I.1 and II.3 in Fig. X.2; in neither case is there any intermediate person.

The members of any generation are written on a horizontal line, and the generation is denoted by a Roman numeral. Each member of the same generation is distinguished by his own arabic number, 1, 2, 3, ...

Full sibs, or *sibs* when there is no fear of ambiguity, are individuals who possess a common pair of parents. *Half sibs* are two individuals who possess precisely one common parent. In Fig. X.2, III.4, III.5, and III.6 are full sibs. It is sometimes convenient to abbreviate a pedigree by writing the numbers in a sibship as subscripts. Thus there might be five males and two females; this can be written $\square_{[5]}$ and $\bigcirc_{[2]}$. In Fig. X.2, III.2 has two unaffected sons and three unaffected daughters.

5. DOMINANT INHERITANCE

The inheritance of identifiable pathological or disadvantageous characters in man is usually carried by genes at a single locus. Sometimes the defective character can be identified as the failure of a single enzyme system; this situation has given rise to the aphorism "one gene, one enzyme." When a single gene or a small number of identifiable genes control a character, the genes are said to be *major genes*. The inheritance of normal characters, such as height, often seems to depend on the action of genes at many different loci; this is called *multifactorial* or *polygenic* inheritance.

At any particular locus, it usually appears to be the case that there is one allele with a high frequency; other alleles are eliminated by selection. But it is sometimes found that a number of alleles have appreciable frequencies—for example, in the *ABO* and *MNS* blood group systems. This state is given the name *polymorphism*. In some cases, the homozygous form of the allele may be dangerous but the allele may have definite selective advantage in the heterozygous state. The gene for sickling of the red cells is a case in point.

A typical pedigree of a defect transmitted by a dominant gene is displayed in Figure X.2. In this pedigree, there is an affected male I.1, who has married a normal female I.2, and their offspring have included normal and

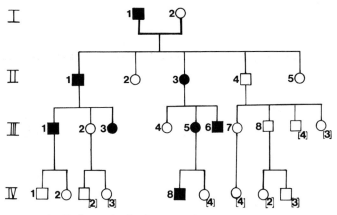

Figure X.2. Pedigree of a dominant gene.

affected individuals. Moreover, every affected person except I.1 himself is seen to have an affected parent.

Dominant genes for defects are rather rare in any population, so that unless the marriage is consanguineous, it can be assumed that the marriage is with a normal. In the case of a marriage between two persons each possessing a dominant gene, the possibility arises that some offspring will be born with two dominant genes; this seems to be a rare event and, in any case, the double dose of the gene often leads to very severe types of the defect. Of course, if anyone with such a defect lives to have a family, all the offspring will possess a dominant gene.

A sibship of n in which one parent carries one dominant gene can be considered. Each sib has a probability of $\frac{1}{2}$ of carrying the dominant by Postulates iv and v (Section X.1), and the probability of a later sib having a dominant gene is $\frac{1}{2}$, independently of the number of dominants passing to the earlier sibs. A case strictly analogous to the tossing of true coins has been reached. The probabilities of the numbers affected are shown in Table X.4. Each line is given by the generating function $(\frac{1}{2} + \frac{1}{2}t)^n$. The mean number of dominants in a sibship of n is $\frac{1}{2}n$. It is easily verified that the probabilities for sibships of size n in Table X.4 are equal to the entries at the corresponding point in Pascal's triangle (Table IV.1), divided by 2^n.

In the consideration of pedigrees, it is usually assumed that *mutations* (i.e., changes in structure of the gene) are not occurring in the individuals included in the pedigree. However, the first member of a dominant line will have been produced by a mutation in the germ cells of the generation prior to him.

We have noticed that dominant genes producing defects tend to be rare in the population. Let us suppose that the defect results in a net reproduction

Table X.4

Matings of Type $Aa \times aa$

Number in Sibship	Number of Sibs Having Dominant Gene, k						
	0	1	2	3	4	5	6
1	$\frac{1}{2}$	$\frac{1}{2}$					
2	$\frac{1}{4}$	$\frac{1}{2}$	$\frac{1}{4}$				
3	$\frac{1}{8}$	$\frac{3}{8}$	$\frac{3}{8}$	$\frac{1}{8}$			
4	$\frac{1}{16}$	$\frac{4}{16}$	$\frac{6}{16}$	$\frac{4}{16}$	$\frac{1}{16}$		
5	$\frac{1}{32}$	$\frac{5}{32}$	$\frac{10}{32}$	$\frac{10}{32}$	$\frac{5}{32}$	$\frac{1}{32}$	
6	$\frac{1}{64}$	$\frac{6}{64}$	$\frac{15}{64}$	$\frac{20}{64}$	$\frac{15}{64}$	$\frac{6}{64}$	$\frac{1}{64}$

rate for the dominants of $(1 - \alpha)R$ and R for normals; $0 < \alpha < 1$. Corresponding to each normal gene there will be R normal genes in the next generation, and corresponding to each dominant gene there will be $(1 - \alpha)R$. After k generations, the normal gene will have R^k descendants and the dominant gene will have $(1 - \alpha)^k R^k$.

It is clear that for any appreciable α, the dominants will tend either to die out or to become notably fewer than the normals. Mutation rates from the recessive to the dominant are of the order of $1/10^4$ generations at a given locus. If $\alpha = 0.8$ and $R = 1$, there will be 0.2 of the mutant strain after one generation, $0.2^2 = 0.04$ after two generations, and so on; each mutation will contribute $1 + 0.2 + 0.2^2 + \cdots = 1/(1 - 0.2) = 1.25$ lives to the population or, more generally, α^{-1} lives. In this example, if the mutation rate were μ, a proportion μ/α of the population would possess the dominant. In many of the pathological cases α is quite high—0.8 would not be unusual—and the proportion in the population would be μ/α or $0.0001/0.8 = 0.000125$ in our illustrative example, if $\mu = 0.0001$.

6. RECESSIVE INHERITANCE

Let us suppose that the gene frequency of a recessive character is q in a given population, which has reached equilibrium at the locus. Then for various values of q we can compute the genotypes as in Table X.5. If q is small, $2pq$ is close to $2q$. The table illustrates this relationship that follows, since p is close to unity.

In a stable population, the conditional probabilities of matings can be computed, given that the offspring is homozygous recessive. The matings must be of the form $Aa \times Aa$, $Aa \times aa$, and $aa \times aa$, since these are the only

Table X.5

HOMOZYGOTES AND HETEROZYGOTES FOR SMALL VALUES OF q

Value of q	Recessive Homozygote Frequency q^2	Heterozygote Frequency $2pq$	Approximate Value $2q$
0.001	0.000.001	0.001.998	0.002
0.002	0.000.004	0.003.992	0.004
0.004	0.000.016	0.007.968	0.008
0.008	0.000.064	0.015.872	0.016
0.010	0.000.100	0.019.800	0.02
0.020	0.000.400	0.039.200	0.04
0.030	0.000.900	0.058.200	0.06
0.050	0.002.500	0.095.000	0.10
0.100	0.010.000	0.180.000	0.20
0.200	0.040.000	0.320.000	0.40

matings in which each parent possesses an a-allele. The probabilities of the matings are $(2pq)^2$, $2(2pq)q^2$, and $(q^2)^2$. The probability that the first type of mating will result in a homozygous recessive is $\frac{1}{4}$, the probability that the second type will result in a homozygous recessive is $\frac{1}{2}$, and it is certain that the final mating will result in a homozygous recessive. The total probability of a homozygous recessive is q^2, the probability that a mating is of form $Aa \times Aa$ and that a homozygous recessive has resulted is p^2q^2; the other probabilities for matings $Aa \times aa$ and $aa \times aa$ are $2pq^3$ and q^4. Given a recessive homozygote, the probabilities that the matings were $Aa \times Aa$, $Aa \times aa$, and $aa \times aa$ are p^2, $2pq$, and q^2. Hence if panmixia holds and q is small, the great bulk of the recessive homozygotes have both parents heterozygous.

Furthermore, if the recessive is rare and if there is a heterozygote, his cousins will have a higher frequency rate than the general population because cousins share a common ancestor from whom the allele can be passed down to both branches of the family. In the pedigree of Figure X.3 there has been a mating of I.1 and I.2, and one of these individuals carries the recessive gene; III.2 and III.3 are cousins and have a homozygous recessive offspring. The mating III.5 and III.6 has resulted in an additional homozygote. The mating of III.7 and III.8 has produced no recessive homozygotes, although there have been five daughters and four sons. It is probable that III.7 and III.8 are not both heterozygotes; if they were, no recessive homozygote in a sibship of nine would have a probability $\left(\frac{3}{4}\right)^9 = 19,683/262,144 = 0.075$—a somewhat rare event.

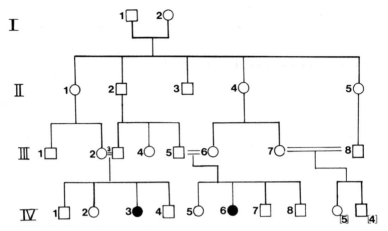

Figure X.3. Pedigree of a recessive gene. The double lines indicate matings between relatives.

The pedigree of a recessive defect may have the same form as a dominant, as in Figure X.4, where the recessive are written black and the heterozygotes with a bar. The barred individuals will be free of any manifestation of the defect. Every individual with the defect has a parent with the defect in this figure. Figure X.4 could well be the pedigree of a dominant. However, if it were known that I.1 was born of a cousin mating and that I.2 was consanguineous, suspicion would be aroused. A mating of the heterozygotes III.2 and III.4, giving rise to the defect, would be conclusive evidence that the gene was recessive.

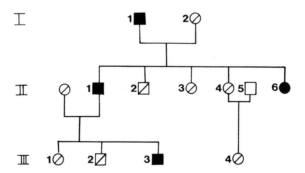

Figure X.4. Incomplete pedigree of a recessive gene imitating that of a dominant gene.

7. SEX–LINKED INHERITANCE

Some genes are carried on the X-chromosome, the female can thus be homozygous recessive, heterozygous, or homozygous dominant. The male with only one X-chromosome can possess only one allele and it may be the dominant or the recessive gene; the male is said to be *hemizygous*, and his phenotype must express the dominant or recessive. Since a male receives his X-chromosome from his mother, the gene is sex linked. Daughters receive one X-chromosome from their father and one from their mother and, if it is a recessive, they show no defect as a rule. Figure X.5 represents an abbreviated pedigree. All cases are males, and each male case can trace his defect back to a single ancestor. Hemophilia yields such pedigrees. Hemophilia has a low gene frequency but the homozygous state is known in females.

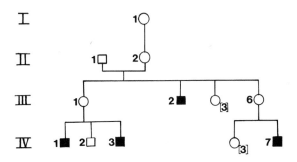

Figure X.5.   Pedigree of a sex-linked gene.

8. THE SEX RATIO IN SIBSHIPS

The sexes in the human species are distinguished by two parallel characteristics: the females possess an XX chromosome pair and the males an XY pair. This is the 23rd or sex chromosome pair. We leave out of consideration here the possibly aberrant pathological cases of the pos-session of combinations XXY, such as appear in Klinefelter's syndrome.

The only possible mating is $XX \times XY$, from which there can result XY and XX zygotes—the male and the female, respectively. It might be expected that XY and XX, male and female, would be equally likely to occur. However, the ratio observed at human birth is $p = 0.513$ males to $q = 0.487$ females, approximately. It has been hypothesized that this is due to differential mortality *in utero*. However, the male ratio is even higher in young embryos.

Table X.6

Sᴇx Rᴀᴛɪᴏ ɪɴ Sɪʙsʜɪᴘs (ᴇᴀʀʟʏ ᴀɴᴅ ʟᴀᴛᴇ)

Males in Excess		Females in Excess	
Completely male sibships		Completely female sibships	
1:—,	$+3.07^a$	—:1,	-4.66
2–4:—,	$+2.78$	—:2–4,	-2.78
5–14:—,	$+0.94$	—:5–15	-1.46
One male in excess		One female in excess	
2:1,	-3.66	1:2,	$+1.33$
3:2,	-4.48	2:3,	$+3.73$
4–10:3–9,	-6.18	3–9:4–10	$+8.22$
Two males in excess		Two females in excess	
3:1,	-4.01	1:3,	$+4.29$
4:2,	-4.48	2:4,	$+3.91$
5–11:3–9	-6.15	3–9:5–11,	$+5.16$
Three males in excess		Three females in excess	
4:1,	-3.15	1:4,	$+1.47$
5:2,	-3.24	2:5,	$+1.97$
6–12:3–9,	-4.42	3–9:6–12	$+4.53$
Four males in excess		Four females in excess	
5:1,	-2.81	1:5,	$+2.55$
6:2,	-4.07	2:6,	$+2.04$
7–12:3–8,	-4.21	3–8:7–12,	$+6.49$
Excess of more than four males		Excess of more than four females	
-4.76		$+4.93$	
Equal numbers of males and females			
1:1		$+1.03$	
3:3 or 2:2		-0.64	
4–11:4–11		-0.87	

[a] Standardized difference between observed and expected male births, $(M - Np)/\sqrt{(Npq)}$.

A problem of interest is whether the p of some parentages differs from that of the mean. It may be noted that p could differ so slightly from the population mean that very large samples would have to be used. A mathematical model may be set up. The following assumptions are made: (1) p is a constant for all parental pairs, (2) p is independent of the age of the parents, (3) the sex of one sib is independent of the sex of those sibs preceding it in the sibship. The probability-generating function for a male birth is thus $(pt + q)$. For a sibship of size n containing no identical twins, the probability-generating function is $(pt + q)^n$. We formulated an example of such a distribution in Table I.7 from Geissler's data as given by Lancaster (1950d). The distributions of the sex ratio in sibships have been the subject of much comment by Gini (1908, 1951), by R. A. Fisher in *Statistical Methods*, and by many other authors. However, few other collections of observations bearing on this problem have been comparable in size to Geissler's.

It cannot be maintained from his data that p is variable between sibships. If this were true, the families with high p would tend to have a higher proportion of males in the earlier births. Thus if we were to consider families with a higher proportion of boys in the early births, we would expect them to have a high proportion in the later births (see Table X.6.) The results are contrary to what we might expect on the hypothesis of variable p.

Another approach is to form tables by a life-table method. Geissler's data enable us to compute the probability that the $(k + 1)$th birth is of a male, conditional on r of the first k births being boys. It is shown in Lancaster (1950d) that the population of sibships, so produced, is consistent with the distributions in sibships of eight neither as recorded nor as obtained by subtracting the ninth child.

9. TWINNING

As Example i of Section IV.6, we have shown that twin births can be analyzed into monovular (monozygous) and binovular (dizygous) types and that the latter can be estimated as being equal in number to twice the number of the unlike-sex twins. Table X.7 presents the statistics for the United States in 1964, by age of mother. We have taken births less the twin confinements as a good approximation to the number of confinements. It is evident from the table that the rate for monovular twinning is little affected by the age of mother, although the binovular twinning rate has a maximum in the 35 to 39 year age group.

A rule, due to C. Zeleny, states that the probability of a confinement resulting in a litter of size n is p^{n-1}, $n = 2, 3, 4, \ldots$; if the probability of a twin confinement is p, the probability of a triplet is p^2. Table X.8 demonstrates approximate satisfaction of the rule. There are reasons for believing that the good approximations for the rule are, in a sense, accidental; for if the rule holds for classes of the population with twinning rates, p_1 and p_2 say, such that $p_1 \neq p_2$, it cannot hold for the whole population.

The use of fertility drugs will render illusory any "biological" significance of the rates for the greater litter sizes.

Table X.7

The Zygosity of Twins in the United States, 1964

Age of Mother	Frequency by Sex of Twins			Total Twin Confinements[b]	Total Twin Confinements Less 2MF	Total Births Less Twin Confinements (thousands)	Frequencies/1000	
	MM	MF	FF				Binovular (Dizygous)	Monovular (Monozygous)
All ages	14,527	12,715	13,888	41,259	15,829	3,986	6.4	4.0
Under 15	26	8	14	49	33	7.767	2.1	4.2
15–19	1,522	869	1,411	3,820	2,082	582	3.0	3.6
20–24	4,563	3,505	4,362	12,465	5,455	1,427	4.9	3.8
25–29	3,807	3,555	3,697	11,104	3,994	996	7.1	4.0
30–34	2,724	2,779	2,506	8,029	2,471	577	9.6	4.3
35–39	1,483	1,663	1,517	4,670	1,344	305	10.9	4.4
40–44	387	327	367	1,084	430	86.5	7.6[a]	5.0[a]
45+	11	7	11	29	15	4.641	3.0[a]	3.2[a]
N.S.	4	2	3	9	5	—	—	—

Data from U.S. National Center for Health Statistics (1967a) and from *Vital Statistics* of the United States (1964) Vol. 1, *Natality*. [a] Frequency depends on smaller numbers of observations. [b] The sex of some twins has not been recorded

Table X.8

Twins and Triplets in the United States, 1964

Age of Mother (years)	Twin Rates/1000 Deliveries	Square of Twin Rate	Observed Triplet Rates/10^6
Under 15	5.8	34	—
15–19	6.3	40	50
20–24	8.5	72	62
25–29	10.9	119	112
30–34	13.7	188	142
35–39	15.0	225	210
40–44	12.2	149	} 165
45+	6.3	40	
All ages	10.1	102	98

Data from Tables C and E, U.S. National Center for Health Statistics (1967a). (See also 1970b.)

10. EVOLUTIONARY ASPECTS OF THE DECLINES IN MORTALITY RATES

The declines in the mortality rates in the later part of the nineteenth century was a new phenomenon in the urbanized states of Europe. Also at this time there were changes in social attitudes, resulting in the abolition of child labor, improvements in working conditions, and some amelioration of the urban environment. Commentators felt that the high levels of mortality were "natural" and gave opinions that any declines in mortality from the levels holding at the end of the nineteenth century would have a disastrous effect on the genetic constitution of the population. This view, which can be found in any of the eugenic writings of Karl Pearson, was one of the guiding themes of the eugenic movement in England. In more modern times, such pessimistic views have been expressed in milder terms by Dubos (1960, 1961) and others.

In favor of the position just described, there are laboratory and field observations showing the selective advantage of some alleles over their competitors under given conditions, and the fear is often expressed that, if those who are more susceptible to infective diseases are treated, the average susceptibility will tend to fall to dangerous levels. Tuberculosis can be specially mentioned here. It is known from experimental work that the ability to resist infections is at least partly genetic; thus it is reasonable to expect that populations tend to become genetically resistant to their own pathogens. It appears necessary to look into possible dysgenic effects of therapy or other medical intervention. However, authors sometimes overlook the very short time that has elapsed since the general decline of mortality began in Europe—perhaps the length of four generations. Can gross changes in genetic composition of the human population have occurred in such a short experience?

Support for a more optimistic view on the long-term effects of control and treatment of disease can be obtained as follows. In general, the declines in mortality have occurred with respect to the infective diseases and the class of violent and accidental injuries. In addition, there has been a certain amount of improvement in the mortality from genetically determined diseases. The position of diabetes is anomalous. The favored theory is that this condition is due to a recessive and has a gene frequency exceeding 0.18. It appears likely that recessive homozygotes have a selection advantage over the dominants under conditions of primitive agriculture, which means that the gene cannot be considered to be unfavorable without qualification. Moreover, the treatment of diabetes has not yet yielded an unusually high number of births to diabetic parents. For other genetic diseases, including hemophilia, treatment is palliative; but the number of such treated cases is not large. It is possible that an equilibrium would be obtained with a somewhat larger gene frequency than would hold without the effective therapy. It has not been claimed that treatment of accident cases has a dysgenic effect.

This leaves us to discuss the treatment of infectious diseases. First, vaccination may be said to be analogous to the appearance of mild variants of a previously dangerous disease; "alastrim" in place of smallpox is a good example. Opportunities to observe such a change in balance between the human population and parasites must be rare. In investigating an epidemic of rabbits, however, Fenner (1959, 1968) and Fenner and Ratcliffe (1965) have demonstrated the evolution of less lethal forms of the virus. This disease, myxomatosis, is spread by mosquito from rabbit to rabbit. The "natural" disease occurs as a persistent skin tumor in the wild rabbit in Brazil. The virus was deliberately introduced into Australia as an acute highly infective disease inflicting a case fatality of over 99.4% in the European rabbit, prevalent in Australia. Since there is little spread by the mosquito during the winter, strains of myxoma virus are favored that do not kill too quickly. In addition, strains of rabbit are favored that are resistant. The combination of these two effects leads to a need for a small number of transmissions over the winter. Incidentally, case fatalities have decreased.

Much of the improvement in human mortality has come about through a diminution of the possibilities of infection (e.g., improved water supply, improved hygiene, and protection of foods). It is a matter of dispute whether this can be thought of as less natural than the high exposure rates of human urbanized populations in recent centuries. Many of the dangerous infections of such communities could not have survived as human diseases in the past. Indeed, some of them (e.g. smallpox and measles) do not have a carrier state in humans; they have only a short infective period, and an attack of the disease confers solid immunity. Such diseases could not have been important causes of human mortality before the foundations of the great city states of the Nile and Mesopotamia. Possibly before that time, man's principal specific pathogens came from related primate groups or domestic animals. Chapter 4 of Cockburn (1963) discusses such problems of the relation of the host and parasite. The author notes that all parasites are descended from free-living ancestors. It is common indeed to find free-living organisms resembling pathogens, for example, *Escherichia coli* and the *Salmonella* genus. Many human infections appear to have come to man as modifications of infections of the primate ancestors or contemporaries. In any case, primitive human groups would be exposed to relatively few infections. With the increase of world population and the opening up of communications, however, the human population became exposed to a greater intensity and variety of infections than ever before. Thus some of our public health measures represent an attempt to redress the balance between human populations and infective organisms.

EXERCISES

1. Imitate 10 tosses of a fair coin by reading the first 10 random sampling numbers from the tables, interpreting an odd digit as a head *H* and an even digit as a tail *T*. The first 10 digits might be 03, 47, 43, 73, 86, and these would be interpreted as *TH*, *TH*, *TH*, *HH*, *TT*; thus there are 5 *H*'s (odds). Draw 20 sets of 10 random sampling numbers from a suitable table. Calculate the mean and variance of these numbers and verify that they approximate to $10 \times \frac{1}{2} = 5$ and $10 \times \frac{1}{2} \times \frac{1}{2} = 2.5$.

2. In a breeding experiment of the form $Aa \times aa$, how many dominant phenotypes would you expect in a litter of five? What would be the variance? Carry out a random sampling experiment that would simulate such a breeding experiment, and compare this with the simulation of coin tossing in Exercise 1.

3. In a pedigree prepared by Dean and Barnes (1955) of a family subject to porphyria, in successive generations there were 5 affected among 10 offspring, 16 among 37, 32 among 59, and 7 among 19. Can this incidence be satisfactorily explained by the hypothesis that the disease is a Mendelian dominant?

4. The probability of the number k of dominants in a sibship of n with parents $Dr \times rr$ is given by the coefficients of t^k in $(\frac{1}{2} + \frac{1}{2}t)^n$ if the parents are first chosen and then their offspring sibship is examined. This is not true if we examine the sibships of size n, including the propositus. This is obviously the case if $n = 1$. We can only find sibships having a single dominant phenotype since, if there is no dominant, there can be no propositus. However, if we take the sibships but do not include the propositus, the number of dominants is given by the terms of $(\frac{1}{2} + \frac{1}{2}t)^{n-1}$.

5. Matings of the form $AaBbCcDdEe \times aabbccddee$ were made by Roberts, Dawson, and Madden (1939). We can record them in a table indicating only the presence of the dominants, A, B, and AB being indicated by the rows, and C, D, E, CD, CE, DE, and CDE being indicated by the columns; thus in the cell at the intersection of the row labeled A and the column labeled DE, we have the number of offspring possessing precisely the dominants A, D, and E.

		Dominants						
		0	1	2	3	4	5	6	7
		I	E	D	DE	C	CE	CD	CDE
0	1	17	13	17	15	16	17	15	15
8	B	19	14	22	16	15	14	24	25
16	A	16	19	15	20	14	19	16	12
24	AB	16	23	17	24	16	20	23	17

How many offspring contain A; how many contain B, ..., how many contain E? Are these numbers consistent with the hypothesis of the form, $\mathscr{P}$ (offspring is an A) = $\frac{1}{2}$?

6. Suppose that the frequencies of the genotypes AA, Aa, and aa are 0.2, 0.6, and 0.2, respectively, in both sexes and that a state of panmixia exists. Construct a table with these numerical values inserted into Table X.3 and verify that the gene frequency of A is 0.5. Verify that the total of the offspring genotypes AA, Aa, and aa are 0.25, 0.50, and 0.25. Verify also that the gene frequency of A in the original population is 0.5 and that the frequencies of the genotypes in the offspring is in accord with the Hardy-Weinberg law.

7. Repeat the computations of the previous exercise with genotype frequencies AA, Aa, and aa equal to 0.2, 0.8, and 0, respectively.

NOTES

Texts on Human Genetics

British Medical Bulletin **25**, (1969) No. 1; Emery, 1970; Gates, 1946; Goodman, 1970; Harris, 1970; Penrose, 1959; Pratt, 1967; Stanbury, Wyngaarden, and Frederickson, 1960; WHO Expert Committee, 1964; WHO Scientific Group, 1964, 1967, 1971.

Genetics Texts

Bailey, 1961; Kempthorne, 1957; Kempthorne (Ed.), 1960; Li, 1955; Mendel, 1965.

Genetics and Clinical Problems

Therapy and Heredity in Diabetes. Aschner and Post, 1956–1957; Steinberg, 1959.
Porphyria. Dean and Barnes, 1959.
Deaf-Mutism. Stevenson and Cheeseman, 1956.
Eugenics. Penrose, 1963; Sutter, 1950.
50 Years of Medical Genetics. Snyder, 1959.

Genetics and Demography

Sutter, 1958; WHO Expert Committee on Human Genetics, 1964; WHO Scientific Group, 1967; WHO Seminar, 1962.

Genetics and Evolution

Crow and Kimura, 1970; Fisher, 1930; Li, 1967; Moran, 1962.

Genetics

Correlation between Relatives. Kempthorne, 1955.
Quantitative Inheritance. Panse, 1940.
Mendelian Ratios. Roberts, Dawson, and Madden, 1939.

Sex Ratio

Lancaster, 1950*d*, Record, 1952; Strandskov, 1942.

CHAPTER XI

Problems of Inference

1. SCIENTIFIC METHOD

We give now a brief and necessarily incomplete description of scientific method, in order to justify and explain some statistical methods of inference. *Scientific method* is defined as the collection of all methods used to obtain a description of the physical world, the general aim being to explain the observations by hypotheses, as few and as simple as possible. The method consists of the accumulation and classification of observations, the construction of general concepts and hypotheses, the refinement of the observations, the testing of the hypotheses, and the construction of further concepts and hypotheses—a circular process, as is well recognized. A science or body of knowledge that can condense the results of many observations into a few general statements or *laws* is said to be highly developed. No "first causes" are sought, and all hypotheses made are tentative; that is, subject to modification after further testing. The theory and history of scientific method is usually described using astronomy and mechanics as examples; for with a few *axioms* (or assumptions or hypotheses) on the laws of motion and the existence of a "force of gravitation," a mathematical model of the solar system can be constructed which enables us to make predictions and to verify them experimentally with a high degree of accuracy. This working out of the assumptions of the theory is the field of applied mathematics. As Bertrand Russell has said, "Mathematics is the art of drawing the necessary conclusions."

We might compare the success of the Newtonian theory of the solar system with the obvious inadequacies of any theory advanced so far to enable us to forecast the future of a simple biological system (e.g., the movement of an amoeba). As opposed to the classical fields of the successful application of mathematics, the biological systems require many features to be entered in the mathematical model as *parameters*—"There are more parameters in an amoeba than in the sun" is a well-known aphorism. But there is an additional difference: in the observations on the motions of the solar system, it is possible (by a multiplication of the observations or refinements of technique) to reduce the importance of the chance variations, thus allowing the investigator to make very accurate observations and predictions.

Example   i. The life table can serve as an example of a mathematical model. Certain aspects of the physical world—namely, the schedule of death rates by age—are abstracted. Then we ask, What will be the average length of life? The commonest age at death? The age distribution of the population when births occur at a constant rate? These all follow by the use of mathematical methods from the initial assumption in the model.

Example   ii. The previous example can be combined with hypotheses on fertility by age to give a description of the growth or declines of populations, the dynamics of population. For many purposes, these simple computations provide a very useful insight into population growth in the real world. Thus the consequences of the low fertility rates in Europe in the 1930s could be deduced. Similarly, the improvements in mortality from the infectious diseases can be shown to lead to certain changes in population size and age distribution. Since there is a tacit assumption in these calculations, that the populations treated are large, random effects tend to be averaged out. This assumption is often realistic; but if the random effects are such as to cause further random effects, the assumption is less realistic (e.g., chains of events can occur as in the progress of an epidemic).

In any case, the random elements in biological and medical applications are sometimes large and cannot always be neglected. The inherent variability of biological systems is one reason for paying attention to random elements, for there are obvious differences in heights and weights and also more subtle differences in the ability of different members of the same species to resist infections; many such varying properties exist. A second reason is that some of the fundamental vital processes are subject to chance effects—that is, some are not completely determined by the initial conditions (e.g., the allele at a locus passing on to a given zygote seems to be "chosen" by a random process, equivalent to the toss of a coin). Such chance (i.e., probabilistic or stochastic) events can also be admitted into the model, but at the cost of more difficult and extensive computations. In any case, to obtain useful (or realistic) results from the model, we need the best estimates possible from the real world. In the construction of a life table, for example, accurate estimates of the mortality by age are required.

Since random effects are common in biological experimentation, the *design of experiments* is concerned with arranging so that the *systematic effects*, in which we are usually interested, can be separated from the *random effects*.

Similarly, random effects must be taken into account when inferences are made from observations. This is the art of *statistical inference*, and examples are presented later.

We mention a special feature of the scientific method, which is often overlooked; *scientific hypotheses are never proved to be correct.* They are retained, always only provisionally, because they summarize existing knowledge and suggest further experiments or observations. The only useful hypotheses are those which summarize existing observations and which can be tested by further observations.

Example   iii. In the rubella example, a hypothesis was made. Rubella is capable of causing congenital defects whenever it attacks the mother at a critical time in the early months of pregnancy; this property is apparent especially in those countries in which infection with rubella is often delayed into adult life. This hypothesis could be tested. There should be a high incidence in geographically isolated countries. This was shown to be the case; consequently, we have more faith or confidence in the hypothesis.

A good elementary account of scientific method has been given by E. B. Wilson (1952). The remarks of the epidemiologist Topley (1942) on "shop pathology" should also be read in a statistical context. Briefly, Topley suggests that much medical research is not testing sufficiently important hypotheses.

2. THE NULL HYPOTHESIS

An experiment or observation can be considered to be relevant to the test of a hypothesis. We must work out the results of such a hypothesis and, in principle at any rate, we must be able to classify all results of the experiment into two classes—those tending to disprove or make less likely the hypothesis, and those favoring it. In order to determine the consequences of a hypothesis, it must be stated exactly. Thus suppose that we have a standard treatment A and a second method of treatment B, and we are interested in testing the hypothesis that B is more effective than A. In general, we would not be interested in the hypothesis that B is inferior to A, for in such a case, we would not be testing B. Our hypothesis to be tested is that A and B are of equal value; this is the *null hypothesis*, usually written H_0. The word "null" is associated with the hypothesis that there is no difference between treatments. Now under H_0, some results will appear to us to be quite probable; other results will appear to us as improbable under the null hypothesis, and these will be called *significant*.

Example. Suppose H_0 specifies that a certain random variable X, observable as a result of an experiment, is standard normal. The most probable value of X is 0, and the values of X have lower probabilities as the distance from the mean becomes larger. Naïvely, we can suggest that large absolute values of X, which appear but rarely, are contrary to the null hypothesis or *significant*. We make precise this notion in Section XI.4.

3. THE ALTERNATIVE HYPOTHESIS

It has often been pointed out that there is no point in carrying out an experiment unless results are possible that suggest either the truth of the null hypothesis or the truth of an *alternative hypothesis* or class of alternative hypotheses. Thus in the example of Section XI.2, the alternative hypothesis might specify that the mean of the normal distribution had been displaced by a distance, μ. This is a simple hypothesis. On the other hand, the alternative hypothesis might specify that the mean was displaced by an amount μ, where the value of μ is not specified but is only said to belong to some class, for example, $\mu > 0$. This is a *composite* alternative hypothesis.

4. THE CRITICAL REGION

It is customary to choose a *level of significance*, often written as α; if the observations fall in a previously determined region, the *critical region*, the observation is said to be *significant*. The critical region A is chosen so that under H_0, the null hypothesis, we have

$$(1) \qquad \mathscr{P}(X \in A | H_0) \equiv \mathscr{P}(X \in A) \leq \alpha.$$

In continuous distributions, the inequality becomes an equality. However, in discrete distributions there may be no subset A, of the space of the points x, such that we have

$$(2) \qquad \sum_{x \in A} p_x = \alpha.$$

In such a case there is controversy about how the critical region should be chosen. If the alternative hypothesis is true, we require the probability

$$(3) \qquad 1 - \beta = \mathscr{P}(X \in A | H_1)$$

to be as large as possible. Here $1 - \beta$ is called the *power* of the test. Therefore, we are obliged to maximize the ratio

$$(4) \qquad \frac{\mathscr{P}(X \in A | H_1)}{\mathscr{P}(X \in A | H_0)}.$$

Maximization requires that we select all those points x for which the ratio $\mathscr{P}(X = x|H_1)/\mathscr{P}(X = x|H_0)$ is high.

Example   i. Let H_0 specify that X is normal with unit variance and variance expectation, and let H_1 specify that X is normal with unit variance and expectation μ, $\mu > 0$. Then for any x we can write

(5)
$$\frac{\mathscr{P}(X = x|H_1)}{\mathscr{P}(X = x|H_0)} = \frac{\exp[-\frac{1}{2}(x - \mu)^2]}{\exp[-\frac{1}{2}x^2]}$$

$$= \exp[\mu x - \tfrac{1}{2}\mu^2],$$

and this *likelihood ratio* becomes larger as x becomes larger. The critical region should contain all the points having large positive x. Therefore, we choose A as the set of points (x_α, ∞), where x_α is such that

(6)
$$\int_{x_\alpha}^{\infty} (2\pi)^{-1/2} \exp(-\tfrac{1}{2}x^2)\,dx = \alpha.$$

Equation 6 is a special case of a *single-tailed* critical region or probability. Sometimes we are interested in departures in either direction; in such cases, the critical region consists of the two tail regions of the forms $(-\infty, -y)$ and (y, ∞). This is a *two-tailed* region. With discrete distributions, the critical region A cannot always be chosen so that the inequality can be used, as we see in Example ii.

Example   ii. Let H_0 specify that X is a binomial variable with parameters p and N, $q = 1 - p$, and let H_1 specify that X is a binomial variable with parameters p_1 and N, $q_1 = 1 - p_1$, $p_1 > p$. Then we have the likelihood ratio, L.R., given by

(7)
$$\text{L.R.} = \frac{\mathscr{P}(X = x|H_1)}{\mathscr{P}(X = x|H_0)} = \frac{\binom{N}{x}p_1{}^x q_1^{N-x}}{\binom{N}{x}p^x q^{N-x}}$$

$$= \frac{(p_1 q)^x q_1{}^N}{(pq_1)^x q^N}.$$

However, this ratio increases as x becomes large; thus A is chosen to contain the points $N, N - 1, \ldots, J$, such that

(8)
$$\sum_{x=J}^{N} \mathscr{P}(X = x) \le \alpha,$$

and J is taken to include as many points as possible. The equality may be impossible to attain.

Example   iii. Suppose that H_0 and H_1 specify Poisson distributions with parameters λ and μ, respectively. The likelihood ratio is

$$(9) \qquad \text{L.R.} = \frac{e^{-\mu}\mu^x/x!}{e^{-\lambda}\lambda^x/x!} = e^{-(\mu-\lambda)}(\mu/\lambda)^x$$

and if $\mu > \lambda$, this is large for large x. Therefore, the critical region is the upper tail of the distribution is the set of integers $J, J+1, \ldots, k, \ldots$, such that J is the least integer for which we can write

$$(10) \qquad \frac{\sum_{x=J}^{\infty} e^{-\lambda}\lambda^x}{x!} \leq \alpha.$$

In all these examples, the choice of the critical region seems to be intuitively correct. Moreover, the general principle due to J. Neyman and E. S. Pearson is of general applicability.

We may note in passing difficulties that arise if the data are discrete and $\alpha - \mathscr{P}(X \in A \,|\, H_0)$ is not small.

5. THE POWER OF A TEST

The results of a test of significance depend on the value of a certain random variable—namely, the test criterion; thus we cannot expect that H_0 will always be *rejected* or said to be significant, when it is not true; an *error of the second kind* is said to occur when the null hypothesis is provisionally accepted, although it is false. In any test at a given level α of significance, the probability of errors of the second kind β must be minimal; alternatively, we require that $1 - \beta$ be large, where β is defined as in (3) of Section XI.4. We refer to $1 - \beta$ as the *power of the test*.

An *error of the first kind* is said to occur when a true null hypothesis is falsely rejected. The probability of an error of the first kind is equal to the significance level if the test criterion is a "continuous" random variable. This kind of error can be controlled by selecting a small significance level, α. However, if α is chosen too small, the power of the test will also be small.

Example.   Let H_0 and H_1 specify normal distributions having unit variances but with expectations zero and μ, respectively, where $\mu > 0$. Let us suppose that we use the following test function:

$$(1) \qquad Y = N^{-1/2} \sum_{1}^{N} X_k,$$

which, under H_0, is normally distributed and has zero expectation and unit variance. Under H_1, the expectation of Y, $\mathscr{E}_1 Y$ is

$$(2) \quad \mathscr{E}_1 Y = \mathscr{E}_1 (N^{-1/2} \sum X_k) = N^{-1/2} \mathscr{E}_1 \sum X_k$$
$$= N^{-1/2} \sum \mathscr{E}_1 X_k = N^{-1/2} N\mu = N^{1/2}\mu.$$

Let y_α be such that $\mathscr{P}(Y > y_\alpha) = \alpha$. Thus y_α is the α-point of the distribution of Y. Now if $\mathscr{E}_1 Y$ were equal to y_α, Y would exceed y_α in 50% of cases or with probability 0.50, since the distribution of Y is symmetric about its mean. Therefore, if we require a power of at least 50%, we shall have to ensure that $N^{1/2}\mu > y_\alpha$. If $\alpha = 0.05$, $y_\alpha = 1.645$; therefore, $N^{1/2}\mu > 1.645$ or $N > (1.645)^2/\mu^2 = 2.706/\mu^2$, approximately. For $\mu = 2, 1.5, 1.0, 0.5, 0.2, 0.1$ standard deviations, N must be not less than 1, 2, 3, 11, 68, and 271, respectively. Thus, to detect small differences or small shifts in the mean, rather large sample sizes N will be required.

6. MULTIPLE COMPARISONS

It is assumed in the theory of significance tests that a single test criterion has been used. If we carried out 20 independent tests of a hypothesis at the 5% level, we would, on an average, reject the null hypothesis once. Similarly, if we carried out k independent tests of a true null hypothesis at the α level of significance, we would accept the null hypothesis in a proportion $(1 - \alpha)^k$ of tests. We would therefore falsely reject the null hypothesis in a proportion $1 - (1 - \alpha)^k$ of trials. It is evident that if $k = 2$, the rejection rate would be $1 - (1.05)^2 = 0.10 - 0.0025 = 0.0975$; if $k = 3$, the rejection rate would be 0.1425, and so on. Therefore, if we wish to avoid rejection rates of the null hypothesis grossly in excess of the stated level of significance, we must modify the tests. The theory of multiple comparisons is still in a controversial state, but some satisfactory solutions can be found in texts of mathematical statistics.

Two general conclusions are worthy of note. First, for any body of observations, the variables to be tested should be few in number and should be distinguished before the observations are made; otherwise, it can be shown that the power of individual tests of significance will be reduced. Second, care should be taken to interpret correctly the following situation. A new treatment B is said to be superior to a standard treatment A. Suppose that 100 observers all test the hypothesis that A and B are equally effective. Four of the observers report their conclusions to the clinical trial—namely, that the null hypothesis has been rejected and that B is superior to A. The 96 other observers do not report their "negative results." Under such conditions, later workers may be tempted to comment that the original statement that B is superior to A is true and that this important finding has been confirmed by the four observers.

7. ESTIMATION

We have already computed age-specific death rates, means, and other measurements. As descriptive measures of the members of a sample, these have an evident meaning. However, it may be asked whether each of these is the best estimate of the parameters in the respective distributions. For example, if we measure the mean height of a properly chosen sample, is it the best estimate of the mean of the population sampled? In all the common distributions (given previously), it appears that this intuitive idea is satisfied. In the theory of estimation, the best estimate is usually the one having the least variance and having an expected value equal to the expectation in the theoretical population or in an existent population being sampled; these requirements are *maximum precision*, or repeatability, and *unbiasedness*.

It is customary to give estimates of a parameter written with a "hat"; for example, $\hat{p}$ is an estimate of the parameter p.

Example i. Let an event occur with probability p at each trial. Suppose that N trials have been made and that the event has occurred m times; then p is estimated by

$$(1) \qquad \hat{p} = \frac{m}{N},$$

and var $\hat{p} = $ var $m/N^2 = Npq/N^2 = pq/N = \hat{p}\hat{q}/N$, approximately. Usually the last approximation is adequate, but if either Np or Nq is small, say less than 5, special devices will have to be adopted. The standard error of the estimate of a proportion is thus $\sqrt{(pq/N)}$ or approximately $\sqrt{(\hat{p}\hat{q}/N)}$.

Example ii. In the Poisson distribution, the best estimate of the expectation λ is

$$(2) \qquad \hat{\lambda} = m,$$

where m is the number observed. Since variance of the Poisson variable is λ, the variance of $\hat{\lambda}$ is λ; if λ is not small, we can write

$$(3) \qquad \text{var } \hat{\lambda} = \hat{\lambda}, \text{ approximately.}$$

Example iii. In the normal distribution with mean μ and variance, σ^2, the estimates from a sample of N independent observations are

$$(4) \qquad \hat{\mu} = \frac{\sum X_i}{N},$$

$$(5) \qquad \hat{\sigma}^2 = \frac{\sum (X_i - \overline{X})^2}{N - 1},$$

having variances σ^2/N, and $2\sigma^4/N$. If the sample size N is not too small, σ^2 and σ^4 can be replaced by $\hat{\sigma}^2$ and $\hat{\sigma}^4$, respectively.

8. ESTIMATION AND TESTS OF SIGNIFICANCE

It is often said that significance tests are not of importance but that estimation is. This is often true in agricultural experiments. However, if treatment B is not shown by a test to be significantly better than treatment A, we will rarely be interested in estimating the value of some parameter, such as the case fatality rate.

In tests of independence between two variables by means of a contingency table, we may be interested only in testing the null hypothesis and, if it is rejected, we will accept provisionally the alternative hypothesis that there is a relation between the variables. New experiments or observations are then planned to determine which one of them is dependent on the other, and why.

It is necessary to avoid the statement that, since the null hypothesis has been rejected at the level α of significance, the probability of the null hypothesis being true is less than α.

CHAPTER XII

Further Distribution Theory

1. RANDOM VARIABLES

Chance events, such as the toss of a coin, are a matter of common experience. We wish to formalize the description of such chance events. A *variable X*, which can take values x as the result of an experiment, is called a *random variable*. It is usually convenient to assume that the values x are real numbers. Thus if X is to represent the random variable for tosses of a coin, it is convenient to say that $X = 1$ when the toss results in a head, and $X = 0$ when the toss results in a tail. We wish to include in the mathematical model of coin tossing the notion that $X = 1$ can be expected to occur on about half the occasions, for there is a certain symmetry in a coin. In the model, we therefore write

$$(1) \qquad \mathscr{P}(X = 1) = \tfrac{1}{2}, \qquad \mathscr{P}(X = 0) = \tfrac{1}{2},$$

which is to be read: "the probability that $X = 1$ is $\tfrac{1}{2}$; the probability that $X = 0$ is $\tfrac{1}{2}$." No other outcome or event is possible, and thus we write

$$\mathscr{P}(X = x) = 0 \qquad \text{if} \quad x \neq 1 \qquad \text{and} \qquad x \neq 0,$$

or

$$\mathscr{P}(X = x) = 0 \qquad \text{for} \quad \text{all other } x.$$

The throwing of a die is also familiar. Here the mathematical model, suggested by the notion that we have no reason to expect one face rather than another, is that

$$(2) \qquad \mathscr{P}(X = k) = \tfrac{1}{6}, \qquad k = 1, 2, \ldots, 6.$$

This is to be interpreted as "the probability that X should take any given value k for any k is $\tfrac{1}{6}$."

At one time, it was customary for statisticians to toss dice or coins in the test of various statistical hypotheses or in the performance of various statistical tests; later it was found more convenient to construct tables of *random sampling numbers*. These are tables of digits arranged in a manner convenient for use and such that if we inspect without foreknowledge the digit at any particular position, the "probability" that it is any particular digit is $\frac{1}{10}$. In common language, it would be a fair wager to pay \$1 and receive \$10 if the number turned out to be the number specified, say 6. Moreover, given the numbers at any specified sites, the probability at any other site does not change. A sequence of five numbers (e.g., 51687) from such a table can be interpreted as a decimal (e.g., 0.51687) on the unit interval [0, 1], zero to unity. (Intervals are written [a, b] if they include both end points, (a, b] if b is included, [a, b) if a is included, and (a, b) if neither a nor b is included.) The lengths of (a, b), (a, b] and [a, b] are the same, and in most cases of practical interest the intervals can be thought of as identical.

The properties of the random sampling numbers are such that, if we choose any interval, 0 to y, a proportion y of the numbers drawn will lie in this interval. Similarly, a proportion $y_2 - y_1$ will fall in the interval $(y_1, y_2]$ where we include y_2 but not y_1 in the interval. Much research has gone into making precise the notion of randomness. The difficulty is that *randomness* is one of the fundamental notions in probability, just as "line" is in geometry. We must assume the existence of a random variable taking values on the unit interval such that if we chose any interval of nonzero length, $(y_1, y_2]$, say, with $y_1 < y_2$, then $\mathscr{P}(X \in (y_1, y_2]) = y_2 - y_1$. There are various ways of producing random numbers—or, better *pseudorandom numbers*—on high-speed computers, and extensive tables have been published. We have chosen for our set the first ten thousand digits of π, which we give as Appendix A.5.

We now show how the experiment of the tossing of a true coin can be imitated. We assign the numbers 0.000...00 to 0.499...99 to the result "head" and the numbers 0.500...00 to 0.999...99 to the result "tail," where we have chosen the length of the decimal to be any arbitrary number, say six decimal places. We now draw a random sampling number. If it is 0.419674, we interpret the result as a head. If it is 0.883764, we interpret the result as a tail, and so on. More complicated cases could be treated. For example, let

$$(3) \qquad \mathscr{P}(X = k) = p_k, \qquad k = 1, 2, \ldots, m, \qquad p_k > 0, \qquad \sum p_k = 1.$$

If the random number Z fell in the interval $[0, p_1)$—that is, if $0 \leq Z < p_1$ —we would say that the event $X = 1$ had been realized; if $p_1 \leq Z < p_1 + p_2$, $X = 2$ had been realized, ..., finally, if $p_1 + p_2 + \cdots + p_{m-1} \leq Z < 1$, $X = m$ had been realized. By an extension of this procedure, all random experiments in the model could be related to the fundamental random variable Z, taking values on the unit interval, $0 \leq z < 1$ to [0, 1). The reference to dice and coins makes probability theory seem rather artificial, but analogous cases appear in genetics, as we have seen in Chapter X.

2. CONDITIONAL PROBABILITY

A common definition of *conditional probability* runs as follows. If A and B are two events and $\mathscr{P}(B) > 0$, the conditional probability of A, given B (or the probability of A conditional on B), written $\mathscr{P}(A|B)$, is defined by

$$(1) \qquad \mathscr{P}(A|B) = \frac{\mathscr{P}(AB)}{\mathscr{P}(B)}.$$

Example. If a true die is thrown, the probability of A, the event "1," conditional on B, "the number of points is not greater than 2," is $\frac{1}{2}$, since $\mathscr{P}(AB) = \mathscr{P}(A) = \frac{1}{6}$. $\mathscr{P}(B) = \frac{1}{3}$. Thus $\mathscr{P}(A|B) = \mathscr{P}(AB)/\mathscr{P}(B) = \frac{1}{6}/\frac{1}{3} = \frac{1}{2}$. This accords with intuition, for if B has occurred, the throw is either "1" or "2," and we have no reason to assign different probabilities to them, since we are working with a true die. This common usage can be regarded as an abbreviation for the following definition:

If X and Y are random variables, the probability of $X \in A$, conditional on $Y \in B$, where A and B are sets, is defined by

$$(2) \qquad \mathscr{P}(X \in A | Y \in B) = \frac{\mathscr{P}(X \in A, Y \in B)}{\mathscr{P}(Y \in B)}.$$

It is easily proved that conditional probabilities so defined have the same kind of properties as ordinary or *unconditional* probabilities. In particular, if A_1, A_2, ..., A_m are mutually exclusive and exhaustive sets, and if $\mathscr{P}(Y \in B) \neq 0$, we have

$$(3) \qquad \sum_{i=1}^{m} \mathscr{P}(X \in A_i | Y \in B) = 1.$$

Conditional probabilities are very common in applied work. Thus we may be interested in the probability of a cure of a disease by certain treatments, conditional on the patient being a male, aged 50 to 54 years, ...

Independence is often defined in terms of conditional probability. Thus X is independent of Y if and only if

$$(4) \qquad \mathscr{P}(X \in A) = \mathscr{P}(X \in A | Y \in B)$$

for every set A and every set B.

Note that (4) implies that

(5)
$$\mathscr{P}(X \in A) = \frac{\mathscr{P}(X \in A, Y \in B)}{\mathscr{P}(Y \in B)}$$

or

(6)
$$\mathscr{P}(X \in A, Y \in B) = \mathscr{P}(X \in A)\mathscr{P}(Y \in B).$$

3. THE POISSON DISTRIBUTION

The Poisson distribution occurs frequently in practical problems, particularly in the study of counting experiments (see Section I.1).

A random variable X is said to have the *Poisson distribution* or to be a *Poisson variable* if it has a frequency given by

(1)
$$\mathscr{P}(X = x) = \frac{\exp(-\lambda)\lambda^x}{x!} \equiv p_x, \text{ say,}$$

where $\lambda > 0$ and $x = 0,\ 1,\ 2,\ \ldots.$ This properly defines a probability distribution, since each p_x is nonnegative and $\sum p_x = 1$ for

(2)
$$\sum_{x=0}^{\infty} p_x = \sum_{0}^{\infty} \frac{\exp(-\lambda)\lambda^x}{x!} = \exp(-\lambda) \sum_{0}^{\infty} \frac{\lambda^x}{x!} = \exp(-\lambda)\exp(\lambda) = 1.$$

Because $x/x! = 1/(x-1)!$, $x(x-1)/x! = 1/(x-2)!$ and since, generally, $x^{(r)}/x! = 1/(x-r)!$, the factorial moments are readily computed:

(3)
$$\sum_{0}^{\infty} xp_x = \sum_{1}^{\infty} \frac{\exp(-\lambda)\lambda^x x}{x!} = \lambda \exp(-\lambda) \sum_{1}^{\infty} \frac{\lambda^{x-1}}{(x-1)!}$$

$$= \lambda \exp(-\lambda) \sum_{0}^{\infty} \frac{\lambda^s}{s!} \qquad s = x - 1$$

$$= \lambda \exp(-\lambda)\exp(\lambda) = \lambda$$

and

(4)
$$\sum_{0}^{\infty} x(x-1)p_x = \sum_{2}^{\infty} \frac{\exp(-\lambda)\lambda^x}{(x-2)!} = \exp(-\lambda)\lambda^2 \sum_{0}^{\infty} \frac{\lambda^s}{s!}$$

$$= \lambda^2,$$

as in the computation of (3).

The mean of the Poisson distribution is thus λ by (3). The variance is also equal to λ, the *parameter of the Poisson distribution*, for

(5) $\mathscr{E}X^2 = \mathscr{E}[X(X-1) + X] = \mathscr{E}[X(X-1)] + \mathscr{E}X = \lambda^2 + \lambda$

(6) $\operatorname{var} X = \mathscr{E}X^2 - \lambda^2 = \lambda^2 + \lambda - \lambda^2 = \lambda,$

which is a special case of the formula $\operatorname{var} X = \mathscr{E}X^2 - [\mathscr{E}X]^2.$

We can write the probability-generating function of the Poisson distribution as

(7) $$P(t) = \sum t^x p_x$$

$$= \exp(-\lambda) + \frac{t \exp(-\lambda)\lambda}{1!} + \frac{t^2 \exp(-\lambda)\lambda^2}{2!} + \cdots$$

$$= \exp(-\lambda)\left[1 + \frac{t\lambda}{1!} + \frac{t^2\lambda^2}{2!} + \cdots\right]$$

$$= \exp(-\lambda + t\lambda).$$

The Poisson distribution arises as a limit when N, the index of the binomial distribution, becomes infinite and p becomes small in such a way that $Np \to \lambda$. A *stochastic process* can be defined as the set of states of a system that is developing in time as a result of random events (e.g., the number of infants born in a city from the beginning of a certain year). Examples are given, following some definitions.

The Poisson distribution can be obtained by considering a *stochastic process* with the following properties:

1. *Stationarity.* The probability of the occurrence of k events in the time interval T to $T + t$ is independent of T.

2. *Absence of aftereffects.* The probability of k events in the time interval T to $T + t$ is independent of the past history of the process.

3. *Orderliness or lack of clustering.* It is assumed that in a short interval of time, the occurrence of more than one event is almost impossible.

The Poisson distribution, given these three properties of the process, is deduced in books on probability theory or statistics.

Example i. Red blood cell counts conform remarkably well to the Poisson distribution if the mean count per small square is less than 4. A good example of such a set of counts appeared in Table I.4. At higher mean counts, the observed variance becomes markedly less than the expected.

Example ii. A radioactive source with a half-life that is not overly small acts like a Poisson process. Counts in successive units of time behave like independently distributed Poisson variables all having the same parameter.

Example iii. The numbers of persons in a given age group dying from a somewhat rare disease can often be regarded as Poisson variables having the parameter in successive years proportional to the numbers at risk. We cite without proof three theorems on the Poisson distribution.

Theorem 1.   *The sum of two mutually independent Poisson variables is again a Poisson variable, having parameter equal to the sum of the two parameters.*

Theorem 2.   *The sum of n mutually independent Poisson variables is Poisson, having parameter equal to the sum of the parameters.*

Theorem 3.   *Let $X_1, X_2, \ldots, X_n$ be independently distributed Poisson variables with parameters $\lambda p_1, \lambda p_2, \ldots, \lambda p_n$, such that $\sum p_i = 1$; then the distribution of $X_1, X_2, \ldots, X_n$ conditional on $S = X_1 + X_2 + \cdots + X_n = s$ is independent of the value of λ.*

Theorem 3 is of importance in the justification for the method of statistical control of counting experiments, introduced in Chapter XV, and it can also be used to give a proof of the distribution of χ^2.

Corollary 3.1.   *If the parameters of the theorem are equal, $p_k = n^{-1}$ for $k = 1, 2, \ldots, n$, and the conditional probability of $X_1, X_2, \ldots, X_n$ given $X_1 + X_2 + \cdots + X_n = S = s$ is*

$$(8) \qquad \mathscr{P}(X_1 = x_1, X_2 = x_2, \ldots, X_n = x_n | S = s) = \frac{s!\, n^{-s}}{\prod_{i=1}^{n} x_i!},$$

the general term of the symmetric multinomial.

4. THE MULTINOMIAL DISTRIBUTION

Lemma   *In the expansion of $(u_1 + u_2 + \cdots + u_m)^N$, the general term is of the form*

$$(1) \qquad \frac{N!}{N_1!\, N_2!\cdots N_m!}\, u_1^{N_1} u_2^{N_2} \cdots u_m^{N_m}, \qquad N_1 + N_2 + \cdots + N_m = N.$$

Proof.   We know this is true for N when $m = 2$ because in Section IV.6, using different notation, we proved that the general term is

$$\frac{N!}{N_1!\, N_2!}\, u_1^{N_1} u_2^{N_2}, \qquad N_1 + N_2 = N.$$

Let us suppose that the lemma is true for $k = m - 1$ and for every N; then the general term in the expansion of $(u_1 + u_2 + \cdots + u_{m-1})^{N-N_m}$ is

$$(2) \qquad \frac{(N - N_m)!}{N_1!\, N_2!\cdots N_{m-1}!}\, u_1^{N_1} u_2^{N_2} \cdots u_{m-1}^{N_{m-1}},$$

The general term in $(u_1 + u_2 + \cdots + u_m)^N$ is also the general term in $([u_1 + u_2 + \cdots + u_{m-1}] + u_m)^N$ or the general term in

(3)
$$\frac{N!}{N_m!(N-N_m)!} u_m{}^{N_m}[u_1 + u_2 + \cdots + u_{m-1}]^{N-N_m}.$$

Thus it is equal to

(4)
$$\frac{N!}{N_m!(N-N_m)!} u_m{}^{N_m} \frac{(N-N_m)!}{N_1! N_2! \cdots N_{m-1}!} u_1{}^{N_1} u_2{}^{N_2} \cdots u_{m-1}^{N_{m-1}}$$

by (2), and this is after cancellation of $(N-N_m)!$ yields (1).

If $Z_1, Z_2, \ldots, Z_m$ take the values $N_1, N_2, \ldots, N_m$ having probabilities equal to the coefficient of $t_1{}^{N_1} t_2{}^{N_2} \cdots t_m{}^{N_m}$, $N_1 + N_2 + \cdots + N_m = N$, in $(p_1 t_1 + p_2 t_2 + \cdots + p_m t_m)^N$, $p_1 + p_2 + \cdots + p_m = 1$, the Z's are said to have the joint *multinomial distribution* with index N and cell probabilities $p_1, p_2, \ldots, p_m$. It is obvious that $(p_1 t_1 + p_2 t_2 + \cdots + p_m t_m)^N$ is the probability-generating function of $Z_1, Z_2, \ldots, Z_m$.

5. THE DISTRIBUTION OF χ^2

Let X be a standard normal variable. Then X^2 is said to have the *distribution* of χ^2 with 1 *degree of freedom*, written shortly 1 d.f.

Let $X_1, X_2, \ldots, X_m$ be mutually independent, standard normal variables and, consequently, let $X_1{}^2, X_2{}^2, \ldots, X_m{}^2$ be m variables having the distribution of χ^2, each distributed with 1 degree of freedom. Then $X_1{}^2 + X_2{}^2 + \cdots + X_m{}^2$ is said to have the distribution of χ^2, having m degrees of freedom. Any variable having the same distribution is also said to have the distribution of χ^2 having m degrees of freedom.

Let us write $Z = X_1{}^2 + X_2{}^2 + \cdots + X_m{}^2$; then we state without proof

(1)
$$\mathscr{P}(Z \le z) = 2^{-m/2}\left[\Gamma\left(\frac{m}{2}\right)\right]^{-1} \int_0^z y^{m/2-1} e^{-y/2} \, dy,$$

and the density function of Z is given by

(2)
$$f(z) = 2^{-m/2}\left[\Gamma\left(\frac{m}{2}\right)\right]^{-1} z^{m/2-1} e^{-z/2},$$

where $\Gamma(a)$ is the Γ-function, $\Gamma(a) = (a-1)!$ if a is a positive integer. The Γ-function has some of the properties of a factorial; for example, $\Gamma(a+1) = a\Gamma(a)$. The distribution of χ^2 is extensively treated in Lancaster (1969).

From the present point of view, there are some theorems important for applications, which we state without proof.

Theorem 1. *If Z_1 has he distribution of χ^2 with m d.f. and Z_2 has the distribution of χ^2 with n d.f., and if Z_1 is independent of Z_2, then $Z_1 + Z_2$ has the distribution of χ^2 with $m + n$ d.f.*

Theorem 2. *If Y is a binomial variable with probability-generating function* $(pt + q)^N$, *the random variable,*

$$X = (Y - Np)/\sqrt{(Npq)}$$

is approximately normal if N, Np, and Nq are all sufficiently large; X^2 is approximately distributed as χ^2 with 1 d.f.

Corollary 1. *We have*

(4)
$$\frac{(Y - Np)^2}{Npq} = \frac{(Y - Np)^2}{Np} + \frac{(N - Y - Nq)^2}{Nq} ;$$

in the binomial distribution

(5)
$$X^2 = \sum \frac{(observed - expected)^2}{expected},$$

where summation is over the two classes and is approximately distributed as χ^2 with 1 d.f.

Theorem 3. *In the multinomial distribution with probability-generating function* $(t_1 p_1 + t_2 p_2 + \cdots + t_n p_n)^N$ *for the cell frequencies N_j, we have*

(6)
$$X^2 = \sum_{j=1}^{n} \frac{(N_j - Np_j)^2}{Np_j},$$

which is distributed approximately as χ^2 with $n - 1$ degrees of freedom.

Remark. This is the famous χ^2-variable of K. Pearson (1900). Equation 6 is a generalization of (4) and (5). It is now customary to write X^2 in place of χ^2 for the empirically observed and calculated values.

Theorem 4. *If the p's in Theorem 5.3 are not given by hypothesis but depend on certain parameters, which must be estimated from the data by setting linear forms equal to zero, the degrees of freedom must be reduced by the number of linear forms set equal to zero.*

Remark. Theorem 5.4 states in an informal manner the modifications in the application of the Pearson χ^2 introduced by R. A. Fisher.

(i) The Symmetrical Multinomial

A set $Y_1, Y_2, \ldots, Y_n$ of blood counts exists on groups of squares in the hemocytometer chamber, the area and hence the expected numbers being the same for each group of squares. Conditional on the total $S = Y_1 + Y_2 + \cdots + Y_n$, the distribution of the Y's is the multinomial with probability-generating function

$$(t_1 n^{-1} + t_2 n^{-1} + \cdots + t_n n^{-1})^N.$$

$$(7) \qquad X^2 = \sum \frac{(Y_j - Np_j)^2}{Np_j} = \frac{n \sum (Y_j - N/n)^2}{N}.$$

Serial Number	Observed Counts, O	Expected Number, E	$O - E$	$(O - E)^2/E$
1	39	36	3	0.2500
2	28	36	-8	1.7778
3	43	36	7	1.3611
4	36	36	0	0
5	34	36	-2	0.1111
Totals	180	180	0	3.5000

In the foregoing tabulation, $p_j = n^{-1} = \frac{1}{5}$; $N = 180$; the expected values are $Np_j = 180 \times \frac{1}{5} = 36$; $\chi^2 = 3.50$ with $(5 - 1) = 4$ d.f. The 5% significance point of χ^2 with 4 d.f. is 9.488. The 50% point of χ^2 is 3.357; therefore, the observed count yields a moderate value of X^2.

An alternative computation can be carried out by noting that (7) can be put in the following forms:

$$(8) \qquad X^2 = \frac{n \sum (Y_j - \bar{Y})^2}{N} = \frac{n(\sum Y_j^2 - \bar{Y} \sum Y)}{N}.$$

Here $\sum Y_j^2 = 39^2 + 28^2 + 43^2 + 36^2 + 34^2 = 1521 + 784 + 1849 + 1296 + 1156 = 6606$, $\bar{Y} \sum Y = 36 \times 180 = 6480$, and $X^2 = 5(6606 - 6480)/180 = 5 \times 126/180 = 630/180 = 3.50$.

(ii) The Poisson Distribution

The red cells are counted over the $400 = N$ small squares of the hemocytometer. If the unknown density of cells in the fluid is such that the expected number on any square is λ, and if the Poisson hypothesis holds, the expected numbers are given by $Np_k = N \exp(-\lambda)\lambda^k/k!$ But if λ is not known it is estimated by setting

$$(9) \qquad N\hat{\lambda} = \sum_k k a_k,$$

where a_k is the number of squares containing precisely k cells. Since $\sum k \exp(-\hat{\lambda})\hat{\lambda}^k/k! = \hat{\lambda}$, $\sum_k (a_k - N\hat{p}_k)k = 0$, thus the estimation procedure sets the linear form $\sum k\hat{p}_k^{1/2}(a_k - N\hat{p}_k)/(N\hat{p}_k)^{1/2}$ in the variables $(a_k - N\hat{p}_k)/(N\hat{p}_k)^{1/2}$ equal to zero. The degrees of freedom are thereby reduced by one.

The counts of Table I.4 can be tested now for goodness of fit, by

Table XII.1

A TEST OF THE GOODNESS OF FIT OF THE POISSON DISTRIBUTION TO AN
OBSERVED RED CELL COUNT BY MEANS OF χ^2

Number of Cells on Square[a]	Observed Frequency, O	Expected Frequency, E	$O - E$	Contribution[b] to χ^2
0	11	10.740	0.260	0.006
1	36	38.851	−2.851	0.209
2	76	70.273	5.727	0.467
3	80	84.737	−4.737	0.265
4	74	76.634	−2.634	0.091
5	58	55.445	2.555	0.118
6	38	33.429	4.571	0.625
7	17	17.275	−0.275	0.004
8	6	7.812	−1.812	0.420
9	3	3.140⎫	−0.804	0.135
10	0	1.136⎬ 4.804		
11	1	0.528⎭		
Total	400	400.000	0.000	2.340

[a] Mean number of cells per square = 3.6175 variance = 3.5308.
[b] X^2 for 8 d.f. = 2.340, $P = 0.97$.

forming Table XII.1, in which there are 10 classes. Since the observed
total and the expected total of the counts are made to coincide, 1 d.f. is
lost. The mean is estimated from the data. There are thus $10 - 2 = 8$ d.f.

(iii)   The Binomial Distribution

In a mating of the form $AaBb \times aabb$, there were 187 offspring having
two dominants, 340 having one dominant, and 174 having no dominant gene.
With the hypothesis that the distribution is a sample from a distribution with
generating function, $N(pt + q)^2$, the expected numbers are $\frac{1}{4}N$, $\frac{1}{2}N$, and $\frac{1}{4}N$.

Number of Dominants	Observed Frequency, O	Expected Frequency, E	$O - E$	Contribution to χ^2
2	187	175.25	11.75	0.7878
0	340	350.50	−10.50	0.3146
1	174	175.25	−1.25	0.0089
Total	701	701	0	1.1113

In the foregoing tabulation, the parameter $p = \frac{1}{2}$ is given. $X^2 = 1.11$ with 2 d.f.—a very good fit, since more than 50% of samples would be expected to yield a larger X^2, than that indicated. However, $\hat{p}$ can be estimated from the data. The expected number of dominants per mating is np, and there are N matings; thus the expected number in all is Nnp. We estimate p by writing $Nn\hat{p}$ = observed number of dominant genes.

$$N = 701, \qquad n = 2.$$

$$701 \times 2\hat{p} = 2 \times 187 + 1 \times 340 + 0 \times 174 = 714.$$

$$\hat{p} = \frac{714}{1402} = 0.507.$$

The expected numbers now $N\hat{p}^2 = 180.191$, $N2\hat{p}\hat{q} = 350.431$, and $N\hat{q}^2 = 170.377$. The X^2 is now $6.809^2/180.191 + 10.431^2/350.431 + 3.623^2/170.377 = 0.2573 + 0.3105 + 0.0770 = 0.6448$. This value of X^2 is distributed approximately as χ^2 with 1 d.f.

(iv) The Normal Distribution

For an empirical distribution of the blood hemoglobin values, expected frequencies have been computed from tables of the normal distribution in such a way that the expected frequencies and the observed frequencies have the same mean and the same variance.

Hemoglobin (g/100 ml blood)	Observed, O	Expected, E	$O - E$	Contribution to X^2, $(O - E)^2/E$
<6.75	20	19	+1	0.053
6.75–7.75	48	47	+1	0.021
7.75–8.75	113	105	+8	0.610
8.75–9.75	151	171	−20	2.339
9.75–10.75	210	201	+9	0.403
10.75–11.75	169	169	0	0.000
11.75–12.75	102	103	−1	0.010
12.75–13.75	50	45	+5	0.556
13.75–14.75	15	18	−3	0.500
	878	878	0	4.492

In the foregoing tabulation $X^2 = 4.492$ for 6 $(= 9 - 3)$d.f, and P is approximately 0.6. This value of X^2 would be exceeded by chance in about 60% of such tests. The fit of expected to the observed frequencies is satisfactory. It is customary to carry rather more significant figures than are given in the expected values listed here.

(v) Contingency Tables

The probability of an observation falling in the ith row is estimated by $\hat{p}_{i.} = a_{i.}/N$, where $a_{i.}$ observations have fallen into the ith row. Similarly, the probability of an observation falling into the jth column is estimated by $\hat{p}_{.j} = a_{.j}/N$, where N is the total numbers of observations, and $\Sigma a_{i.} = N = \Sigma a_{.j}$. The hypothesis usually of most interest to us is that of independence. The probability of observation falling into the ith row and that jth column is then

$$(9) \qquad \hat{p}_{ij} = \hat{p}_{i.}\,\hat{p}_{.j}$$

and the expected numbers are

$$(10) \qquad \mathscr{E}a_{ij} = N\hat{p}_{ij} = N\hat{p}_{i.}\hat{p}_{.j} = \frac{a_{i.}\,a_{.j}}{N}$$

The value of X^2 can be computed in the usual way by Σ(observed —expected)^2/(expected). The number of degrees of freedom is now $(r - 1)(c - 1)$, where r and c are the numbers of rows and columns, respectively. There are, indeed, rc classes; but one linear restriction is imposed by Σ(observed $-$ expected) $= 0$, $r - 1$ are imposed by the estimations $\hat{p}_{i.} = a_{i.}/N$, and $c - 1$ by the estimations $\hat{p}_{.j} = a_{.j}/N$. We give now an example of the computation of X^2 in a 2×5 contingency table describing the duration of studies of nurses.

| | Years | | | | | |
	0–1	1–2	2–3	3–4	4+	Totals
Observed,[a] O	516	107	105	93	115	936
Expected, E	682.587	85.973	64.827	49.573	53.040	
$O - E$	-166.587	21.027	40.173	43.427	61.960	
$(O - E)^2/E$	40.660	5.143	24.895	38.043	72.380	
Observed, O	1453	141	82	50	38	1,764
Expected, E	1,286.413	162.027	122.173	93.427	99.960	
$O - E$	166.587	-21.027	-40.173	-43.427	-61.960	
$(O - E)^2/E$	21.573	2.729	13.210	20.186	38.406	
Total	1,969	248	187	143	153	2,700

[a] Number of Mantoux reactors. $X^2 = 277.225$ for 4 d.f.

(vi) The Fourfold Table

In the fourfold table, which is a 2×2 contingency table, X^2 can be computed as in the example just given. The formula can also be written

$$(11) \qquad X^2 = \frac{N(a_{11}a_{22} - a_{12}a_{21})^2}{a_{1.}a_{2.}a_{.1}a_{.2}}.$$

This can be represented as the square of the difference between two proportions divided by its standard error, as well; namely

(12)
$$X = \frac{(a_{11}/a_1. - a_{21}/a_2.)}{\sqrt{(\hat{p}\hat{q}/a_1. + \hat{p}\hat{q}/a_2.)}}.$$

where $\hat{p} = 1 - \hat{q} = a_{.1}/N$.

6. CONTINGENCY TABLES

Comparisons of percentages, homogeneity of distributions, or independence of random variables can be tested by the application of the χ^2 test to contingency tables.

We now describe the 2×2 or the *fourfold table*, which appears very frequently in medical statistical work, and the sampling models under which it can arise. The theory is readily generalized to tables of r rows and c columns.

Model 1. *Unrestricted bivariate sampling.* We suppose that there is a set of probabilities as already defined and that N independent observations are made, where $\mathscr{P}(X = i, Y = j) = p_{ij}$ at each observation, the set of p_{ij} being fixed. We consider random variables A_{ij}, the numbers of times the pair of values (i, j) of X and Y has occurred. The variables $A_{11}, A_{12}, A_{21}, A_{22}$ are jointly distributed in the multinomial distribution from the hypotheses made with parameters p_{ij}. The actual values taken by the random variables A_{11}, A_{12}, A_{21}, and A_{22} can be displayed in either of the following forms:

a	b	$a + b$	a_{11}	a_{12}	$a_{1.}$
c	d	$c + d$	a_{21}	a_{22}	$a_{2.}$
$a + c$	$b + d$	$a + b + c + d = N$	$a_{.1}$	$a_{.2}$	$a_{..} = N$

Model 2. *The comparative trial.* In this model, the rows or the columns, but not both, are fixed by the design of the experiment. Without loss of generality, let $a_{1.}$ be chosen in the first row and $a_{2.}$ in the second row. It is supposed now that the probability of an observation falling into the first column is p and that successive observations are independent:

(1)
$$\mathscr{P}(a_{11}|a_{1.}, p) = \frac{a_{1.}!}{a_{11}! \, a_{12}!} p^{a_{11}} q^{a_{12}}, \qquad p + q = 1.$$

(2)
$$\mathscr{P}(a_{21}|a_{2.}, p) = \frac{a_{2.}!}{a_{21}! \, a_{22}!} p^{a_{21}} q^{a_{22}}.$$

Hypothesis H_0 specifies that the observed number a_{11} and a_{21} are mutually independent; thus we have

(3) $$\mathscr{P}(a_{11}, a_{21} | a_{1.}, a_{2.}, p) = \frac{a_{1.}! \, a_{2.}! \, p^{a_{.1}} q^{a_{.2}}}{a_{11}! \, a_{12}! \, a_{21}! \, a_{22}!},$$

the product of (1) and (2). The conditional probability of $\{a_{11}, a_{12}, a_{21}, a_{22}\}$ given $a_{.1}$ can now be computed, since $a_{.1}$ is the binomial variable with index $N = a_{.1} + a_{.2}$ and probability of falling into the first column p.

Under Model 1 (unrestricted bivariate sampling), we can write

(4) $$\mathscr{E}(a_{ij}) = Np_{ij}.$$

Thus if the p_{ij} are given by hypothesis, a χ^2 test of the hypothesis is obtained by setting

(5) $$X^2 = \sum_i \sum_j \frac{(a_{ij} - Np_{ij})^2}{(Np_{ij})},$$

which is often appropriate in genetic examples. However, often the theoretical values of p_{ij} or $p_{i.}$ or $p_{.j}$ are not given and must be estimated from the data. Under the hypothesis of independence, we have

(6) $$p_{ij} = p_{i.} \, p_{.j},$$

and the probabilities are estimated by

(7) $\hat{p}_{i.} = a_{i.}/N, \, p_{.j} = a_{.j}/N,$ $i = 1, 2, \ldots, r;$ $j = 1, 2, \ldots, c,$

and

(8) $$\hat{p}_{ij} = \hat{p}_{i.} \hat{p}_{.j}.$$

Under Model 2, p and q in (3) are estimated by $\hat{p}_1 = a_{.1}/N$ and $\hat{p}_2 = a_{.2}/N$, respectively and then

(9) $$X^2 = \sum_i \sum_j (a_{ij} - a_{i.} \hat{p}_j)^2 / (a_{i.} \hat{p}_j).$$

In both models with fixed marginal totals (i.e., with the unknown parameters estimated from the data), the expected numbers take the form $a_{i.} a_{.j}/N$ and so the computations of X^2 are identical in the two models; furthermore, in the 2×2 table with parameters estimated from the data, there is one degree of freedom.

An exact test of significance is possible. We take as our random variable, Z, the entry at position $(1, 1)$. A conditional distribution for Z can be obtained by dividing the expression on the right of (3) by $\binom{N}{a_{.1}} p^{a_{.1}} q^{a_{.2}}$, since under the hypotheses made the number of entries in the first column is a binomial variable with parameters, N and p. The quotient obtained can be written as

$$(10) \qquad \mathscr{P}(Z = z) = \frac{a_1.\,!\,a_2.\,!\,a_{.1}\,!\,a_{.2}\,!}{z!(a_1. - z)!\,(a_{.1} - z)!\,(N - a_1. - a_{.1} + z)!\,N!}$$

by setting $a_{11} = z$, the values of $\mathscr{P}(Z = 0)$, $\mathscr{P}(Z = 1)$, … can be computed. We suggest how this can be done in the exercises.

Furthermore, $\mathscr{E}Z$ and var Z can be computed and a test criterion

$$(11) \qquad X = (Z - \mathscr{E}Z)/\sqrt{(\text{var } Z)}$$

can be determined. It is possible to show that X^2 of (11) is equal to Pearson's $\sum (O - E)^2/E$ test criterion, multiplied by a factor $(N - 1)/N$.

7. STUDENT'S *t* TEST

Theorem. *Suppose that $X_1, X_2, X_3, \ldots, X_N$ are mutually independent and normally distributed having expectation α and variance σ^2. Then the mean $\overline{X} = (X_1 + X_2 + \cdots + X_N)/N$ is also normally distributed with expectation α and variance σ^2/N.*

Remark. We are not able to prove Theorem 1 without going beyond the bounds we have set for the book. The general meaning of the theorem is that, for independent and normal variables, the expectation of the mean is the true expectation, and the scatter or variance of the observed means about the true result is inversely proportional to the sample size. The standard deviation of the mean, $\sigma/\sqrt{N}$, is often referred to as the *standard error of the mean*, and some authors always use "standard error" as an elliptic or shortened version of this phrase.

These statements about the expectation and standard error of the mean are not special properties of the normal distribution; rather, they are appropriate to all distributions that possess a finite variance. Of all such distributions, however, the normal alone possesses the property that the mean has the same distribution as the individual components $X_1, X_2, \ldots$ except for a scale factor.

Theorem 2. *Suppose that $X_1, X_2, \ldots, X_N$ are mutually independent random variables, each having an expectation α, variance σ^2, and the same form of distribution. Then the mean $\overline{X}$ has the same expectation α and a variance σ^2/N. Furthermore, if N is large, the distribution of $\sqrt{N}\overline{X}$ is approximately normal with mean $\sqrt{N}\alpha$ and variance unity.*

Remark.   This is a special form of the *central limit theorem* of probability theory. Its practical importance is that the approximation is surprisingly good for small values of N. Thus let random variables X_1, X_2, ..., take values on the unit interval $(0, 1)$, and $\mathscr{P}(X < a) = a$, $0 \le a \le 1$. Then the graph of the density of $2^{-1/2}(X_1 + X_2)$ is a triangular area, the graph of the density of $3^{-1/2}(X_1 + X_2 + X_3)$ is bell-shaped, and the graphs of $4^{-1/2}(X_1 + X_2 + X_3 + X_4)$, $5^{-1/2}(X_1 + X_2 + \cdots + X_5)$, and standardized means having higher values of N cannot be distinguished graphically from the normal variable having the same expectation and variance.

Now the common variance of X_1, X_2, ... can be estimated from the data by (1) of section III.10, which we repeat in the following form:

(1)
$$\hat{\sigma}^2 = \frac{\sum(X_i - \bar{X})^2}{N - 1}.$$

With large value of N, $\hat{\sigma}^2$ in practical cases will approximate closely to σ^2. The foregoing theorem 1 shows that $(\bar{X} - \alpha)$ is distributed normally with zero mean and variance σ^2/N, hence

(2)
$$Y = \frac{\bar{X} - \alpha}{(\sigma^2/N)^{1/2}} = \frac{N^{1/2}(\bar{X} - \alpha)}{\sigma}$$

is distributed normally, having an expectation of zero and unit variance.

Let us now write

(3)
$$t = \frac{N^{1/2}(\bar{X} - \alpha)}{\hat{\sigma}};$$

if N is large, $\hat{\sigma}$ is a good approximation to σ, and t is approximately normal, having an expectation of zero and unit variance. It had been the custom to use (3) as an approximation to (2) until W. S. Gosset (1876–1937), who wrote under the pseudonym of "Student," showed that the variable t of (3) had a distribution that could be tabulated for low values of N to give exact tests. This enabled comparisons to be made between small numbers of variables, an essential facility in many fields in which it is impossible or impractical to collect a great number of observations.

8.   THE BIVARIATE NORMAL DISTRIBUTION

Random variables, X and Y say, can be (1) mutually independent, (2) such that a knowledge of one of them determines the other, or (3) such that although Y is not determined by X, a knowledge of X enables an improved estimate of Y to be made (e.g., if X and Y are heights and weights of men in some human population, there will be a tendency for tall men to weigh more than short men; similarly, heavy men will tend to be taller than light men). Pairs of variables possessing this type of relation are said to be *correlated*. Many pairs of correlated variables conform approximately to the normal form of correlation, which we introduce after the manner of Francis Galton.

We assume that X is standard normal and that its frequency function is

$$(1) \qquad g(x) = (2\pi)^{-1/2} \exp\left(-\tfrac{1}{2}x^2\right).$$

We assume that the distribution of Y for a fixed x is normal, having mean ρx and variance $1 - \rho^2$

$$(2) \qquad h_x(h) = (2\pi)^{-1/2}(1 - \rho^2)^{-1/2} \exp\left(\frac{-\tfrac{1}{2}[y - \rho x]^2}{[1 - \rho^2]}\right).$$

The joint density is then obtained

$$
\begin{aligned}
(3) \quad f(x, y) &= g(x)h_x(y) \\
&= (2\pi)^{-1}(1 - \rho^2)^{-1/2} \exp\left(\frac{-\tfrac{1}{2}[x^2 - 2\rho xy + y^2]}{[1 - \rho^2]}\right), \\
&\qquad -\infty < x < \infty, \qquad -\infty < y < \infty
\end{aligned}
$$

by a multiplication of the conditional density of Y, $h_x(y)$, by $g(x)$ the density of X.

In this approach, $\mathscr{E}X = 0$ and var $X = 1$, since X is standard normal. We can evaluate $\mathscr{E}XY$ by considering the expectation of $\mathscr{E}[X(Y - \rho X)]$. For every fixed value of X, $\mathscr{E}(Y - \rho X)$ is zero, since Y is distributed conditionally, having mean ρX. For each value of X, we multiply the conditional value of $\mathscr{E}(Y - \rho X)$ by X, to obtain zero. Finally, $\mathscr{E}[X(Y - \rho X)] = 0$; thus $\mathscr{E}XY - \rho\mathscr{E}X^2 = 0$, $\mathscr{E}XY = \rho$.

The form of $f(x, y)$ is symmetrical, which shows that we could equally well have begun with Y normal and the conditional distribution of X for a given y normal, having mean ρy and variance $1 - \rho^2$.

We may summarize. The *standard joint normal distribution* is given by (3), and its properties are as follows:

(i) $\mathscr{E}X = \mathscr{E}Y = 0,$ var X = var $Y = 1,$

(ii) $\rho = \mathscr{E}XY,$

(iii) $\mathscr{E}(Y \mid X = x) = \rho x$ and $\mathscr{E}(X \mid Y = y) = \rho y.$

The lines of regression pass through the origin and are straight lines.

(iv) The points of equal probability density lie on ellipses, given by

$$(4) \qquad x^2 - 2\rho xy + y^2 = \text{constant}.$$

(v) The probability distribution of $Y - \rho x$ conditional on $X = x$ is the same for every x. Similarly, the probability distribution of $X - \rho y$ conditional on $Y = y$ is the same for every y.

(vi) If $\rho = 0$, X is independent of Y, and conversely. Note that the hypothesis is not that X is normal and Y is normal and $\text{corr}(X, Y) = 0$ but that X and Y are jointly normal, $\rho = 0$.

These properties can all be related to the general joint bivariate normal distribution by making the transformation

$$(5) \qquad\qquad x = \frac{x' - a}{\sigma_1} \qquad y = \frac{y' - b}{\sigma_2}.$$

(i) $\mathscr{E}X' = a$; $\mathscr{E}Y' = b$; $\text{var } X' = \sigma_1{}^2$, $\text{var } Y' = \sigma_2{}^2$.

(ii) $\text{cov}(X', Y') = \sigma_1\sigma_2\rho$; $\text{corr}(X', Y') = \rho$.

9. REGRESSION IN MATHEMATICAL MODELS

The *line of regression of Y on X* is the set of all points $(x, \mathscr{E}(Y|X = x))$; similarly, the line of regression of X on Y is the set of all points $(\mathscr{E}(X|Y = y), y)$. Let us consider the regression of Y on X. A line can be drawn joining the points with neighboring values of x. For every x, there is precisely one point, since $\mathscr{E}(Y|X = x)$ is determined and unique if $\mathscr{P}(X = x)$ is not zero. Therefore, the graph is nowhere vertical, and it can be horizontal. Indeed, if Y is independent of X, $\mathscr{E}(Y|X = x) = \mathscr{E}Y$, a constant, independent of x. The line of regression can be straight. In this case, Y is said to be *linearly regressed on X*.

Regression can also be defined in an empirical distribution of points. As a rule, equal weights are assigned to the points. The data considered might be a collection of readings on heights and weights. For a given value of X there may be only one value of Y, which means that the conditional distribution method of definition breaks down to a triviality if X and Y are continuous. The straight line can be chosen such that for any x the best estimate of Y can be made. Various methods of specifying "best" could be given, but the following has gained general acceptance.

Let points (x_1, y_1), (x_2, y_2), ..., (x_N, y_N) be given and assigned equal weights. The general point is written (x, y). A method of estimation of Y conditional on $X = x$ by a straight-line formula

$$(1) \qquad\qquad \hat{y} = \beta x + \alpha,$$

will be said to be *best in the least-squares sense* if the sum of squares of the residuals

(2)
$$\sum (\hat{y} - y)^2 = \sum (\beta x + \alpha - y)^2$$

is as small as possible for all possible choices of α and β. The line given by (1) is then called the *linear least-squares regression line*. Let us write $x = \xi + \bar{x}$, $y = \eta + \bar{y}$, where $\bar{x}$ and $\bar{y}$ are the means of the x's and y's respectively. Then we have, for example,

(3)
$$\beta x + \alpha - y = \beta \xi - \eta + (\alpha + \beta \bar{x} - \bar{y}) = \beta \xi - \eta + A.$$

Now we must minimize $\sum (\beta \xi - \eta + A)^2$ by choices of β and A. Since $\sum \xi = 0$, $\sum \beta \xi A = 0$, and similarly $\sum \eta A = 0$. Thus the sum of the squares in (2) has become

(4)
$$\sum (\beta \xi - \eta + A)^2 = \beta^2 \sum \xi^2 - 2\beta \sum \xi \eta + \sum \eta^2 + NA^2$$
$$= \sum \xi^2 \left(\frac{\beta - \sum \xi\eta}{\sum \xi^2} \right)^2 + NA^2 + \sum \eta^2 - \frac{(\sum \xi\eta)^2}{\sum \xi^2},$$

where we have added and subtracted the same quantity $(\sum \xi\eta)^2/\sum \xi^2$. Now the first two terms are necessarily nonnegative, and $\sum \eta^2 - (\sum \xi\eta)^2/\sum \xi^2$ does not contain any parameters. Equation 4, hence (2), is minimized by setting $A = 0$ and $\hat{\beta} = \sum \xi\eta/\sum \xi^2$. It is customary to write the unknown parameters as Greek letters α, β, ... and the estimated values as $\hat{\alpha}$, $\hat{\beta}$, ... or as the corresponding latin letters a, b, ... We now have

(5)
$$\hat{\eta} = \left[\frac{\sum \xi\eta}{\sum \xi^2} \right] \xi,$$

(6)
$$\hat{y} - \bar{y} = \frac{\sum (x - \bar{x})(y - \bar{y})}{\sum (x - \bar{x})^2} (x - \bar{x})$$
$$= \frac{\text{cov}(X, Y)}{\text{var } X} (x - \bar{x})$$

There are many variations on the problem as stated. First, it is possible that not all the x's and y's will be distinct if we are dealing with an empirical distribution. In this case we write f_{xy} for the frequency with which the pair (x, y) occurs, and the summations are of the form $\sum x^2 f_{xy}$, $\sum xy f_{xy}$, ..., but the formula of the second line of (6) remains unchanged. Alternatively, we may be dealing with a bivariate theoretical distribution, which means that we have $f_{xy} = \mathcal{P}(X = x, Y = y)$. In the previous discussion we did not introduce any hypotheses about the errors in the variables X and Y; such hypotheses are necessary if we wish to give the sampling distributions of $\hat{\alpha}$, $\hat{\beta}$, ... the estimates of α, β, ...

From either (5) or (6), it is evident that the *least-squares linear regression line* passes through the mean of the distribution. Note also that a regression line of X on Y could be computed, as follows:

(7)
$$(\hat{x} - \bar{x}) = \frac{\text{cov}(X, Y)}{\text{var } Y}(y - \bar{y}).$$

Since the regression line (7) also passes through the mean $(\bar{x}, \bar{y})$ of the distribution, the two regression lines meet at the point $(\bar{x}, \bar{y})$.

The product of the two regression coefficients is

(8)
$$\frac{\text{cov}(X, Y)}{\text{var } X}\frac{\text{cov}(X, Y)}{\text{var } Y} = [\text{corr}(X, Y)]^2.$$

EXERCISES

The Multinomial Distribution

1. Assume that the probability-generating function of the multinomial variables $X_1, X_2, \ldots, X_m$ is $(p_1 t_1 + p_2 t_2 + \cdots + p_m t_m)^N$. Prove that the probability-generating function of any one of them, X_k say, is $(q + pt)^N$ by setting $t_k = t$, all other $t_i = 1$, and $p_k = p$ and $q = 1 - p$. (The marginal distributions of the multinomial distribution are thus all binomial.)

2. Compute the terms of the joint probability-generating function $(\frac{1}{3}t_1 + \frac{1}{3}t_2 + \frac{1}{3}t_3)^3$, simplifying the arithmetic by considering this expression to be multiplied by $27 = 3^3$. Obtain the marginal distribution of one of the variables by setting $t_1 = t$, $t_2 = t_3 = 1$ in the expression computed.

3. D. Harvey Sutton [*Med. J. Austral.*, **1** (1945) 611–613], gives figures for births each hour as follows, beginning at 6–7 p.m.:

92	97	117	97
102	136	80	93
100	151	125	100
101	110	87	93
127	144	101	131
118	136	107	105

Test the null hypothesis that the distribution of births is uniform throughout the 24 hours. Carry out a similar test by grouping the hours in each column. Comment.

The Poisson Distribution

4. The numbers of squares on the hemocytometer containing 0; 1, 2, 3, 4, 5; 6, 7, ..., 10; 11, ..., 15; 16, 17 cells were, respectively, 0; 1, 5, 8, 29, 49; 65, 76, 51, 42, 36; 15, 12, 6, 1, 3; 0, 1, total 400. Compute the mean and variance using 7 as the arbitrary origin [mean = 7.3175, variance = 6.0267].

5. With the same notation used in Exercise 4, the numbers of squares were 79; 132, 96, 62, 18, 10; 2, 1 and the total, 400. Compute the mean and variance using 2 as an arbitrary origin [mean = 1.6375, variance = 1.6839].

6. Fit Poisson distributions to the frequency distributions of Exercises 4 and 5 by computing the expected numbers with the aid of (1) of Section XII.3: namely, $400 \exp(-\hat{\lambda})\hat{\lambda}^x/x!$, where $\hat{\lambda}$ is the observed mean in each case. Construct a table with the observed numbers and the expected numbers for each x. If necessary, pool the terminal classes to obtain an expected number greater than 5 for each class. Compute (observed-expected) for each class and, finally, X^2. Test the significance of the X^2 so determined, noting that the degrees of freedom are 2 less than the number of classes.

7. It is often thought that the Poisson distribution is the law of small numbers. However, the following data can be obtained from P. Plum [*Acta Med. Scand.*, **90** (4) (1936), 342–364]. In 17 successive fillings of the hemocytometer chamber, the total counts over the 400 small squares were 1868, 1992, 1868, 1883, 1867, 1822, 1830, 1837, 1807, 1769, 1860, 1864, 1867, 1813, 1807, 1756, 1799; total 31,309. Treat these as a sample from the multinomial with each $p_i = 1/17$ [$X^2 = 22.13$ for 16 d.f.].

8. An observer counts on sets of 80 small squares of the hemocytometer and obtains the results that can be tabulated as follows:

Experiment	Number of Replicates	Arbitrary Origin	$\sum x$	$\sum x^2$	X^2
1	10	390	28	134	0.1415
2	10	390	−2	28	0.0708
3	10	390	35	129	0.0165
4	10	390	31	101	0.0125

Calculate the X^2 of the 10 replicates in each case, noting that $X^2 = \sum_1^{10} (x_i - \bar{x})^2/\bar{x}$. Interpret these surprisingly low values of X^2. [Data cited from C. Smith, *Arch. Int. Med.*, **47** (1931), 206].

9. In a genetic experiment, 551 matings of the form *AaBbCcDdEe* against *aabbccddee* were made. The number of dominants present were five in 17 offspring, four in 104, three in 180, two in 152, one in 81, and none in 17. Are these results consistent with the independent segregations at the five loci? [*Hint*. Calculate the expected numbers as the terms of 551 $(\frac{1}{2}t + \frac{1}{2})^5$ and calculate X^2.]

10. Calculate $\mathscr{P}(X = x)$ for $x = 0, 1, 2, \ldots$ to four decimal places when X has the Poisson distribution with parameter $\lambda = 1, 0.9, 0.8, 0.7, 0.6, 0.5, 0.4,$ and 0.3.

11. Suppose that bacterial cultures are being subcultured with an inoculum of such a size that the mean number of cells per inoculum is λ. Assume that Poisson distribution obtains. Calculate the approximate upper limit to the value of λ such that, if the subculture takes, it has grown with probability greater than 0.9 from one cell.

Contingency Tables

12. In (10) of Section XII.6, write $\mathscr{P}(Z = z) = p_z$ and prove the recurrence relation

$$\frac{p_{z+1}}{p_z} = \frac{(a_{1.} - z)(a_{.1} - z)}{(z + 1)(N - a_{1.} - a_{.1} + z + 1)},$$

where p_0 simplifies to $a_2! \, a_{.2}! / N! (N - a_1 - a_{.1})!)$, and each term can be calculated by the recurrence relation. But it is often more convenient to set $p_0 = c$ before computing $p_1 = ca_{1.} a_{.1} / [1(N - a_{1.} - a_{.1} + 1)]$ and then $p_2, p_3, \ldots$ by the recurrence relation. Since the sum of the probabilities is unity, c is then determined. This is a simple routine on a desk calculator. (First rearrange the table so that $a_{1.} \leq a_{.1} \leq a_{.2} \leq a_{2.}$ by renumbering the rows and columns and, if necessary, transposing the table.)

13. Compute the probabilities of the fourfold table using the methods of Exercise 12 when $a_{1.} = 7$, $a_{.1} = 8$, $a_{.2} = 9$, and $a_{2.} = 10$.

14. At Caesarian section, the site of the *corpus luteum* was noted. When a male child was born, the corpus was in the right ovary 23 times and in the left 16 times; for female children, the corpus was in the right ovary 13 times and in the left 12 times. Set these findings up as a fourfold table and make the null hypothesis, the independence of ovary side and sex of child. Calculate X^2. [Data from J. W. Williams (1921), *Bull. Johns Hopkins Hosp.*]

15. Calculate X^2 for the following table:

Sex of First-born of Family	Sex of Second Child	
	Male	Female
Male	17,341	16,518
Female	16,797	16,232

Test the null hypothesis that the sex of the second child is independent of that of the first child.

16. Nurses were tested for tuberculosis by the Mantoux skin reaction. Of those reporting less than 10 years' residence in a city environment, 99 had a positive and 452 a negative Mantoux reaction. Of those reporting more than 10 years' residence in a city environment, 208 had a positive and 568 a negative Mantoux reaction. Test by X^2 whether length of residence in the city is an important factor in the rate of infection with tuberculosis. [The examples on tuberculosis incidence of nurses are drawn from a series of articles by D. Anderson, *Med. J. Austral.*, commencing at **1** (1940), 747.]

17. Mark in the positions of the six cells of a 3×2 table. Write in marginal totals $a_{1.}, a_{2.}, a_{3.}, a_{.1}$, and $a_{.2}$, which are to be taken as fixed. Show that the values of any two cells not in the same row determine the contents of every cell. [The 3×2 table has $2 = (3 - 1)(2 - 1)$ d.f.]

18. The following 3×2 table is the result of a tuberculosis-sensitivity survey of nurses.

Age	Positive Mantoux Reaction	Negative Mantoux Reaction	Totals
17 to 19	285	983	1268
20 to 24	172	401	573
25+	59	69	128
	516	1453	1969

Calculate the expected values in the cells by means of the formula $a_{ij} = a_{i.}\,a_{.j}/N$. Hence compute $a_{ij} - a_{i.}\,a_{.j}/N$, the difference (observed $-$ expected). Hence compute also $(a_{ij} - \mathscr{E}a_{ij})^2/\mathscr{E}a_{ij}$ the contribution to X^2 for each cell and sum to find the total X^2 with 2 d.f.

19. In repeated examinations of untreated carriers of *Entamoeba histolytica*, an observer found positives and negatives as follows: 5 and 17, 12 and 1, 8 and 0, 3 and 17, 1 and 22, 3 and 11, 11 and 4, 6 and 15, 22 and 21, giving in all 71 positives and 108 negatives. By the use of a 9×2 contingency table, show that the probability of obtaining a positive (demonstrability) varies with the carrier. See Section XV.8.

20. In a certain period, the frequencies of congenitally deformed infants born in seven areas were noted, as well as the corresponding number of the total births; and the results appear in the following table:

Area	Number of Congenital Abnormalities	Total Number of Births
1	61	1736
2	36	1496
3	28	945
4	36	1309
5	48	1323
6	34	1386
7	52	1668
Total	295	9863

By using the technique of X^2 in a 7×2 contingency table, test the hypothesis that the proportion of congenitally deformed infants is independent of the area.

21. A follow-up of patients suffering from cancer of the breast who submitted to radical mastectomy gave the following results:

Age Group	Survivors after 5 Years	Total Number of Patients
15–24	0	1
25–34	6	17
35–44	64	132
45–54	106	221
55–64	88	210
65–74	43	107
75+	5	14

Test whether age has any effect on the prognosis.

22. The experience of certain forces with respect to inoculation against typhoid has been summarized by Topley and Wilson *The Principles of Bacteriology and Immunity* (1936) p. 1224] as follows:

	Not Attacked	Attacked	Total
Inoculated	10,322	56	10,378
Not inoculated	8,664	272	8,936
Total	18,986	328	19,314

Calculate X^2 on the hypothesis that inoculation is ineffective. Consider whether any test is justified on such data, which represent a mixture of the experience of troops from very diverse areas. For example, in some places the inoculated and uninoculated may have run no risk at all. The experiences of two areas, in neither of which was the inoculation effective, might be as follows:

50	50	100	950	50	1000
500	500	1000	95	5	100

Combined these figures give rise to the table

	Not Attacked	Attacked	Total
Inoculated	1000	100	1100
Not inoculated	595	505	1100
Total	1595	605	2200

Show that the X^2 of this table, regarded as the results of observations, is high. Comment on how you would avoid this effect if you were designing an experiment to test the efficacy of inoculation.

23. In a field trial on the effectiveness of B.C.G. inoculation against tuberculosis, we have the following data:

| | B.C.G. | | |
Result	Inoculated	Control	Total
Alive after 6 years	1516	1397	2913
Died of tuberculosis	4	28	32
within 6 years			
Died of other causes	30	32	62
Total	1550	1457	3007

Calculate the expected values in each class on the hypothesis of independence between inoculation and death. This yields a X^2 for 2 d.f. Compute also X^2 for the comparison between those dying from tuberculosis and all others. This value is significantly high.

24. In a campaign against cholera, results were as follows:

	Not Attacked	Attacked	Totals
Inoculated	276	3	279
Not inoculated	473	66	539
Totals	749	69	818

Test the efficacy of treatment by X^2.

25. In such experiments as Exercise 24, the results in a single series may not be significant, perhaps because the number of observations was not sufficiently large. However, the X^2 of a number of experiments may be available. Suppose that the X^2 with 1 d.f. for each experiment was 1.92 in the first experiment, 2.96 in the second, 3.52 in the third, and 4.67 in the fourth. Assume the independence of these results and take the sum. It is X^2 with 4 d.f. Is it significant at the 5% level?

26. In a number of countries, the average income per head in dollars and the infant deaths per thousand live births were measured. The results were: (country) 1, income 346, infant death rate 79; 2, 679, 25; 3, 216, 77; 4, 582, 57; 5, 125, 97; 6, 296, 140; 7, 40, 115; 8, 92, 92; 9, 482, 56; 10, 89, 82; 11, 183, 50; 12, 86, 76; 13, 100, 111; 14, 44, 96; 15, 300, 120; 16, 250, 115; 17, 101, 29; 18, 36, 68; 19, 264, 41; 20, 146, 102. These results are all in the form (k, x_k, y_k). Compute $\sum x_k$, $\sum x_k^2$, $\sum y_k$, $\sum y_k^2$, $\sum x_k y_k$. Hence obtain the variances of the form $[\sum x_k^2 - (\sum x_k)^2/20]/19$, and the covariance $[\sum x_k y_k - \sum x_k \sum y_k/20]/19$. Estimate the coefficient of correlation by $\rho = \text{cov}(X, Y)/\sqrt{(\text{var } X \cdot \text{var } Y)}$.

27. Plot the observations of Exercise 26 as a spot diagram. Plot the least-squares regression line of Y on X, namely,

$$\hat{y} - \bar{y} = \frac{\text{cov}(X, Y)}{\text{var } X} \cdot (x - \bar{x}),$$

where $\bar{y}$ and $\bar{x}$ are the means of the Y and X observations. [In such a diagram the distances of the observed y-values from the corresponding regression values $\hat{y}$ are small if $\hat{\rho}$ is large (i.e., if $1 - \hat{\rho}^2$ is small).]

28. In a "growth" survey, 336 boys aged 7 were examined and the following constants were determined:

	Height, X (in.)	Weight, Y (lb)
Mean	48.29	52.76
Variance	4.1514 in²	2.4970 lb²
Covariance	2.4636 in.-lb	

Using the formula

$$\hat{y} - \bar{y} = \frac{\text{cov}(X, Y)}{\text{var } X}(x - \bar{x})$$

and a similar one, estimate the line of regression of heights on weights, and vice versa.

Plot the lines graphically.

Calculate the standard error of the mean of both height and weight for this age group.

Student's t Distribution

29. The following deviates were obtained in an experiment: 1.28, 1.16, 0.16, 1.66, 1.26, -0.05, 0.18, 0.68, 0.58, and 2.48. Suppose that the null hypothesis is that the mean is zero and the variance is unknown. Calculate the mean and variance of the sample. (The sample mean divided by the sample standard deviation is distributed as Student's t.) Test its significance, using as your alternative hypothesis that the mean has some positive value.

30. Using the same hypotheses employed in the previous exercise, calculate the sample mean and variance and Student's t, the observed deviations being 1.20, 2.31, 1.35, 1.74, and 1.27.

31. A random sample of 15 men have the following heights:

Heights (cm)				
172.5	165.0	171.5	176.5	165.0
171.5	162.5	167.5	180.0	166.0
172.5	177.5	167.5	172.5	185.0

Calculate the arithmetic mean and test the hypothesis that these values are a random sample from a normal population having mean 175 cm, using the 5% level of significance.

32. A group of subjects were tested for their ability to remember certain material; their scores before and after training were 20 and 17; 14 and 20; 13 and 17; 17 and 22; 18 and 22; 19 and 25; 18 and 23; and 17 and 18. Calculate the mean and standard deviations of the set of differences $17 - 20 = -3, 20 - 14 = 6$, etc. Now make the null hypothesis of the form of Exercise 29 and carry out the test of Student's t.

NOTES

This chapter is an informal introduction to the use of tests of significance. We explained in Section IV.8 how the normal curve can be used to calculate the probabilities in the binomial distribution. Here we suggest that the same can be done for the multinomial distribution, in which many classes replace the two classes—successes and failures of the binomial. This leads us to the test of significance in the symmetrical multinomial; and in distributions in which the class probabilities p_i are given by hypotheses that there is an underlying Poisson, binomial, normal or other distribution. We also introduce and treat contingency tables as a special case of the multinomial with fitted parameters. In Section XII.6 we give the sampling distributions for the contingency tables, paying special attention to the simplest case, the fourfold table. Student's t distribution is presented in Section XII.7. This and the χ^2 test are very versatile and useful tests.

Notions of correlation and regression have been introduced very briefly. Lacking a more detailed presentation of the underlying mathematics and statistical theory, which is beyond our present aims, it is difficult to go much further. Moreover, there are now many elementary texts on probability and statistical theory. For example, Whitworth (1948), a reprint of a classic of 1867, requires little prior mathematical knowledge. Feller (1957) is an elementary introduction that contains many applications to genetics and other fields. Riordan (1958) and Ryser (1963) go more deeply into the combinatorial side of probability and design of experiment. Armitage (1971) gives an extended treatment of the topics of the present chapter.

CHAPTER XIII

The Control of Laboratory Measurements

1. PRECISION AND ACCURACY

There are two qualities of laboratory readings, such as the routine estimation of blood hemoglobin, which seem desirable. First, we should be able to reproduce the results; second, the results of our estimates should average out to the true results. Thus the readings should be *precise* and *unbiased*; if so, they may be said to be *accurate*.

The mathematical model of the measurement of an unknown magnitude C can be set up as follows. We suppose that C has a true value γ which is capable of exact measurement. We suppose that a measurement by some means is X. We consider the case where a number of independent measurements $X_1, X_2, \ldots, X_N$ could be performed on C. We can think of the measurements as N independent observations of a random variable X. The X is assumed to possess a mean μ and variance σ^2, and we have

(1)
$$\mathscr{E}X = \mu,$$

(2)
$$\mathscr{E}(X - \mu)^2 = \sigma^2.$$

In those unusual cases without a finite mean or variance, we would not be able to determine any useful information about C by taking the mean of observations. We define

(3)
$$\hat{\mu}_N = \frac{X_1 + X_2 + \cdots + X_N}{N},$$

where $\hat{\mu}_N$ is the estimator of μ and is the mean of the N values of $X_1, X_2, \ldots, X_N$. The *estimates* are the particular values assumed by the estimator. The absolute difference between the estimate $\hat{\mu}_N$ and μ will be small if N is large, and this is a desirable property. If the variance σ^2 is large, we should find that the difference would be prone to fluctuate and not to "settle down" to a series of values $\mu_N, \mu_{N+1}, \mu_{N+2}, \ldots$, all close to μ.

Given the foregoing assumptions, if successive values of the mean μ_N are plotted as the ordinate against N as the abscissa, the lines $y = \mu + \xi$ and $y = \mu - \xi$, can be drawn and it is almost certain that all points $(k, \hat{\mu}_k)$ will lie between these lines, after a sufficiently large number of observations have been taken for any positive ξ.

The *precision* of a measurement method is measured by the spread of the readings—their repeatability or consistence. In the mathematical model, the precision is measured by the variance of the random variable X. The smaller the expected variance, the greater the precision. It is convenient and possible to define the precision by a single number because the *central limit theorem* states, in this special case, that $\hat{\mu}_N$ is approximately normal, having expectation μ and variance σ^2/N. Since the normal distribution is completely specified by its mean and variance, no other information on the distribution of X is required. It is found in practice that the observed means $\hat{\mu}_N$ can be treated as if they were normal for N not very large.

Example i. Suppose that X has the rectangular distribution on the unit interval; then X has a mean $\mu = \frac{1}{2}$, and variance $\sigma^2 = \frac{1}{12}$; $\hat{\mu}_4$ would have an expectation $\mu = \frac{1}{2}$ and a variance $\frac{1}{4}\sigma^2$ or $\frac{1}{48}$. Its distribution can be readily determined and, when the frequency function is plotted, it is indistinguishable by eye from the normal frequency function having the same mean and variance.

The variance of an estimator of the mean can also be estimated by repeated trials, for if $\hat{\sigma}^2$ is defined by

(4)
$$\hat{\sigma}^2 = \frac{(X_i - \hat{\mu}_N)^2}{N - 1},$$

$$\hat{\mu}_N = \bar{X} = \frac{X_1 + X_2 + \cdots + X_N}{N},$$

then

(5)
$$\mathscr{E}\hat{\sigma}^2 = \sigma^2.$$

The precision of the estimator $\hat{\mu}_N$ can be increased by taking more measurements, since the variance of the mean is σ^2/N and this evidently becomes smaller as N increases. A measurement X is said to be an *unbiased estimate* of C if $\mathscr{E}X = \gamma$. This is a variation on a statistical definition of an estimator, which is *unbiased* if its expectation is equal to the true value of the parameter being estimated.

Thus X is *unbiased* if its expectation $\mu = \gamma$. If its variance is small, it is *precise*. If it is precise and unbiased, a measurement can be said to be *accurate*.

Example ii. It was desired to estimate the variance of hematocrit readings, six readings on a single sample taken from each of ten subjects being made and recorded as in Table XIII.1. The sum of squares about the mean was computed for each subject, and this sum had an expectation of $5\sigma^2$. The results from the different subjects were added to give a total sum of squares with an expectation of $50\sigma^2$. The estimate of σ^2 is then $\hat{\sigma}^2 = $ (total of the sums of squares about the respective mean)$/50 = 0.08$.

Table XIII.1

VARIATION BETWEEN REPEATED HEMATOCRIT ESTIMATIONS ON 10 BLOOD SAMPLES

Sample	Replicate Hematocrit Readings						Sample Mean	Sums of Squares about Sample Mean
1	49.1	49.0	49.1	49.3	49.0	49.0	49.08	0.0683
2	49.3	49.5	49.0	49.0	48.2	49.2	49.03	1.0133
3	42.0	42.0	41.8	42.0	41.7	41.8	41.88	0.0883
4	43.0	43.0	42.5	42.5	42.0	42.3	42.55	0.7750
5	48.2	48.0	48.0	48.0	48.0	48.2	48.07	0.0533
6	39.0	38.5	38.7	38.8	38.5	39.0	38.75	0.2550
7	45.2	45.6	46.0	45.9	45.5	45.5	45.62	0.4283
8	44.0	43.8	43.5	44.0	43.2	43.5	43.67	0.5133
9	42.3	42.2	42.5	41.7	42.2	42.2	42.18	0.3483
10	40.8	40.5	40.2	40.8	39.9	40.5	40.45	0.6150
							Total	4.1881

Degrees of freedom of total of sums of squares $= 5 \times 10 = 50$.
Estimated variance $= 4.1881/50 = 0.08376$
Estimated standard deviation $= 0.29$.
Estimated standard error of a sample mean of six readings $= 0.12$.

It must be noted that in Example ii we estimated the variance of the measurement, the hematocrit reading, after the blood had been collected. There would be a greater variance if we were to take separate samples of blood from each individual; we leave the computations to the Exercises. The estimate of the variance would then be 0.7991.

Errors in measurements are often classified into *systematic* and *accidental*. It is often said that a systematic error is one which affects uniformly all determinations or measurements made by a given method under standard conditions. In the foregoing analysis, the systematic error is $\mu - \gamma$. Accidental error is due to the sum of all the variations that enter into the experimental determination or measurement of the unknown quantity; for example, inabilities to bring the level of blood in a pipette to the desired mark or to read a scale to an arbitrary level of exactitude, uncontrollable small changes in carrying out the observations, or uncontrollable variations in the quality of chemicals used.

The three devices to test measurement procedures are: the measurement of known materials, comparison with other measurement procedures, and comparison with modifications of the measurement. Let us briefly discuss each of these.

(i) The Measurement of Known Materials

If it is desired to test the amount of glucose in blood, known concentrations of glucose can be added to blood samples and the resultant measurements can be checked to see that the differing added concentrations are reflected in the measurements.

(ii) Comparison with other Measurement Procedures

There may be available known, accurate methods of determining the quantities to be measured. Samples are then tested both by the known accurate method, yielding a measurement Y, and by the ordinary laboratory method, yielding measurements X. If the methods agree closely within acceptable limits, nothing need be done. If it happens that X behaves as though it were a function of Y (e.g., a linear function), corrections must be applied to the readings typified by X; for example, a constant may have to be added to X, or it may be revealed that the corrected reading is of the form $aX + b$. The measurement of X can be said to be *calibrated*.

(iii) Comparison with Modifications of the Measurement

The procedures for taking the measurement may be varied. For example, if urea concentration in the urine is being measured, it would be possible to compare the readings with those taken when the urine is diluted with an equal volume of water.

2. COUNTING EXPERIMENTS

In this section we consider the statistical control of laboratory measurements, analogous to the quality control of industrial processes. The aim of such control is to detect deviations from ideal conditions and to suggest improved techniques. A good example of the use of this type of statistical control method is provided by counting techniques, and so we begin with a detailed consideration of control of red cell counting. The blood is diluted 1/200 with saline and thoroughly mixed; the cells are allowed to sediment out of a layer 0.1 mm thick onto a glass slide ruled into squares of 0.0025 mm^2, whereupon they are counted, commonly over five sets of 16 squares.

Next a mathematical model is set up to explain (a) the distribution of the cells in the fluid above the squares in the sedimenting chamber and (b) their distribution on the squares of the slide. We make the assumption that the red cells have a negligible volume, which means that the presence of one red cell in the volume above a square has a negligible effect on the probability of the presence of another cell. This is not unrealistic, since the volume occupied by the red cells of a normal subject is about 0.2% of the fluid dilution. We make the following assumptions in the mathematical model

1. The probability of a red cell appearing in any unit of volume is proportional to the volume.

2. It is impossible for more than one cell to occupy a very small volume.

3. The number of cells in any unit of volume is independent of the number in any other unit of volume.

These assumptions can be made more precise in a formal mathematical setting, as in Section XII.3, and they lead to the conclusion that the appropriate distribution is the Poisson. In Table XII.1, we displayed the large sample test of goodness of fit of the Poisson distribution. It would be an impractical method in applied work. However, the test given under the heading of the symmetrical multinomial in Section XII.5 is practicable, since technicians usually record their counts over five sets of 16 small squares. If their technique is good, we should expect the differences between parallel counts to approximate to those suggested by theory. A system of quality control of counts can be set up as follows.

In Table XIII.2 we give sample computations of X^2 in a few red cell counts; X^2 is computed by (8) of Section XII.5. Results of the quality control of two experienced technical assistants A and B, appear in Table XIII.3.

From tables of the theoretical χ^2 distribution, we find that in 100% of all occasions, the X^2 of (3) will exceed zero, it will exceed 1.064 in 90%, 2.195 in 70%, 3.357 in 50%, 4.878 in 30%, and 7.779 in 10%. These values of χ^2 are to be used as the boundaries of classes 1.0 to 0.9, corresponding to χ^2 values of 0 to 1.064; 0.9 to 0.7, corresponding to χ^2 values of 1.064

Table XIII.2

STATISTICAL CONTROL IN HEMATOLOGY BY X^2

Counts on Blocks of 16 Hemocytometer Squares					Total	Σy_i^2	Sample χ^2 or X^2	Probability Class by Size of χ^2
24	14	31	25	32	126	2701	8.21	0.1–0
17	26	34	19	29	125	2896	7.92	0.1–0
26	18	28	32	31	135	4126	4.59	0.5–0.3
26	32	21	23	32	134	3268	3.84	0.5–0.3
22	26	28	27	33	136	4939	2.31	0.7–0.5

Table XIII.3

QUALITY CONTROL OF BLOOD CELL COUNTING

Probability Class	Red Cell Counts of A	White Cell Counts of A			Red Cell Counts of B	
		October	January	February	First Series	Second Series
1.0–0.9	15	8	3	8	24	13
0.9–0.7	23	6	17	17	25	31
0.7–0.5	24	12	14	19	24	22
0.5–0.3	11	20	19	14	25	20
0.3–0.1	18	20	25	33	2	7
0.1–0	9	34	22	9	—	7
Total counts	100	100	100	100	100	100
Total X^2	360.96	542.04	423.18	336.42	173.28	316.82
Degrees of freedom	400	300	300	300	400	400

to 2.915, and so on. Moreover, 10% of all sets of counts can be expected to fall into the first and last of the classes and 20% into each of the other four classes. The methods can be applied to white cell counting, for which four *parallel* or *replicate* counts are available. There are now 3 d.f., and the values of χ^2 dividing the classes are 0.584, 1.424, 2.366, 3.665, and 6.251. One observer had his white cell counts distributed over the six classes as

follows: 8, 6, 12, 20, 20, 34, giving too many sets of counts having high X^2 and dispersion. With modifications of technique (increasing the acetic acid strength of the diluent), sets were obtained with 3, 17, 14, 19, 25, and 22, and later, 8, 17, 19, 14, 33, and 9 (which were more in accord with theory). One technician yielded 24, 25, 24, 25, 2, and 0 in the six classes in red cell counting. This technician evidently attempted to pick closely agreeing groups of 16 squares. This subjective choice does not lead to a more accurate determination of the mean. J. Berkson and his colleagues have shown how arbitrary selection of areas for counting yields unsatisfactory or poor estimates of the mean.

Once an observer or technician begins to obtain satisfactory results as shown by a distribution of counts over the probability classes, in accord with theory, he can dispense with further quality control if the laboratory conditions and his technique remain constant.

3. THE CONTROL OF ROUTINE MEASUREMENTS

Some general points can now be made about the routine measurement of the common laboratory variables; we take our examples from hematology.

Errors can be *systematic*—that is, the mean of the readings do not tend to be closer to the true value if the number of observations is made arbitrarily large. Systematic error occurs, for example, when the capacity of a pipette has not been correctly standardized. This problem is overcome by checking on all such laboratory instruments before use, by introducing a suitable factor into later calculation, or by buying equipment known to have been submitted to appropriate standardization. Similarly, the depth of the hemocytometer chamber may not be within the certified range. Errors introduced by such defects can be reduced to negligible proportions by calibration.

The pipettes, even if accurately calibrated, cannot be filled exactly. There will always be difficulty in correctly aligning the meniscus against the mark on the pipette. The error thus introduced is usually small and is (or can often be) reduced by having the reading made at a thin neck of the apparatus.

The material to be examined must be representative in some sense. For example, estimations of blood sugar are made under standard conditions of fasting and consumption of sugars.

In some fields, personal errors are apt to be high. In certain forms of estimation, the human observer can be replaced by a photoelectric cell. Individuals vary in their ability to read a scale and, especially, in their ability to estimate fractional parts between the lowest divisions of the scale. Some of these errors are distributed uniformly, but numerous authors have reported on the biases of laboratory workers in reading a scale. According to the studies of Berkson, many technicians give systematically low counts of the red cells. In the past, a disturbing factor in the red cell counting particularly has been a preconceived notion of an ideal "accuracy," which evidently biases many observers' counts. Some commonly used procedures often diminish the precision of the results. Thus if an observer is counting red cells and attempts to determine which sets of 16 small squares are most nearly in agreement, subjective bias is almost certain to be introduced. If he counts on two sets and looks for other sets that agree with the first pair, he is effectively basing his results on the counts of the two sets.

EXERCISES

1. Five hematocrit estimations were made on each of eight subjects and the results were recorded as follows:

Total Error of Hematocrit Determination

Subject	Hematocrit Readings for Replicate Samples					Mean for Subject	Sums of Squares about Mean
1	42.0	41.8	41.2	40.0	40.0	41.00	3.68
2	48.0	47.2	47.1	46.8	45.4	46.90	3.60
3	45.0	44.8	44.2	43.7	42.6	44.06	3.71
4	48.5	49.0	48.5	47.6	46.8	48.04	3.07
5	44.8	44.6	44.0	42.8	44.0	44.04	2.43
6	47.0	47.0	46.6	46.0	44.5	46.22	4.37
7	45.2	45.0	44.5	44.0	43.8	44.50	1.48
8	46.0	46.0	45.2	45.2	43.8	45.24	3.23
						Total	25.57

Degrees of freedom of total of sums of squares; $4 \times 8 = 32$.
Variance $= 25.57/32 = 0.7991$.
Standard error $= 0.894$.

Estimate the variance and standard deviation of such an estimation. Note that this variance includes more possible sources or error than that determined in Table XIII.1.

2. From 10 samples of blood, each collected from a different person, replicate determinations of the blood sedimentation rate were made as follows (Walsh et al., 1953):

Sample	Replicate Values of the Sedimentation Rate (mm after 60 min)						Sample Mean	Sums of Squares about Sample Mean
1	15.2	14.0	14.0	14.0	15.5	15.0	14.62	2.41
2	11.0	11.5	11.5	11.0	12.0	11.0	11.33	0.83
3	11.0	13.0	11.0	12.5	14.5	14.0	12.67	10.83
4	2.2	2.8	3.0	3.0	2.9	2.8	2.78	0.45
5	18.8	19.2	20.0	20.2	20.1	21.0	19.89	2.98
6	9.0	10.0	9.8	10.0	9.4	11.0	9.87	2.29
7	1.5	2.0	2.0	2.0	2.0	1.5	1.83	0.33
8	24.5	23.8	26.0	31.0	31.5	26.2	27.17	54.21
9	4.8	5.0	6.0	5.5	5.8	5.5	5.43	1.05
10	1.5	1.5	2.0	2.0	1.8	1.9	1.78	0.27
							Total	75.64

Determine the variance for each sample. Note the tendency for the mean and variance to be correlated.

3. Interpret $\sum (X - \bar{X})^2/(N - 1)$ as the sample variance in Exercise XII.7, where $N = 17$. Show that this variance is of the same order as the variance computed under the hypothesis of Poisson variation. Therefore, other sources of variance, such as the varying hemocytometer depth from experiment to experiment, must be of small magnitude.

4. It is often impossible to carry out numerous replicates on one test. Prove that, in such cases, it is more efficient to estimate variances from 20 sets of triplicate than from 30 sets of duplicate readings. (*Hint.* Count the degrees of freedom in the two cases.)

NOTES

The account in Section XIII.1 owes much to the handbook of Ku (Ed., 1969), which contains articles by such authors as C. Eisenhart, W. S. Connor, H. H. Ku, and W. J. Youden. A general account of the theory of measurement has been given by Pfanzagl (1968). In the medical field, the reader can refer to Mainland (1938) and Glasser (1944). For the application of quality control methods to hematology, we cite the works of Berkson (1944);

Berkson, Magath, and Hurn (1935, 1940); Magath, Berkson, and Hurn (1936); Lancaster (1950c); and Walsh, Arnold, Lancaster, Coote, and Cotter (1953).

The distribution named after S. D. Poisson (1781–1840) has been rediscovered by many other authors, especially H. Boltzmann (1844–1906), E. Abbe (1840–1905), and W. S. Gosset ("Student") (1876–1937). The large bibliography of Haight (1967) is available. The use of statistical control in counting experiments, as expounded here, is due to Fisher, Thornton, and McKenzie (1922). A very fine survey article on bacteriological counting problems has been published by Eisenhart and Wilson (1943).

On the technical side of red cell counting, J. Berkson and his colleagues have done very good work. A full bibliography of red cell counting by Stavem (1964) is available. Lancaster (1950c, 1953b) has considered some problems of fitting the Poisson model to the observations; one paper in particular, (1950c) discusses the "crowding effect" first noted by Berkson and shows that this effect can be neglected when comparing sets of 16 hemocytometer squares. The "crowding effect" is negligible for mean red cell counts of less than 3.5 per small hemocytometer square, but it leads to a variance of about 80% of the expected value at counts of 7 or 8 per small square, as Berkson first pointed out. For notes on frequency counts of particle size, see Kottler (1950).

CHAPTER XIV

Clinical Trials and Observations

1. INTRODUCTORY

The vast polemic and apologetic literature that exists on the conduct of clinical trials may be a transient feature best explained by a brief historical introduction. Few effective remedies were available in clinical medicine before 1850. After excluding the purges from consideration, we might admit that opium, the salicylates, and digitalis were valuable palliatives; but we would be able to find few remedies that exerted direct action on the causal agent of any disease. With the rise of chemical technology, a greater range of chemicals, especially of organic compounds, became available. The microbial theory of infectious disease suggested that a direct attack on the causal agent might be possible, and Joseph Lister (1827–1912) successfully treated wounds with phenols as antiseptics. But he and many others saw the need for drugs that would be more specific in their action, being effective against the causative organism without unduly harming the tissues of the host. To meet such a need, Paul Ehrlich (1854–1915) examined systematically the therapeutic value of many compounds, specially synthesized. As a result, the organic arsenicals were introduced into clinical medicine in 1904. Other chemical agents followed. Methods of active and passive immunization were also devised. Gerhard Domagk (1895–1964) introduced the sulfonamide compounds into clinical practice in the middle 1930s; other chemotherapeutic agents and then the antibiotics next came into use.

At first, there was much *in vitro* bacteriological evidence in favor of the new agents, and they were so effective in some diseases that few clinical trials were needed. However, other diseases did not yield fully to the various remedies, and there were often competing remedies for the same disease. Thus, after the unequivocal early results, the need for clinical trials became increasingly obvious. Clinical trials had not been common before World War II. Indeed, until the new agents had come into use, most of the results would have been discouraging to all concerned. In particular, the statistician would have been in the difficult position of declaring, almost invariably, that the proposed remedy did not perform significantly better than the control. This may explain the lack of followers of the pioneers in the use of numerical methods in clinical medicine such as Pierre Charles Alexandre Louis (1787–1872) and Louis Denis-Jules Gavarret (1809–1890). Doubts might well occur to them about the worth of the efforts required to collect information under such unfavorable conditions for the retrospective analysis of clinical treatment.

Another factor of importance was the development of the statistical methods appropriate for analysis of data and the testing of hypotheses in a biological field. Beginnings were made by Francis Galton (1822–1911), W. F. R. Weldon (1860–1906) and, particularly, Karl Pearson (1857–1936). An extensive general theory of experimentation in conditions, under which uncontrollable variables played a large part, was first developed by Ronald Aylmer Fisher (1890–1962). Fisher and his school at Rothamsted, England, and elsewhere, devised efficient methods for the design and analysis of experiment in agriculture and veterinary science and set forth a general theory that could be readily transferred over to medical fields. It may be remarked, in passing, that much of Fisher's work was motivated by a profound interest in human genetics and evolution.

Before the Fisherian methods could be successfully applied to the theory of clinical trials, however, a number of special problems had to be resolved. First, compared with the typical laboratory animal, man is large and long-lived; treatment of him or experimentation on him is often very expensive, and sometimes the duration of observation must be long. In addition, there are always costly administrative expenses associated with human experimentation. It is evident that part of the cause of the failure of the followers of Louis or Gavarret was the lack of an efficient administrative structure in the primitive hospitals of their times.

Second, ethical problems, which may not arise in agriculture or veterinary practice, are of prime importance in medical practice and must be solved in an acceptable manner. The rights and best interests of the patient must be preserved, as must his relations with medical and nursing attendants, mutual continued respect and cooperation being essential for successful clinical experimentation. The difficulties are real; for example, the need for the process of randomization of treatments takes the responsibility for the assignment of treatment out of the hands of the regular physician.

Third, on a purely practical level, medicolegal problems must be avoided. As an example of difficulties, let us note that the use of a remedy that prevented the deaths from a disease in 10 % of those treated but caused blindness in 1 % of the patients would be regarded as a very successful cure in veterinary practice but would cause great ethical and legal problems in medical practice.

Fourth, the adoption of scientific modes of thought has lessened the effects of the "style" of the physician. There is now, perhaps, wide agreement on the general principles of treating a given disease apart from the specific remedies. This circumstance may make it easier for a physician to recommend that his patient be submitted in a trial to either penicillin or aureomycin, for example, without making the choice himself, because he is assured that the rest of the treatment will be in accord with his own ideas. In any case, he may well have ordered either remedy for the particular case. We can conclude that given an increased insight into the causes of disease, as well as the improved administrative and technical resources at hand, it is now possible to carry out clinical trials in an acceptable manner. The necessary changes of attitude and practice have been brought about by many physicians and statisticians, but we can say that the cautious approach of the British school of medical statisticians under Austin Bradford Hill (1897–   ) has done much to make the experimental methods in clinical trials acceptable to physicians and to the community, alike.

The experimental method in clinical trials is sometimes justified by reference to the progress of science. However, the findings are often quite devoid of wider scientific interest, and it would be equally logical to carry out clinical trials on any other species, if this were the aim. The aim is to benefit the patient, both present and future, and the human community in general. The justification of the formal clinical trial is that useful experience and information of high quality will not be wasted but will be included in the general body of medical knowledge, that it will furnish the clinician with heightened insight, and that it will lead to more effective treatment of patients.

2. CONDUCT OF THE CLINICAL TRIAL

A clinical trial cannot begin in the absence of the availability of substantial amounts of clinical information, such as the cause of the disease, its incidence by age and sex, and the results of past treatments. For definiteness, we suppose that we are to test the effectiveness of various agents A, B, C, ... against the *Pneumococcus* causing lobar pneumonia. It will be known that A, B, C, ... are effective in reducing the growth of pneumococci *in vitro* (i.e., in artificial cultures) and that A, B, C, ... are effective against the pneumococci in suitable laboratory animals such as mice. It will also be known that the pneumococci do not constitute a homogeneous class but that some types are more dangerous to man than others. Our general aim will be to reduce the mortality from pneumonia in the human population at large, by the choice of the appropriate remedy from A, B, C, ...

The first step is to specify what cases are to be admitted to the trial. We might insist, as evidence of the presence of the disease, on the patient possessing the following characteristics:

1. Clinical temperature above 103°F (39.4°C).
2. Radiological findings suggesting the beginnings of a lobar pneumonitis.
3. The isolation of a *Pneumococcus* from the sputum. (The treatment, of course, is to be initiated immediately after the sputum has been suitably collected. The case must be deleted from the trial if no *Pneumococcus* is isolated by the bacteriologist.)

Since it is impossible to prove a scientific hypothesis, such as: treatment A is more effective than treatment B, we must proceed indirectly. Our aim is to carry out an experiment so that if A is indeed more effective than B, we have the best chance of making any other hypothesis appear unlikely. We set up a hypothesis H_0 that treatments A and B are equally effective against the disease. Our results will be recorded as in Table XIV.1 and the analysis will be based on Model 2 of Section XII.6. Using the notation of that section, we have assigned 200 cases to Treatment A and 200 to the Treatment B; thus $a_{1.} = a_{2.} = 200$. Under the null hypothesis, our best estimate of the mortality is given by $\hat{q} = 33/400 = 0.0825$. The observed ratios for Treatments A and B are 3/200 and 30/200, and the difference is 27/200. The standard error of the difference is

$$(2.1) \quad \sqrt{(\hat{p}\hat{q}/200 + \hat{p}\hat{q}/200)} = \sqrt{(\hat{p}\hat{q}/100)} = \sqrt{(0.0825 \times 0.9175)/10} = 0.0275$$

$$(2.2) \quad \frac{\text{difference between rates}}{\text{standard error of the difference}} = \frac{0.135}{0.0275} = 4.91.$$

Table XIV.1

THE TREATMENT OF PNEUMOCOCCAL PNEUMONIA[a]

	Deaths	Survivals	Total
Treatment A	3	197	200
Treatment B	30	170	200
Total	33	367	400

[a] Analyzed as the difference between two binomials:

$$\chi = \frac{\text{difference between means}}{\sqrt{\hat{p}\hat{q}/200 + \hat{p}\hat{q}/200}} = \frac{27/200}{1/10\sqrt{\hat{p}\hat{q}}} = \frac{0.135}{0.275} = 4.91.$$

Analyzed by the χ^2 test:

$$\chi^2 = 400 \frac{(3 \times 170 - 30 \times 197)^2}{33 \times 367 \times 200 \times 200} = 24.0.$$

This result is clearly significant at the 1%, or even 0.1%, level by Table A.2 of the appendix. Note also in Table XIV.1 that $4.91^2 = 24.0$.

Our results are to be analyzed as though conditions in the two classes of patients have been as much alike as possible except in the type of treatment. *Randomization* is the solution here. Every case entering the trial is given equal chances of being assigned to either treatment series. In the simple case with two classes, which we are considering, randomization is a process equivalent to the toss of a coin—"heads" resulting in the patient being assigned treatment A and "tails" resulting in him being assigned to treatment B.

Subjective methods of grading the patients and alloting them to treatment and control have been found to be subject to bias—if the observer wishes very strongly to see one treatment proved effective, he may assign the more favorable cases to the "more effective" treatment. Alternatively, he may wish to make sure that all the less favorable cases get the "good" treatment, since they need it most. Randomization avoids the introduction of such biases.

Of course, it would be inconvenient to spin a coin for the assignment to treatment classes as the patient entered the clinic. Before the trial has begun, therefore, we assign the serial numbers of the future cases to the various treatments by processes equivalent to the toss of a coin or the spin of a roulette wheel. This randomization may be unrestricted—which means that we might end the trial with unequal numbers in the treatment and control classes. To avoid this, methods can be devised to ensure that the numbers are equalized at, say, every eighth case. One way of achieving this is to take random permutations of the first eight integers (e.g., 5 3 6 1 8 4 2 7) and replace the odd numbers by treatment A, the evens by treatment B to obtain AABA, BBBA. Such "random permutations" are available in the common books of statistical tables. It is known that, if the effects of the two treatments are different, the most powerful method for distinguishing their results is to assign equal or approximately equal numbers to the classes. Often it is desirable to have the instructions for the assignment for each case enclosed in a sealed envelope, but in many cases this is quite unnecessary.

Let us conclude this description of a very simple trial by supposing that we have agreed to accept as a patient in the clinical trial every individual displaying certain well-defined criteria; either treatment A or treatment B is assigned to any given patient. The proportions benefiting from each treatment are compared, and the difference between the proportions is tested by an agreed statistical test. The verdict of the trial might be: treatment A is superior, treatment B is superior, or there is no significant difference between treatments.

3. DESIGN OF EXPERIMENT

General principles of design can be laid down as follows:

1. *Statement of the problem.* It is required to test two treatments, and both are believed to be effective against the disease agent.

2. *Possible interpretations of the experimental results.* The possible results of the experiment have been considered, and the interpretations that will be given to them have been agreed on.

3. *The null hypothesis.* An appropriate null hypothesis has been set up— namely, the treatments are equally effective—and a suitable test of the hypothesis has been devised. This procedure avoids the possibility that some special feature might be chosen as the test criterion after the experiment had been carried out. Such experimental procedure would render all probability statements illusory.

4. *Randomization.* The patients have been assigned to the two treatments by a randomization process. The severer cases might still be predominantly assigned to one treatment, but this effect is allowed for in the statistical analysis.

5. *Size of the test.* It can be anticipated that results would be freer of chance effects if the numbers in the two groups were made large. This is true. However, resources of time, hospital beds, manpower, or even cases, are usually limited and thus a compromise is generally necessary. As a rule, using larger groups will enable smaller differences to be detected.

6. *Generality of the results.* A typical conclusion might be that treatment A is superior to treatment B in the treatment of lobar pneumonia in humans as presenting in the particular clinic.

7. *Stratification.* Both patients and disease agents could have been further analyzed. It might be desirable to test separately in children, adults, and the elderly, and to consider the sexes separately. We might consider the groups of patients as *strata*, as follows: children under 15 years, males 15 to 64 years, females 15 to 64 years, males over 65 years, and females over 65 years. The patients in each stratum would constitute the subjects of a single experiment.

8. *Refinement of the problem.* There might be grounds for believing that different pneumococcal types behaved differently. Separate trials could be carried out on each type or on certain agreed subclasses of types of the pneumococci.

4. SPECIAL POINTS OF TECHNIQUE

Clinical trials do not always have the simplicity of the test of antibacterial agents, as in the example broadly sketched in the preceding Section. Some leading principles can be stated.

Treatments to be given should be laid down in general terms before the commencement of the trial. Rules must also be formulated regarding what is to be done if the patient decides to leave the trial (this is less important in investigations of an acute disease than in studies of chronic ailments). Before the patient can be accepted into the trial, a clinical assessment of the existence and severity of the stated disease must be made. This must be done before it is known what treatment the patient is to receive; otherwise there may enter various biases, conscious or unconscious.

Criteria of cure must be laid down. In an acute disease such as pneumonia, survival is usually the important criterion; however, speed of recovery, absence of complications such as empyema, and length of stay in hospital, may also be important. Usually it is best to consider these separately. Certainly, in cases of grave diseases survival is apt to be the leading criterion; but if the disease is rarely lethal, other criteria of cure or of the value of the therapy are often appropriate. These criteria can be considered separately, or often they can be combined.

The criteria of cure should be assessed by someone who does not know which treatment has been given. Sometimes the control patients can be given a "dummy" that cannot be distinguished by patient or medical attendants from the treatment being tested; sometimes the measurement can be performed so that bias cannot enter (e.g., measurements of blood sugar or blood hemoglobin and other biochemical tests can be carried out by laboratories whose members are not involved in the trials). Chest X-rays can be presented to the assessor identified only by numbers. On occasion, it may be quite impossible to conceal from the assessor the treatment class of the patient, however; in these cases, an independent assessor is desirable.

Sometimes the patient can serve as his own control. For example, in an experiment involving skin lesions, we might treat the right side of the body with a treatment lotion and the left side of the body with a control lotion; in this example, we would randomize side of body, since dextrality might affect the treatment of the symptoms differently on the two sides. On the other hand, treatment and control of long-standing diseases often can be applied in alternate periods. Here also we would do well to randomize, thus ensuring that treatment and control have equal probability of being the first on the right side.

In the foregoing paragraphs, we have introduced the notion of control groups. Sometimes it is difficult to decide whether the group is a control or another treatment group. Perhaps the word "control" in this context is an anachronism. As a rule, modern trials involve a disease for which there is a standard accepted treatment, and any new treatment will be expected to perform better than the standard treatment; thus the comparison is usually between treatments rather than between a treatment and no treatment.

5. ALTERNATIVES TO THE CLINICAL TRIAL

It is sometimes believed that there exist acceptable alternatives to the clinical trial, and this is true in a few cases. If a disease has been invariably fatal in the past (e.g., tuberculous meningitis or certain forms of acute bacterial endocarditis), and if under a new drug, known to be active against the organisms *in vitro*, several cases survive, the drug can be assumed provisionally to be efficacious. Further experience sometimes puts the matter beyond reasonable doubt.

However, we are on less certain ground if we try to apply the same principle to a disease such as lobar pneumonia, which had a mortality in the past of, say, 20% in young adults. The type of the causative organism may vary from year to year, for example; hospital policy may change, increased interest in the disease may lead to the admission of milder cases to hospital, or the use of radiographical diagnosis may result in the inclusion of cases formerly not diagnosable as lobar pneumonia.

Sometimes investigators hope to compare the patients of two physicians who have different methods of treatment, or the patients in two hospitals. The same kind of objection applies to each category; it is by no means certain that the two groups are comparable in age, sex, severity of disease, or other relevant attributes.

6. ETHICS OF CLINICAL TRIALS

Some ethical principles concerning the conduct of clinical trials have been accorded wide agreement.

As a rule, the inclusion of the patient in a clinical trial calls for the consent of the patient or of one standing in the relation of a parent to him. There is a requirement for the consent of the individual's hospital physician, and sometimes that of his referring physician (who may have sent him to the hospital for a specific form of treatment). Experiments should not be performed on dependent classes of the community, such as prisoners, the chronically ill, and the insane, who cannot be said to give free consent.

The procedures in the trial should be in accordance with the best ideals of the community at large, especially as represented by the nursing and auxiliary hospital staff, editors of medical journals, and the medical profession generally.

The experiment must be directed toward solving a worthwhile problem in therapy, for which no alternative solution is available. Here let us note that only studies on patients can determine or verify the best method of treating human disease. Moreover, exercises directed toward improving the methodology of clinical trials mut be avoided.

Unnecessary risk and pain should be avoided.

The standard of the general medical and nursing attention devoted to those participating in the trial should not be inferior to those not in the trial.

Information obtained from the trial should be made freely available for the guidance of future therapy and as preliminary information for the conduct of other trials.

Many such maxims could be laid down for the conduct of clinical trials. Further readings on the ethical aspects are suggested in the notes to this chapter.

It is unethical to claim success for new treatments before they have been adequately tested. Much energy has been wasted in the past by introducing new but ineffective remedies that have become widely adopted because of false claims, perhaps made by highly-regarded authorities, influenced by the best of motives.

7. CLINICAL AND EPIDEMIOLOGICAL OBSERVATIONS

It is often stated that progress in medical science can come only as a result of controlled experimentation. However, many advances have been made by observation. In the following examples, the results have been established by a statistical type of argument.

Example   i. Chapters I and XVI present full discussions of the investigations into the causation of congenital defects by rubella. Clinical observations and a study of the official statistics were used. Essentially, the argument to establish the connection is as follows: (a) congenital cataract is a rare disease; (b) in certain years there are many more cases than is reasonable to assign to a chance mechanism operating equally in every year; (c) in the years in which there are many cases, a history taken shows that in a very high proportion of cases, the mother of an affected infant has had rubella in the first trimester. The evidence seems to be so clear-cut that it is not generally recognized that a probabilistic argument is being used. However, what would medical and statistical opinion have been if Gregg's original series had consisted of only one or two cases?

Example   ii. Pulmonary diseases, or as the miners called it *Bergkrankheit* or mountain sickness, had long been known to exist in the mines at Schneeberg, in the Erzgebirge, forming the border between Saxony and Bohemia. According to Lorenz (1944), however, Harting and Hesse (1879) were the first to show that the disease was lung cancer. It was known that the disease affected miners who had worked more than 10 years in the mines. Surveys of deaths in the area were carried out in 1913. The principal grounds for considering a mineral to be the cause of the lung cancers were the length of the miners' exposure and the absence of the disease in the other inhabitants of the villages; 40% of the deaths of miners were indeed caused by the disease, and it could not be considered as a chance association of lung cancer deaths in one area. Doubts with respect to which constituent of the uranium or other ore was the cause have persisted, and radon is now favored. However, the observation was of historical importance in showing that chemical substances could cause cancer. An earlier example was the scrotal cancer of chimney sweeps, described by Percival Pott (1714–1788).

Example   iii. It is of interest to compare Example ii with that of Chapter 25 of Hill (1962*b*), which tells of a much smaller group of deaths due to lung cancer, as investigated by Hill and E. Lewis Faning. In this case, inorganic compounds of arsenic were believed to be the activating cause. Those having closer contact with the compounds, such as engineers and packers, had higher rates of lung cancer mortality than other workers in the factory or in the neighboring town.

Example   iv. McCloskey (1950) was able to obtain the histories of 31 persons who had been injected with vaccines against pertussis, alone or in combination, within 90 days of suffering paralyses from poliomyelitis. In 30 of the patients developing paralyses, out of 45 limbs inoculated, 33 were paralyzed and 12 were unaffected; of uninoculated limbs, 18 were paralyzed and 57 were unaffected. Such a result would be very rare under a null hypothesis that the site of paralysis is independent of the site of inoculation. See also Hill and Knowelden (1950) for a similar experience.

Example   v. The observations of John Snow (1813–1858) on the incidence of cholera in London are classical and have been recounted in the address of Hill (1953) on "observation and experiment" in the *New England Journal of Medicine* (**248**, 995), reprinted as Chapter 16 of Hill (1962*b*). Briefly, the customers of two companies supplying water to the southern suburbs of London suffered high death rates from cholera in 1849. By 1853 one company had begun to receive its water from a reach of the River Thames not contaminated by the sewage of the city of London. In one area supplied by one company alone, there were no deaths. Snow followed up this lead in an epidemic in 1854, and ascertained that 286 deaths had occurred in 40,000 houses supplied by one company and 14 deaths in 26,000 houses supplied by a second company. Here Snow was able to obtain a satisfactory control series because nearby houses in some suburbs were supplied by different companies. The argument is that given an equal probability of a consumer being infected from the water of either company, a concentration of cases in the consumers of one company has occurred; this would be a very rare event, under the null hypothesis of equal probabilities, and therefore, the null hypothesis is rejected.

The observations of John Snow are typical of the conclusions that could be drawn by careful field observations, which would enable effective preventive measures to be taken against a disease in his day (i.e., when the etiology had not always been established).

Example vi. We may mention once more the observations on smoking and cancer of the lung, especially the survey of Doll and Hill (1950) on smoking and cancer of the lung. Here again, the important points were (*a*) the making of observations on the lung cancer cases and on controls, and (*b*) the demonstration that the cancer patients smoked more tobacco than the controls.

Example vii. Lancaster and Nelson (1957) carried out a similar type of survey by questionnaire, concentrating on patients suffering from melanoma. However, it was a far more difficult task to measure the degree of insolation in the cases and controls. Nevertheless, it was possible to establish that the degree of insolation was as great in the melanoma patients as in skin cancer patients, and both groups had experienced greater insolation than controls drawn from patients suffering from other cancers.

NOTES

Texts on Clinical Trials. Armitage, 1960, 1971; Harris and Fitzgerald, 1970; Herdan, 1955; Hill, 1962b, 1963, 1971; Witts (Ed.), 1959.

Texts on Design Techniques. David, 1963; Fisher, 1935, 1970; Kempthorne, 1952; Wilson, 1952.

Texts on Clinical Observation. Kessler and Levin (Ed.), 1970; Morris, 1957; Witts (Ed.), 1959.

Prospective Methods of Comparison and Follow-Up Methods. Berkson, 1962; Doll and Hill, 1964.

Clinical Trials, Historical. Bull, 1959.

Criticism and Theory of Retrospective Inquiries. Mantel and Haenszel, 1959; Myers, 1963; Sheps, 1958.

Ethical Aspects of Human Experimentation. Fox, 1959; Hill, 1951, 1958, 1971; *News and Comments*, 1964; Shimkin, Guttentag, Kidd, and Johnson, 1953; Witts (Ed.), 1959.

Observation. Hill, 1953, 1962*a*.

Drug Safety. WHO Scientific Group, 1966.

CHAPTER XV

Special Techniques

1. OPERATIONS RESEARCH

Operations research (often shortened to OR) is a term introduced during World War II to describe the inquiries or researches into the special problems of military operations; for example, given various resources, what is the best strategy to use against the submarine? An essential feature of operations research is the application of scientific methodology to the problem at hand. The distinction between scientific investigations and operations research, therefore, lies not in the difficulty of the problem nor in the methodology, but in the type of solutions or answers to be expected.

For example, that a certain application of the resources available is probably the most effective against the enemy submarines in 1943 is a hypothesis lacking in the generality of a good scientific hypothesis. However, in other cases, the validity of this dichotomy into operations research or scientific research is not so evident; for example, the inquiries into the causes of invalidity, hindering the construction of the Panama Canal, might have a technological aim, but they could also produce information of scientific interest.

Good examples of operations research in medicine are provided by inquiries into the treatment of patients from street accidents, the handling of large disasters, the surgery of peptic ulcer, and clinical trials in general. A difficulty about operations research as an academic subject is the lack of widespread applicability of the methods, for they are dictated by the special field of study; thus the appropriate methods for the follow-up of treated cancer patients and for the handling of casualties from large disasters will be quite different. However, a common procedure is the construction of a mathematical model suitable to the problem, from which can be determined the effects of different treatments on some factor in the model. This is a useful procedure, since often it would be unethical or very expensive to set up an experiment in the real world to determine the best strategy. Sometimes an answer can be obtained by direct mathematical reasoning. In other cases, such a solution may not be possible. Section·XV.3 suggests how modern computers enable workers to obtain solutions in such cases by way of simulation.

2. THE USE OF COMPUTERS

Mechanical aids, such as the abacus, have long assisted clerks and mathematicians in the common operations of arithmetic. The cog-and-wheel principle used in clocks was adapted to the construction of a hand-driven computer in the seventeenth century. In our century, desk calculating machines powered by electricity were made. In the early 1940s, however, the need arose in technology and science for a means of making more extensive computations at high speed. It was found that high speed could be attained only if the actions were automatic and if the system of wheels were abandoned; in modern machines, the cogs and wheels are replaced by electric circuits. An essential feature is the presence or absence of an electric charge at various points. For maximum efficiency, therefore, it is necessary to carry out the computations in the scale of 2, the binary scale, rather than in the previously familiar decimal scale. We note that the rules of addition in the binary scale are very simple: $0 + 1 = 1$, $1 + 0 = 1$, $1 + 1 = 0 +$ "carry 1." The numbers 0, 1, 2, ..., 9 are written in binary scale as: 0, 1, 10, 11, 100, 101, 110, 111, 1000, 1001. Multiplication is simple and can be written out in a table, as in the following examples:

$$
\begin{array}{ll}
2 \times 3 = \begin{array}{r} 11 \\ 10 \\ \hline 00 \\ 110 \\ \hline 110 = 6 \end{array}
&
3 \times 3 = \begin{array}{r} 11 \\ 11 \\ \hline 11 \\ 110 \\ \hline 1001 = 9 \end{array}
\end{array}
$$

$$
7 \times 7 =
\begin{array}{rl}
111 & \\
111 & \\
\hline
111 & = 1 \times 7 \\
1110 & = 2 \times 7 \\
\hline
10101 & (= 3 \times 7) \\
11100 & = 4 \times 7 \\
\hline
110001 & = (1 + 2 + 4)\,7 = 7 \times 7,
\end{array}
$$

as required for $110001 = 100000 + 10000 + 1 = 2^5 + 2^4 + 1 = 32 + 16 + 1 = 49$.

Subtraction and division, can also be carried out readily in the binary scale.

The computer is designed to combine several simple operations to yield answers to complicated problems. The computer is fed data and instructions, the *input*, sometimes by direct punching but more commonly by preliminary punching onto tapes or cards. There are arrangements in the machine, collectively known as the *control*, for performing the computations, and a *memory* into which information and instructions can be fed and stored and from which it can be recalled when required. After the instructions have been completed, the results or *output* are available, usually in the form of punch cards or printout.

It should be noticed that the computations within the machine are carried out very rapidly and with a high degree of accuracy.

Example   Let $t, u, v, \ldots, y, z$ be a set of k anthropometric measurements for which we want to find the means, variances, covariances, and correlations in a sample of N persons. We must feed the kN measurements into the computer once, verifying that we have transcribed each measurement correctly. When a suitable set of instructions has been fed in, no further human intervention is necessary. On a desk computer, the N values of t must be entered for each correlation involving t (or, for each pair of variables, there will be $2N$ numbers to be entered). Since there are $\frac{1}{2}k(k-1)$ pairs, $k(k-1)N$ numbers must be entered on a desk machine. This means that input is less in the computer by a factor of $(k-1)$.

However, it should be noted that large inputs and outputs in the computer are expensive. The gains come whenever extensive computations are to be performed on the input. In many other cases no great advantage is obtained by the use of the machines. For suppose that we are calculating a mean and a standard deviation; we must record the information—namely, the observations $x_1, x_2, \ldots, x_N$ on a tape—and each step will have to be checked. This takes approximately the same time as putting $x_1, x_2, \ldots, x_N$ onto a desk machine and performing the check computations. Electronic machines are relatively inefficient in classifying and ordering data. Thus if bibliographies are constructed by the use of computers, it is several hundred times more expensive to feed the details into the computer than to make out an ordinary library catalog card. Similar considerations apply to simple survey material. Often, however, the use of the computer can be justified when many operations are to be carried out.

3. SIMULATION

Sometimes medical research, technology, or management generates problems that can be clearly formulated and for which a mathematical model can be constructed. Indeed, complete mathematical solutions are available in certain cases. However, the solution may be of a form too general for easy comprehension. In such cases, it is often possible to obtain a clearer appreciation by a study of worked examples, and desk machines or electronic computers may be needed for this purpose. If chance is involved, the problem may be more difficult to solve. For example, if a stream of patients suffering from a particular disease were to enter the hospital at a determined rate, it would be easy to determine the resources needed to cope with them. If, however, their entry were determined by chance, the hospital would be faced with the more difficult task of determining what resources were needed to keep the waiting time for treatment or admission down to acceptable levels. In such cases, it may be possible to obtain approximate solutions that are sufficient for practical purposes. In the example mentioned previously, the data to be fed into the machine would be the probability of a new patient arriving per unit of time. The computer would carry out a random sampling experiment to determine whether a patient had arrived in any unit of time. It would then work out the consequences of the arrivals and give a summary of a number of such *simulated* experiences.

Example i. A clinical trial can be planned, and we can give anticipated rates of cure in the various subclasses of patients in the treated series A and B. A *simulation* of a trial, whereby the entries to the trial in the mathematical model are imitated, is then possible. Since the computer can operate very rapidly in such simulations, the investigators will be enabled to compute the percentage of trials in which the null hypothesis of the equality of the effects of the two treatments is rejected. (This is the power of the test; see Section XI.5). The assumed proportions of cures under the two treatments can be allowed to vary from trial to trial, and suitable tables can be constructed. (In this example, direct analytic solutions might also be obtained.)

Example ii. If we know the probability of an accident (road or otherwise) at any time within a given geographic unit, and also the facilities available, how large will the reserves of staff and of hospital facilities have to be in order to prevent unacceptable delays before treatment occurs or before a hospital bed has been obtained? It is obvious that in this example we cannot carry out an experiment—namely, observations made using different levels of staff as a variable—but, by a random sampling experiment, we could imitate the accident incidence or other features. We could then estimate the needs for staff and other facilities if various situations are not to occur, say, more than once in a thousand days.

Example iii. We may wish to establish the best rules for admitting patients for interview to a medical clinic, with a view to minimizing time wasted by patients in waiting for the physician or by the physician in waiting for the next case. Rules established or suggested can be tested in this case by simulation, with the inclusion in the model of some probability laws for the rate of arrival of patients, the length of time for an interview by the physician, the losses of time by the patient, the use of hospital facilities, and other relevant factors.

4. THE USE OF CARD SYSTEMS IN CLINICAL RESEARCH

The use of recording cards in hospitals is familiar. We consider here their design and use for the purposes of clinical research, such as in follow-up or epidemiological surveys. Some criteria for their design can be laid down as follows:

1. *The card should have a heading giving the title of the hospital and perhaps the director of the project.* The project's purpose usually can be described in a heading, although sometimes it is better described in non-committal terms, to avoid releasing information that might distress or otherwise harm the patient.

2. *The card should satisfactorily identify the patient.* In some cases, if the survey is only a single interview or examination, the entering of personal details is avoidable. As a rule, however, it is necessary to record the full name, sex, age, marital status, and next of kin; in follow-up studies, it is often desirable to record also the name of any other person to whom inquiries may be directed if the patient should lose contact with the clinic.

3. *The card should be as simple as possible, consistent with the purposes of the inquiry.* It is worthwhile to devote some thought on the purposes of the inquiry, for there is often a tendency to leave the goals undefined and to collect information under too many headings, hoping that new leads will be obtained during the survey. Usually a good deal is known about the subject, however, and it is possible to select a few relevant questions or observations. It is useful to consider how the project would be described at its completion. It is obvious that only a limited number of topics can be discussed in such an article or report, and the whole survey and the design of the card should be planned with the final description in mind.

4. *The mechanics of card sorting should be as simple as possible.* The simplest form of card enables the investigator to have the cards entirely under his control. In a survey of heights and weights of school children, for example, the name, sex, and age, can be entered on a plain piece of cardboard, and the heights and weights can be recorded. The card can be sorted manually by sex and age, and each age–sex group can be subsorted by heights and weights, producing a series of two-dimensional contingency tables. From these frequency tables, additional tables of interest (e.g., the

changes of heights and weights with age) can be constructed without any further sorting. The distribution of the heights with age for either sex, for example, is readily obtained by transcribing the heights distribution from the table for each age.

5. *The design of the card should be as simple as possible.* Blank white cards would be adequate for the survey of heights and weights just mentioned. However, a printed card would be more convenient. It is almost always known that the answers to any question or the results of a measurement will be finally assigned to a determined set of classes. It is desirable in such cases to have the possible results classified by means of numbered boxes in which a cross, tick, or other mark can be inserted. If the boxes are numbered, the results can be transcribed or punched readily onto Hollerith-type cards for mechanical sorting. Punched cards of the Hollerith type have been very useful and versatile. It is possible to punch the numbers 0, 1, 2, ..., 9 at each of 80 or 120 columns, allowing the investigator to make a classification on each of a number of different criteria. Classifications in one variable can be made easily by an automatic sorting procedure on one column of the cards; subclassifications on other variables or classifications can then be made. The possibility of using Hollerith cards makes it desirable to give each set of boxes a location number, which guides the eye of the puncher in the operation of punching from the clinical card to the Hollerith card or special punch tape.

The Hollerith cards can be sorted mechanically; the information from either the Hollerith cards or the punch tape can be fed into an electronic computer—sometimes this is desirable, particularly if it will be necessary to perform additional computations, such as of the coefficients of correlation. It should be mentioned that although the great advantage of the electronic computer lies in these computations, the results of many surveys can be completed more cheaply and rapidly by simpler means, such as hand sorting.

Example i. A clinical survey to determine whether solar radiation is an important cause of melanoma would require a series of questions: the clinical card would have to contain not only the usual identification details and the sex, age, and marital state, but it would also need to have spaces for the answers to questions eliciting data on exposure to the sun.

Example ii. More extensive data are required if the disease being investigated is characterized by a low fatality rate. We may cite *The National Halothane Study: A study of the possible association between halothane anesthesia and postoperative hepatic necrosis* of the National Research

Council (1969). Since hepatic necrosis is not a common complication, it was necessary to investigate the results of hundreds of thousands of anesthetics from a great number of hospitals. It would have been difficult to carry out this investigation in the total absence of mechanization.

5. CANCER REGISTRIES

Cancer registries can be very useful in testing the reliability of mortality cancer statistics. For example, using data on known cancer patients in the registry, we can determine the proportion in which a diagnosis of cancer appeared on the death certificate. Equally, given a diagnosis on the certificate, the registry can be used to check the cancer diagnosis. According to Gordon, Crittenden, and Haenszel (1961, p. 133), mortality statistics fell into disrepute in the 1930s. However, later inquiries based on a state-wide registry system in Connecticut by Dorn (1944), Dorn and Cutler (1954), and Griswold, Wilder Cutler, and Pollack (1955) have shown that mortality statistics in the United States have tended to give a fairly accurate picture of cancer incidence, and we are inclined to agree with this view.

Registries can provide a good deal of information about the incidence and prevalence of the cancers. Owing to the existence of special factors affecting individual hospitals, one hospital seldom has an experience typical of the whole geographic unit, whether it be a city, province, or state. Such comprehensive coverage can only come by pooling information from the various hospitals and clinics serving the geographic unit.

Registries can be very helpful to individual hospitals in the follow-up of treated patients. Their staffs will have special technical knowledge to assist in follow-up inquiries; the registry will be of assistance in tracing patients, moving within its particular area but changing clinics or hospitals, and in tracing patients who move to other areas. Such a central body can also monitor death lists from the statistical offices, such as the office of the Registrar-General (England and Wales). Cancer registries can be expected to produce or assist in producing much useful information on incidence, effectiveness of therapy, and so on, which is essential if treatment is not to degenerate into an unthinking sequence of operations, radiotherapy, chemotherapy, and other treatments.

A central cancer registry can provide lists of patients for studies on the patients' attitudes to cancer, on the reasons for the delay in seeking treatment, on the economic and family aspects of cancer, and on many other sociological factors. The mechanism by which such research might be carried out is a random sampling of the cases on the registry files, followed by inquiries directed to the persons chosen in the sample.

In summary, cancer registries can be of great value in assessing the results of therapy and in inquiring into social aspects of it. The epidemiology of human cancer has its own peculiar problems and must be studied in man. Such studies can be greatly assisted by a registry and, in the past, many etiological insights have followed epidemiological studies.

6. HOSPITAL RECORDS

Records are an essential part of hospital or clinic management. Their uses include:

1. Hospital management.
2. Hospital reports to the management board and local, state, or federal departments of health.
3. Medicolegal requirements.
4. Follow-up studies.
5. Morbidity estimates.
6. Epidemiological studies.

(i) Hospital Management

The patient must be satisfactorily identified, and the details must be entered. In larger hospitals, it is economic to make a template, or "plate" or "disc" as it is known in commerce, which the ward can use for ordering pathology tests, diets, consultations, and so on. This information can be arranged so that it can be transferred automatically to a computer, if required.

(ii) Hospital Reports

If the diagnosis and other details are available in the storage of a computer (i.e., on magnetic tape), the statistics such as admissions by age, sex, and provisional diagnosis, and discharges by age, sex, diagnosis, and state of cure, can be obtained readily. However, much of this information is also easy to obtain by hand or by Hollerith sorting.

(iii) Medicolegal Requirements

In the event of legal proceedings, it will be necessary to have the original documents, which will always have more secure legal standing than recorded information on machines.

(iv) Follow-up Studies

Often the medical records can be used for retrospective analysis of case-fatality or survival rates. If it is known that follow-up studies are to be made, it is always more satisfactory to have a special card completed for each patient and kept in a special file.

(v) Morbidity Estimates

If the admissions to every hospital are known, and if the condition being studied leads to admission to hospital, the combined records can serve to furnish estimates, or at least minimum estimates, of the disease incidence or prevalence.

(vi) Epidemiology Studies

Hospital records can be used in epidemiological studies, particularly retrospective studies. To avoid missing details on important relevant factors, a specially designed card is very useful (the principles underlying its design were discussed in Section XV.4).

7. INVESTIGATION OF AN UNEXPECTED EPIDEMIC

As an example of some of the methods suggested previously, let us consider the investigation by Bundesen, Connolly, Rawlings, Gorman, McCoy, and Hardy (1936)—*Epidemic amebic dysentery: The Chicago outbreak of 1933*. The Century of Progress Exposition held from May 27 through November 12, 1933, had attracted more than 8 million visitors to Chicago. In mid-August 1933, among other cases of amebic dysentery reported, there were two cases from a Chicago hotel "X." It later was found that most cases had been guests at two hotels "X" and "Z." Many of the conclusions of the investigating team were made by statistical types of reasoning.

We may comment on the questionnaires, which could serve as models of tact and brevity. The Chicago Director of Health sent a covering letter stating that he was making a report "which has to do with the vitally important phase of the general health of the visitors," and the questionnaire contained only five questions:

1. Were you courteously received ... ?
2. Have you any suggestions for better future control ... ?
3. Did your observations show that food and dishwashing were handled in a sanitary way?
4. Did you or any of your family develop any sickness while in Chicago or after you returned home?
5. If any illness did develop, please state below the exact nature of first symptoms.

It may be remarked that no question was asked suggesting that the patient may have had symptoms of amebic dysentery.

To those replying positively to the first questionnaire, a second was sent, along with a covering letter including a request for the name and address of the individual's physician. This time, increased specificity was possible, and the following data were elicited:

1. Dates of arrival in and departure from Chicago.
2. Name of hotel or address of home.
3. Name of each place at which meals were eaten.
4. Name of hotel or restaurant at which most meals were consumed.
5. Name and address of each physician consulted in Chicago.
6–9. Questions on symptoms and course of the disease.
10. Patient's opinion on the source of the illness.

The third questionnaire, sent to the physician, asked questions aimed at establishing the nature of the illness. As a control, copies of the first questionnaire were sent to the visitors to four other hotels. As a result of these questionnaires, it was learned that 256 guests out of 9919 at Hotels X and Z and 3 guests out of 12,380 at the four control hotels had developed amebic dysentery—clearly suggesting that risk of infection was relatively higher at Hotels X and Z. Additional information obtained revealed that the risk was particularly high for the months August to October, 1933. Since numerous persons had only spent a few days in Chicago, valuable information could be obtained on the incubation periods of the disease, the period between onset and consultation with a physician, difficulties of diagnosis, and many other points.

8. INTERPRETATION OF SURVEYS

Hotel employees and others were repeatedly examined in connection with the epidemic of amebic dysentery mentioned in the preceding section, and the problem is a rather general one. It can be formalized as follows. A *carrier* is defined as a person who carries the parasite of interest at the time of examination (regardless of whether it is detected and whether the carrier exhibits symptoms). A group of N persons is examined by a laboratory test (e.g., an examination of the stools by microscopy). Not all carriers are detected at the first examination, but only a number X_1. These X_1 will not be reexamined, but only the remainder $N - X_1$; X_2 will be found positive at the second examination; ... X_i will be found positive at the ith examination. After an indefinite number of examinations, it can be assumed that all carriers, X in number, have been detected:

$$(1) \qquad\qquad X = X_1 + X_2 + X_3 + \cdots.$$

It is required to estimate X from a knowledge of the first few examinations.

Let us suppose that a given carrier can be detected with a probability p, called the *demonstrability*. Rarely is p equal to unity. Let us suppose that this carrier is examined repeatedly. He will be detected for the first time at the first, second, third, ... examinations, with probabilities p, pq, pq^2, ..., and $p + pq + pq^2 + \cdots = \sim 1$ approximately for any finite series.

If X persons having the same demonstrability are examined, approximately Xp, Xpq, Xpq^2, ... carriers will be detected for the first time at the first, second, third, ... examinations. In the analysis of a survey, we could set

$$(2) \qquad\qquad X_1 = X\hat{p} \quad\text{and}\quad X_2 = X\hat{p}\hat{q}.$$

Thus

$$(3) \qquad\qquad \hat{q} = \frac{X_2}{X_1} \quad\text{and}\quad \hat{p} = \frac{X_1 - X_2}{X_1}.$$

Now this estimate of $\hat{p}$ can be used in (2) to obtain

$$(4) \qquad\qquad X = \frac{X_1}{\hat{p}} = \frac{X_1{}^2}{X_1 - X_2}.$$

However, if p varies between carriers, estimates of X given by the estimate (4) are too small, as a rule. The carriers showing higher demonstrability will tend to be detected at the earlier examinations (see Table XV.1). Thus the mean demonstrability of the carriers, undetected after $k - 1$ examinations, will fall as k increases.

Table XV.1

REPEATED EXAMINATIONS OF SUSPECTED AMEBIC CARRIERS

Examination	Number Examined	Number Positive	Proportions Positive
First	1176	203	0.172619
Second	867	123	0.141869
Third	670	56	0.083582
Fourth	558	33	0.059140
Fifth	454	32	0.070485
Sixth	202	8	0.039604
Seventh	24	2	0.083333
Total specimens examined	3951	457	—

Data from Table 10 of Bundesen et al. (1936).

The problem is treated in full by Lancaster (1950b). The analysis of such data is complicated because individuals may drop out of the survey. Corrections can be made with the aid of life-table methods. The theory suggests that estimates of carrier rates reported for various parasites have almost always been too low. Exercise XII.19 presents evidence that p varies from carrier to carrier.

NOTES

Additional references include the following.
Automation. U.S. Department of Labor, 1962.
Computers and Medicine. Finney, 1965; Ledley, 1962; Ledley and Lusted, 1960; Medical Research Council, 1965.
Follow-Up. Armitage, 1959; Berkson, 1962.
Simulation. Shubik, 1960.
Use of Records. Acheson, 1967; Bachi and Baron, 1969; Reid, 1957.
Operations Research. Flagle, Huggins, and Roy, 1960.

CHAPTER XVI

Statistical Epidemiology

*1. STOCHASTIC PROCESSES

Most of the problems considered in classical statistical theory deal with samples of a fixed finite size—for example, the distribution of the number of successes in N mutually independent trials having constant probability of success equal to p. However, an account of the development in time of the successes cumulated up to the Nth trial might be required. For simplicity, we consider the case $p = \frac{1}{2}$. We might want to know not only the probability of the successes being equal to half the number of trials after $2m$ trials, but also whether there is a positive probability that this equalization is never achieved. This apparently artificial example, typified by tosses of a coin, has led to much interesting but difficult mathematical theory, with applications to many physical and biological problems.

The botanist Robert Brown (1773–1858) observed the constant and erratic motion of small particles under the microscope, now known as the Brownian motion. Albert Einstein (1879–1955) was not aware that such motion had been already observed and that it was, in fact, well known to microscopists; he was anxious to find a physical phenomenon that would make evident the existence of molecules. He deduced that bombardment of microscopic particles by the molecules of the liquid would result in such a type of movement, since the impacts of the molecules were chance effects, which meant that from time to time there would be such a succession of impacts from one side that the particle would move. A simplified mathematical model is as follows.

Time is divided into a number of small intervals of equal length. In each interval, the particle moves one unit of length to the left with probability $\frac{1}{2}$, or one unit to the right with probability $\frac{1}{2}$. The resulting motion—the simplest "random walk"—is one-dimensional. If the process were realized by the position of a light on a line having equal intervals between successive positions, and if the resulting events were photographed and projected at increased speed, we could indeed reproduce the appearance of Brownian movement constrained to one dimension. If three similar processes were carried out in three dimensions—that is, along axes at right angles—a good imitation of Brownian movement would be obtained. Of course, a more complete theory would allow, as did Einstein, for time to be continuous and for the impacts to vary in magnitude.

Models of the development of gene frequencies in a population can also be considered in the theory of *stochastic processes*, that is, the development of a sequence of random events in time. A simple problem is the approach to homozygosity in small populations; for example, suppose that we have $2N$ mice, N males and N females, breeding and select by a chance procedure N offspring of each sex to form the next generation. Suppose further that at a certain locus there are alleles A or a. What is the probability that either A or a is lost to the population, which becomes homozygous at the locus? It is known that one of the genes will be lost with a probability near to unity before the elapse of kN generations, where k is a small positive number.

A variant of this problem is of great importance in the attempt to study the migration of human populations by measuring gene frequencies, usually of the blood groups. A rather naïve approach is sometimes used, whereby the random event that an individual should possess a gene A is independent of the event that a second individual in the population should possess one. However, all the individuals in a population of a given area may well have obtained their genes from quite a limited number, say 100 or even 20 ancestors who first settled in the area. Consequently, all measurements of gene frequencies will be a sampling of the genes of the limited number of first settlers; thus considerable differences may exist in gene frequencies in two such areas, although the populations have descended from a common stock.

*2. POPULATION SIZE AND EPIDEMICS

The phenomena of the waxing and waning of epidemics and the not-unusual disappearance of the infective agent from the host population have been leading preoccupations of epidemiologists. Thus annual numbers of deaths from measles in Sweden are now available for about 200 years, and records of the deaths from measles in England have been kept since the first half of the nineteenth century. Similar statistics are available in other countries for smallpox, scarlatina, plague, and other acute infective diseases.

As a typical example of acute infective disease, let us devote detailed consideration to measles. The modern study of measles can be said to have begun with the description of Panum (1846) of an intense epidemic of measles in the Faeroe Islands in that year. In an era before the laboratory investigations of the infectious diseases, Panum was able to establish that measles was infective from person to person and that an incubation period of about 14 days elapsed between infection and the appearance of an exanthem (i.e., rash) when the patient was infective. He believed that the immunity provoked by the disease was long standing and that elderly persons, who had had the disease at the time of an epidemic in 1781, were immune. It is now known that a second attack of measles is comparatively rare.

Since Panum's time, it has been established that the disease is due to a filter-passing virus. His main conclusions were correct, and they sufficiently characterize the disease for our purposes. A convenient source of further references is Volume 103 (1962) of the *American Journal of Diseases of Children.*

The properties of high infectivity, fixed incubation period, and immunity to subsequent attack can be included in the mathematical model of the progress of an epidemic. Such early workers as Sir Ronald Ross (1857–1932) devised a *deterministic model* of an epidemic. For simplicity, a community is supposed to consist of N susceptible persons, and there is introduced into it, a single case of the disease. Since each person in the community is assumed to have a constant probability of infecting any susceptible member of the community, the number of new infections is proportional to the product of the number of infected cases and the number of susceptibles. In this model it is also supposed that N is so large that we can treat the number of new cases per unit of time as equal to the expected proportion. Let y now be the number of infected persons at time t and let λ be the rate at which the interaction between one infective and one susceptible individual leads to the susceptible becoming infected. We now have

$$(1) \qquad \frac{dy}{dt} = \lambda y (N - y),$$

or equivalently

$$(2) \qquad \frac{N \, dy}{y(N - y)} = N\lambda \, dt,$$

or

$$(3) \qquad \frac{dy}{y} + \frac{dy}{N - y} = N\lambda \, dt.$$

Equation 3 yields

$$(4) \qquad \log y - \log(N - y) = N\lambda t + C,$$

where C is a constant determined by the initial conditions $y = 1$ when $t = 0$; therefore, $C = -\log(N - 1)$, and we can write

(5)
$$\frac{y}{N - y} = \frac{\exp(N\lambda t)}{(N - 1)},$$

or

(6)
$$y[(N - 1) + \exp(N\lambda t)] = N \exp(N\lambda t),$$

or

(7)
$$y = \frac{N}{1 + (N - 1)\exp(-N\lambda t)}.$$

The defect of this model is its implication that every member of the population will become infected. Indeed, $y = N$ when $t \to +\infty$. Models can be constructed in which the susceptibles become infected, remain infective for a limited period, and become immune from further attack or, alternatively, die. Thus it is possible to construct models that imitate characteristic features of any individual disease. For example, the transmission of the disease agent through a cycle in an alternative host could be allowed for in the model. However, as the conditions are elaborated, the mathematical treatment becomes more difficult.

A. G. McKendrick (1876–1943) and W. O. Kermack (1898–1970) saw the need to introduce a stochastic element into the mathematical model of an epidemic. It is common experience that an infective case does not infect all susceptibles with whom he comes in contact. There is a probability p, $0 < p < 1$, that such a contact will result in an infection. Moreover, as the epidemic progresses there will be an increasing proportion of immunes, and thus an infective case will have a lower expectation of cases infected from him as the epidemic progresses. In populations of a finite size, therefore, there will be a stage in the epidemic during which the number of new cases begins to fall and the epidemic terminates.

Let us consider the minimum size of a population that would be required to support a measles epidemic if it were under our control. The period of incubation can be assumed to be 14 days and the period of infectivity 3 days. There will be needed one new case every 14 days. However, it is by no means certain that the appropriate infection will occur in the meeting of the case and the susceptible, and there is a distinct probability that the epidemic chain will be broken. For these reasons, we might make a provision against such a break in the chain by infecting two cases at each link in the chain. Thus about 50 new cases will be required every year to maintain the epidemic with a reasonable probability of success. In addition, 50 new births per annum will be needed, or a population of about 2000 persons. In a natural epidemic, more cases will be needed at each link of the chain, for the cases may not meet suitably susceptible contacts. This means that the actual number needed to maintain an epidemic is much greater than 2000 persons under natural conditions; further, from time to time there will be epidemics which use up the susceptibles at too fast a rate. Thus measles will tend to die out in island communities.

Simulation experiments on the minimum size of population required to maintain an epidemic of measles under natural conditions have suggested 250,000 as an adequate size. However, data from Australia suggest that the minimum size in actual populations may be much larger. This should not surprise us, since the total population of the world has failed to maintain epidemic influenza, for serological evidence suggests that each new pandemic is the result of an introduction of a new strain of the influenza virus, which cannot be isolated from the population after the pandemic has ceased.

A mathematical model of an epidemic might then be devised as follows. At time $t = 0$, there are n susceptibles and 1 infective. There is mixing of the population such that, in any given unit of time, every infective case has an equal probability of infecting any susceptible in the population. New cases become infective after a specified time (incubation period) and remain so for a specified time (infective period); after which they are no longer infective and are immune to further infection.

Mathematicians have worked out the consequences of such models and have revealed that they exhibit many of the properties of epidemics as observed. Their special value lies in showing that certain special hypotheses made to explain the behavior of real epidemics are unnecessary. For example, there is no need to postulate changes in the infectivity of the organism to explain why epidemics die out before all susceptibles have been attacked, because in the model the same phenomenon can be observed when the corresponding parameter—the probability of a case infecting a susceptible—is held constant.

3.   EPIDEMIC BEHAVIOR

The mathematical model of an epidemic suggested in Section XVI.2 appears to describe what might happen when measles is introduced into a small population. The observations of Panum (1846) in the Faeroe Islands, of Gordon (1875), Squire (1875–1877) and others in Fiji, and of Fog-Poulsen (1957) in Greenland, are but a few of the many that could be cited.

It is clear from such observations that measles could not have persisted in the small human populations of the Old Stone Age, and it has been suggested that measles has been introduced into the human populations as a mutation from a virus in an animal population such as canine distemper, whose virus is closely related to the virus of measles.

Some viruses can persist in the human population by lying dormant in the body cells such as the virus of *herpes simplex*, which may become activated at the time of a common cold, or *herpes zoster*, due to the virus of *varicella*, which can lie latent in the nerve tissues for decades, and then multiply to become responsible for the cutaneous lesions, allowing it possible access to further susceptibles. A virus possessing this property of dormancy can cause an epidemic of indefinite length on an island of small population.

The considerations of the importance of the size of the population have thrown new light on the epidemic behavior of plague. There have been a number of pandemics of plague due to *Pasteurella pestis*, and the pandemic has died out in every country in which it has been epidemic—except in its classical endemic foci around the Himalayas and in Ethiopia and in its recently acquired endemic foci elsewhere in Africa and North America. In these foci, plague is responsible for subacute infections in wild rodents.

The occurrence of a pandemic can now be described. The infection has persisted as an endemic in the wild rodents and then, for reasons not clearly understood, the infection spreads to the field rat *Rattus norvegicus* and to the domestic rat *Rattus rattus*. Once it becomes established in *Rattus rattus*, the infection can spread along the human routes of communication, in vessels carrying grain or in other ships, for example, perhaps subsequently infecting the rats in many cities to cause a pandemic. However, the epidemic is unstable with respect to *R. rattus* and *R. norvegicus*, because the disease is acute in these animals, killing the rat or leaving it immune from further infection. Thus we find that the disease has failed to obtain a permanent footing outside the "natural" habitat in the areas about the Himalayas and in Ethiopia and in the acquired habitats in Africa and North America.

4. RUBELLA EPIDEMICS AND CONGENITAL DEFECTS

We are now in a position to offer an explanation of the epidemics of deafness and other congenital defects that have occurred in Australia (see tables in Chapter I).

Measles and rubella have similar properties: both are virus diseases having no carrier state, and second infections are rare because each virus provokes a high degree of immunity in those infected. In the large aggregations of populations in Europe and North America, measles, and presumably also rubella, were diseases of childhood. They caused infection in a high proportion of the population passing through childhood, and adults were generally immune to both measles and rubella in the areas cited.

The striking statistics of Stocks (1942) and the annual reports of the

Registrar-General for England and Wales suggest that the great bulk of the population were indeed infected with measles in the first three years of life. Possibly the same held with rubella. In contrast to these findings, there is evidence that measles had died out several times in the Australian colonies and New Zealand, for in these places, during certain recorded years, there were no deaths from measles. Such an absence of deaths from measles suggests that no more than 100 or 150 cases could have appeared in the year in question, and even that the infection had died out—for it is unlikely that as few as 100 or 150 cases would be arranged in a nice chain to keep the epidemic in being. Moreover, the reports of the official statisticians state that measles epidemics did in fact die out. Additional confirmation of this hypothesis comes from the age distributions of the cases and deaths in the Australian and New Zealand epidemics of measles. Specifically, a far higher proportion of the deaths occurred in adults in those places than in England, which indicates that many adults may not have been exposed to measles infection during childhood.

It is a plausible inference that rubella epidemics also died out, and this is the opinion of experienced practical epidemiologists of the period. Females thus passed through childhood without becoming immune to rubella. When rubella was reintroduced into Australia, epidemics with many adult female cases occurred, and a proportion of women in the first semester of pregnancy were infected with rubella. Thus it seemed that the Australian and New Zealand populations, rather than the rubella virus active in them, were unique. The observations of Sigurjonsson (1961, 1962) are important in that they suggest that every epidemic of rubella in Iceland was followed by congenital malformations and that epidemics of congenital deafness occurred in Iceland only when there had been a preceding epidemic of rubella there. Rutstein, Nickerson, and Heald (1952) were able to demonstrate that the births of babies suffering from congenital heart disease had a seasonal incidence that could be attributed to the seasonal incidence of rubella infections.

Much interest was aroused by the original report of Gregg (1941), and it was hoped and even anticipated that a large proportion of congenital defects would be shown to be due to infective agents. However, it appears that rubella plays a role, exceptional among the infective agents, in producing congenital defects.

NOTES

Epidemiology Texts.   Bailey, 1957; *British Medical Bulletin*, 1971; Burnet, 1953; Chiang, 1968; Cockburn, 1963; Creighton, 1891, 1894; Fletcher, 1963; Fox, Hall, and Elveback, 1970; Greenwood, 1932, 1935, 1936*b*,

1946; Haenszel (Ed.), 1966; Kessler and Levin (Eds.), 1970; May (Ed.), 1961; Morris, 1957; Paul, 1966; Rolleston, 1937; Taylor and Knowelden, 1964; Topley and Wilson, 1936; Westergaard, 1881.

Bibliographies of Epidemiology. Ovenall, 1965; Serfling, 1952.

General Texts of Bacteriology. Rahn, 1939; Topley and Wilson, 1936.

Infections. Dauer, Korns, and Schuman, 1968; Dietz, 1967; Grainger, 1958; Lancaster, 1952*a*, 1952*b*, 1953*a*, 1954*b*, 1963, 1964*a*, 1967; Siegel and Fuerst, 1966.

Population Size and Epidemics. Bartlett, 1957, 1960*a*, 1960*b*.

Epidemic Waves. Ransome, 1880. Bartlett, 1956.

Herpes. Hope-Simpson, 1954, 1965.

Measles. Black, 1966; Fog-Poulsen, 1957; Gordon, 1875; Panum, 1846; Peart and Nagler, 1954; Rolleston, 1937; Squire, 1875–1877.

Rubella and Congenital Deafness. Aycock and Ingalls, 1946; Fraser (1964*a*, 1964*b*) Hay, 1949, 1953; Hopkins, 1946, 1949; Ingalls, Babbott, Hampson, and Gordon, 1960; Lancaster, 1951*a*, 1954*a*, 1964*b*; Lancaster and Pickering, 1952; Lundstrom, 1962; Manson, Logan, and Loy, 1960; Sigurjonsson, 1961, 1962; Swan, Tostevin, and Black, 1946; Swan, Tostevin, Moore, Mayo, and Black, 1943.

Epidemiology of Noninfective Diseases. *British Medical Bulletin*, 1971; Haenszel (Ed.), 1966; Reid, 1960.

Ecology. Clegg, 1968; Gordon, 1966; Kartman, 1967; Pavlovsky, 1963; Rogers, 1960.

Geographical Pathology. Chaklin, 1962; Doll (Ed.), 1959; Steiner, 1954; Zelinsky, 1962.

Stochastic Processes. Bartlett, 1961, 1968; Chiang, 1968; McKendrick, 1926.

Surveillance of Communicable Diseases. Langmuir, 1963.

Congenital Defects. Shapiro, Ross, and Levine, 1965; Stevenson, Johnston, Stewart, and Golding, 1966; Siegel, Fuerst, and Peress, 1966; Warkany and Kalter, 1961.

CHAPTER XVII

Problems of Classification

1. INTRODUCTORY

Classification problems arise in many different fields. First, at an early stage in a science such as botany or zoology, the objects of study have to be arranged in sets with common properties, the *taxa* (singular, *taxon*). Historically in medicine, the states of ill-health had first to be classified into *disease syndromes* or *diseases.* We may call this the *taxonomy* problem. Second, once a classification had been established (i.e., when the taxa have been defined), there is a need to determine the taxon to which a given individual belongs. This is the *diagnosis* problem. Third, the method of diagnosis that is most economical in time and energy and yet efficient has to be determined. Fourth, norms for good classification have to be established.

Closely related to the four problems just named is the classification of factual material or *information* in such a way that it can be readily retrieved—the problem of *information retrieval*.

2. ELEMENTARY SET THEORY

In presenting the classification problems, let us introduce some elements of elementary set theory. The individuals to be classified belong to a collection or *set*, U. The set is just this collection, thought of as a whole or unit. A *subset* of U is any collection of individuals belonging to U. It may contain every individual, in which case it is called *improper*. It is necessary also to define the *empty set* or *null set*, which contains no member. To every subset A there is a *complement* or *complementary* subset containing precisely those members of U which do not belong to A. The *union* of two subsets A and B is written $A \cup B$; to the *union* belong those individuals x which belong to A or to B or to both and no other individual. The union sign has the force of "and/or." The *intersection* of two subsets is written $A \cap B$ or, usually, more shortly AB. To AB belong those individuals, which belong both to A and to B, and no other individual. The intersection sign has the force of "and." A *classification* is a set of rules by which individuals in U can be assigned to subsets $A_1, A_2, \ldots, A_m$. A classification is mutually exclusive if $A_i A_j = \varnothing$ whenever $i \neq j$. A classification is *exhaustive* if $A_1 \cup A_2 \cup \cdots \cup A_m = U$, so that every individual in U is assigned to at least one set.

If the classification is exhaustive, so that we have

(1) $$U = A_1 \cup A_2 \cup \cdots \cup A_m,$$

and mutually exclusive, so that we have

(2) $$A_i A_j = \varnothing \qquad \text{if} \quad i \neq j,$$

it is called a partition of U.

The complement of A is written $\bar{A}$, and $A\bar{A} = \varnothing$ and $A \cup \bar{A} = U$. A classification by a criterion A into the two mutually exclusive and exhaustive sets A and $\bar{A}$ is often called a *dichotomy*. Since there may be more than one criterion for classification A, B, C, $\ldots$, we obtain $U = A \cup \bar{A}$, $U = B \cup \bar{B}$, $U = C \cup \bar{C}$. These criteria can also be applied simultaneously to obtain partitions such as

(3) $$U = AB \cup A\bar{B} \cup \bar{A}B \cup \bar{A}\bar{B}.$$

Given two criteria A and B, each yielding a dichotomy of U, we have $2 \times 2 = 2^2 = 4$ *ultimate classes*. If each criterion yields a dichotomy of U and we have k criteria, we will have $2 \times 2 \times 2 \times \cdots \times 2 = 2^k$ classes. These are the *ultimate classes* or *ultimate sets*.

It is possible also to define *positive* classes. The positive class A contains all individuals having that property. The positive class AB contains all individuals possessing the two properties, and so on. Since every individual has at least zero properties, U itself can be said to be a positive class. With n criteria, there are 2^k positive classes; for example, when $k = 3$ there are $2^3 = 8$ positive classes, namely: U, A, B, C, AB, AC, BC, ABC. Let us write $n(U)$ for the total number of individuals, $n(A)$ for the number of individuals with the property A, $\ldots$, $n(AB)$ for the number of individuals with both A and B, $n(A\bar{B})$ for the number of individuals with A but not B, $\ldots$. There are relations between the ultimate class numbers and the positive class numbers, such as the following examples:

(4) $$n(U) = n(A) + n(\bar{A})$$

(5) $$n(U) = n(B) + n(\bar{B})$$

(6) $$n(\bar{A}) = n(U) - n(A), \qquad \text{from (4)}$$

(7) $$n(\bar{B}) = n(U) - n(B), \qquad \text{from (5)}$$

(8) $n(A\bar{B}) = n(A) - n(AB)$

(9) $n(\bar{A}\bar{B}) = n(\bar{A}) - n(\bar{A}B)$
                        $= n(U) - n(A) - n(B) + n(AB).$

The partitions by A, B, C, ... are said to be *set theoretically independent* if no ultimate class is empty. Unfortunately, set theoretically independent partitions are almost unknown in nature. Classifications by different criteria A, B, C, ... into the ultimate classes is often termed *hierarchical*.

Example   i. Let U be the set of all animal species. Let A be the species with backbones and B be the species which ferment glucose. Then $A\bar{B}$ is empty. Thus the A classification and the B classification are not set theoretically independent.

The example shows that neat hierarchical classifications are usually not available in biology. To subdivide the vertebrates, criteria will be needed quite different from those appropriate for the subdivision of the bacterial species.

We give without proof the following theorem.

Theorem 1.   *Suppose that there are N individuals (or taxa), x_1, x_2, ..., x_N in a set and that there is a collection of M criteria, such that for every pair of individuals x_i and x_j, there is a criterion which distinguishes them: then at most $(N - 1)$ of the criteria will be needed to classify (or identify) the individuals.*

Example   ii. A set of individuals can be classified by a collection of criteria as follows

| | Individuals | | | | |
	x_1	x_2	x_3	x_4	x_5
A	$\bar{A}$	A	A	A	A
Properties B	B	$\bar{B}$	B	B	B
C	C	C	$\bar{C}$	C	C
D	D	D	D	$\bar{D}$	D

The same schema could also be written as

| | Individuals | | | | |
	x_1	x_2	x_3	x_4	x_5
A	$-$	$+$	$+$	$+$	$+$
Properties B	$+$	$-$	$+$	$+$	$+$
C	$+$	$+$	$-$	$+$	$+$
D	$+$	$+$	$+$	$-$	$+$

In this form, we could insert a unit after each plus or minus sign. Note that x_1 and x_4 can be distinguished by either A or D, x_2 and x_3 can be distinguished by B and C. However A, B, and C combined cannot distinguish x_4 from x_5, and it will be found that no three of the four criteria are sufficient to distinguish x_5 from each of the other individuals.

Since k criteria define 2^k classes, in favorable cases—that is, no class is empty and there is set theoretical independence between the criteria—2^k individuals can be distinguished by k criteria. Therefore, we can assert the following theorem.

Theorem 2.   *Given N individuals* (*or taxa*), *the number of criteria necessary to classify them is not less than the integral part of* $log_2(N-1) + 1$ *and not greater than* $(N-1)$.

Example   iii. If $N = 7$, $2^2 < 6 < 2^3$. Thus $2 < log_2 6 < 3$, the minimum number of criteria required is 3, and the maximum number is 6.

Example   iv. Let $N = 16$, $2^3 < 15 < 2^4$. The minimum number of criteria required is 4 and the maximum number is 15.

It might be thought that the number of criteria required would often be of the order of $log_2 N$. In practical problems such as the diagnosis of bacterial species, however, the number required seems rather to be of the order of N. Thus in bacteriology, the diagnosis of 512 bacterial species seems to require not $log_2 512 = 9$ tests but, rather, a number of the order of hundreds, as is evident from a consideration of the numbers of species and tests given in any text [e.g., Topley and Wilson (1936)].

3. THE TAXONOMY AND DIAGNOSIS OF DISEASES

We consider the classification problems of the establishment of disease entities (the taxonomy problem) and the diagnosis of diseases. There are available to us properties or criteria or signs and symptoms of disease, which have been established by clinicians and other researchers over many centuries; we refer to all these as signs of disease. A sign $\mathscr{A}$ must classify the population of patients into more than one class, if it is to be of any value. A sign taking numerical values is potentially able to define an infinite set of classes, but this is never realized, owing to measurement errors. Thus a sign $\mathscr{A}$ can define a partition into m classes, $m \geq 2$. In what follows we assume for convenience that $m = 2$ so that each sign yields a dichotomy of the universe. This is not a loss of generality, however, since we can always represent a partition into m classes as a series of dichotomies.

Example   i. Classes defined as containing patients having (*a*) no fever, (*b*) fever lasting less than a week, and (*c*) fevers lasting more than a week constitute a partition of the universe U of patients into three classes. We write the classes of those with or without fever as A and $\bar{A}$, respectively. We write the class of those having fever lasting more than a week as B and the class of those who have no fever or a fever lasting less than a week as $\bar{B}$. Then AB is the class of those who have fever more than a week, $A\bar{B}$ is the class of those who have fever lasting less than a week, $\bar{A}B$ is empty, and $\bar{A}\bar{B}$ is the class of those who have no fever.

We assume that we have a series of signs $\mathscr{A}$, $\mathscr{B}$, $\mathscr{C}$, ..., or $\mathscr{A}_1$, $\mathscr{A}_2$, $\mathscr{A}_3$, ..., each one yielding a dichotomy of the universe U of patients, allowing us to write

(1) $$A \cup \bar{A} = U = B \cup \bar{B} \cdots = U = C \cup \bar{C} \cdots,$$

or

(2) $$A_1 \cup \bar{A}_1 = U = A_2 \cup \bar{A}_2 = \cdots A_k \cup \bar{A}_k = \cdots.$$

Certain signs or criteria are said to be *pathognomonic* of a disease. Under the dichotomy by the sign $\mathscr{C}$, the classification of a patient into C is sufficient for the disease. A stronger condition would be that classification into C is necessary and sufficient for the diagnosis of the disease. In the diagnosis of the disease, pathognomonic signs are seldom sought in the early stages, because it is more economical in time to consider general diagnostic signs (e.g., fever, pain, losses of function) which reduce the total number of possibilities to a restricted number. In making a differential diagnosis between the possibilities in this restricted class, pathognomonic signs are valuable.

The process of diagnosis is sequential because various signs $\mathscr{A}_1$, $\mathscr{A}_2$, ..., $\mathscr{A}_m$ are applied to the patient presenting with signs, and it is determined that the patient belongs to a class $A_1\bar{A}_2\bar{A}_3A_4 \cdots A_m$, say. Clinical training then suggests that various signs $\mathscr{B}_1$, $\mathscr{B}_2$, $\mathscr{B}_3$, ..., $\mathscr{B}_n$ should be applied, and this narrows the possible diagnoses to a few diseases. Special signs known to differentiate these diseases are applied next; often only one possibility remains, and a provisional diagnosis is made. To confirm this diagnosis, the possible diseases causing the leading symptoms say, A_1 and A_4, are listed and it is asked whether each could have been the cause of the signs; often these possible diseases can be eliminated because other signs characteristic of them are not present.

The foregoing formalization of the diagnosis problem enables investigators to perform diagnosis by way of computer. Of course, something is lost in the procedure—the machine method requires that observations be made on a number of signs $\mathscr{A}$, $\mathscr{B}$, $\mathscr{C}$, ... which are known to be useful in clinical diagnosis, and the case is found to fall in the class $A\bar{B}\bar{C}D\cdots$. In the memory of the computer, $A\bar{B}\bar{C}D \cdots$ corresponds to a certain disease or to a restricted number of diseases; if the latter is true, the computer printout will recommend certain additional tests to obtain a more precise diagnosis.

Probabilistic considerations enter diagnosis more than is usually recognized, although there is the well-known aphorism that rare diseases should be diagnosed rarely. Because of the need for rapid diagnosis, because of the expense, or for other reasons, it is clearly impossible in any given case for diagnosis to obtain all the information that might be obtained. In addition, it may be impossible or impractical to secure information, for example, on the state of a particular internal organ in the diagnosis of the "acute abdomen." In such a case, prior probabilities may enter into the making of the diagnosis.

Example ii. The differential diagnosis of the causes of enlarged cervical lymph nodes is well known. In an area where glandular types of tuberculosis are common, it will be common to make a provisional diagnosis of tuberculous disease of the lymph nodes that has a high probability of being correct, whereas the same signs presenting in a community not susceptible to tuberculous infection of the lymph nodes would not be diagnosed with the same degree of confidence. The clinician uses Bayesian techniques, named after Thomas Bayes (1702–1761).

Example iii. Let the first urn contain a proportion p_1 of white balls and a proportion $1 - p_1$ of black balls, and let the second contain proportions p_2 and $1 - p_2$. Let it now be supposed that a ball is drawn from the first urn with probability $\frac{1}{2}$ or from the second, also with probability $\frac{1}{2}$. If a white ball is observed at the drawing, what is the probability that it was drawn from the first urn? The probability of obtaining a white ball is $\mathscr{P}$ (sampling first urn) $\mathscr{P}$ (white ball being drawn from the first urn) $+ \mathscr{P}$ (sampling second urn) $\mathscr{P}$ (white ball being drawn from the second urn) $= \frac{1}{2}p_1 + \frac{1}{2}p_2$. The probability that the white ball came from the first urn is thus $\frac{1}{2}p_1/(\frac{1}{2}p_1 + \frac{1}{2}p_2)$. If the ratio p_1/p_2 is large, the probability is high that the white ball was drawn from the first urn.

This is a simple example of the probability of hypothesis, whereby if we are given a priori (or prior) probabilities for various hypotheses and conditional probabilities for each hypothesis, we can assign a posteriori (or posterior) probabilities to the hypotheses after the experiment has been carried out. In a medical context, if a sign is common in one disease and rare in another, its appearance favors a diagnosis of the first disease.

Example iv. In a certain country, let it be supposed that a case X presents for diagnosis, and let us call the probabilities that X has the disease D_1 or D_2, $\mathscr{P}(X \in D_1)$ and $\mathscr{P}(X \in D_2)$, respectively. Suppose that $\mathscr{P}(X \in A | X \in D_1) = p_1$ and $\mathscr{P}(X \in A | X \in D_2) = p_2$, where A is a certain sign and p_1 and p_2 are the demonstrabilities. The total probability that the case X should have the sign is then $p_1 \mathscr{P}(X \in D_1) + p_2 \mathscr{P}(X \in D_2)$. Conditional on the presence of the sign A, the probability that it arose as a result of disease D_1 is

$$(3) \qquad \mathscr{P}(X \in D_1 \,|\, X \in A) = \frac{p_1 \mathscr{P}(X \in D_1)}{p_1 \mathscr{P}(X \in D_1) + p_2 \mathscr{P}(X \in D_2)}$$

If p_1 and p_2 are both close to unity, we should choose the disease with the higher prior probability, $\mathscr{P}(X \in D_1)$ or $\mathscr{P}(X \in D_2)$, as the cause.

4. INFORMATION RETRIEVAL

It is a familiar fact that books can be classified in such a way that nearby volumes on a library shelf refer to related topics. In most cases, a satisfactory position on the shelf can be found for every book. A general form of this idea is that *information*—that is, knowledge or information in the common meaning—can be classified in such a way that the classification will indicate whether any given item or book is relevant, say, to epidemiological theory. Customarily, the results of this classification have been stored on index cards, printed bibliographies, and the like. However, the information is not on instant call. In some technological fields (e.g., in patent registration, in military operations, or in the field of poison antidotes), it is convenient and desirable to be able to obtain the information instantly. It is feasible to achieve this end by storing the information in the modern computers, usually on magnetic tape. For more strictly academic work, these computer methods are probably too expensive for general adoption. A general review of this problem, accompanied by many references, has been given by Lancaster (1970).

NOTES

Texts on problems of classification are Ainsworth and Sneath (1962), Ledley (1962), Sokal and Sneath (1963), and Vickery (1958).

Computational aspects of medical diagnosis have been discussed by Hollingsworth (1959), Ledley (1962), and Ledley and Lusted (1960). For screening, see Federer (1963).

CHAPTER XVIII

Medical Statistics

1. THE HISTORY OF MEDICAL STATISTICS

The history of medical statistics can be said to have begun with the observations of John Graunt (1620–1674) on the *Bills of Mortality of the City of London*, as we mentioned in Section VI.1. For further readings on Graunt, the reader may consult Glass (1950, 1963, 1964), Graunt (1662), Greenwood (1941–1943), Hull (1899), Lancaster (1962), Ptukha (1937), Sutherland (1963), and Willcox (1937). Graunt's great achievement was to show that important conclusions about disease and mortality could be drawn from observations on the population as a whole or, as we should say now, from official statistics.

Graunt may well have discussed the *Bills* with his friend William Petty (1623–1687), whose lively imagination was restrained by rather less self-criticism than was Graunt's. However, Petty saw the need for censuses and the routine collection of information of vital statistical events, which were not to be available in his country for another hundred years. Greenwood (1941–1943), Hull (1899), and Strauss (1954) relate further details on Petty's work.

After Graunt had suggested the idea of a life table, the astronomer Edmond Halley (1656–1742) realized that better data on population and deaths were essential; these he obtained from Breslau. The idea of an age-specific mortality rate seems to be due to Halley. In his construction of a life table he used a notion equivalent to that of the stable population. Johan de Witt (1625–1672), John Finlaison (1783–1860), and Pehr Wilhelm Wargentin (1717–1783) also worked on the life tables.

In official statistics in Great Britain, the next great figure was William Farr (1807–1883), a medical graduate who became Compiler of Abstracts in the Central Registry Office in London. He developed procedures for the standardization of the death rates and an effective method of classification which was later included in or taken over by the classification of Jacques Bertillon (1851–1922), thus beoming the basis of the *International Classification* of the causes of death. Farr compared the mortality in the "healthy districts" with that in the industrial areas and concluded that it was possible to lower the rates in the latter. This notion of an *élite* mortality has proved to be very productive. Farr's statistics were useful also in the work of the sanitarians of the latter part of the nineteenth century—for example, Florence Nightingale (1820–1910) and Charles Booth (1840–1916).

An account of the work of Graunt, Petty, Halley, Farr, and others has been given by Greenwood (1942, 1943, 1948). This is the official statistics aspect of medical statistics, with the emphasis on mortality, morbidity, and natality. It may be said that we still lack a sufficiently broadly based history, even of this limited aspect of medical statistics. For example, there is no easily accessible account of the impact of some of the great French mathematicians on vital statistics, although Irénée-Jules Bienaymé (1796–1878) and Jean-Baptiste-Joseph Fourier (1768–1830) were official statisticians at various stages of their careers, and Pierre-Simon Laplace (1749–1827) worked on demographic topics.

The official type of medical statistics is related to many other fields that are of historical interest. We may mention the political arithmetic of Petty, Charles Davenant (1656–1714), Gregory King (1648–1712), and Richard Price (1723–1791), as well as the later speculations on population by Johann Peter Suessmilch (1707–1767) in 1742 and 1761–1762 and Thomas Robert Malthus (1766–1834). Malthus drew attention to the possibilities of population growth and the relations between population and resources, a problem that is of great importance today. Leonhard Euler (1707–1783) had already obtained an exponential (or geometric) rate of population increase, but the problem had to wait until recent times for the general solution offered by Alfred James Lotka (1880–1949).

Among those who have contributed to the study of epidemics and great plagues, Friedrich Prinzing (1858–1938), Harald Westergaard (1853–1937), and Major Greenwood (1880–1949) are especially to be mentioned.

There has long been interest in the applications of numerical methods to the study of the effectiveness of therapy. Thus Daniel Bernoulli (1700–1782) attempted the assessment of the value of smallpox inoculation. Later Pierre Charles Alexandre Louis (1787–1872) tried to determine factors useful in the treatment and prognosis of tuberculosis by a systematic collection of data, mentioned in Greenwood (1936a). It seems likely that the leads of Louis and Louis-Denis-Jules Gavarret (1809–1890) were later abandoned because of the absence of effective remedies. In Section XIV.1 we briefly sketched the historical background of the modern developments of statistical methods, as applied to clinical trials.

In the nineteenth century much interest was shown in anthropometry; here Lambert Adolphe Jacques Quetelet (1796–1874), an astronomer, and later Francis Galton (1822–1911) played leading roles. Similarly, Gregor

Mendel (1822–1884) introduced combinatorial and statistical ideas into genetics, and Galton began his studies on the inheritance of characters in man. These investigations were followed by those of Walter Frank Raphael Weldon (1860–1906) and Karl Pearson (1857–1936), who developed more advanced technical methods of analysis. Ronald Aylmer Fisher (1890–1962) later reconciled the two approaches to inheritance—the combinatorial type of Mendel and the continuous type of the English biometric school—by demonstrating that the characters studied by the biometric school depended on genes at many different loci.

The foregoing discussion is a mere fragment of a history of medical statistics—almost every branch of theoretical statistics finds an application in the study of man, and the theory of medical statistics becomes but a part of the general theory of statistics, on the history of which there has been as yet no satisfactory monograph. For references to biographies and bibliographies of individuals making contributions to the field, the reader can consult the *Bibliography of Statistical Bibliographies* by Lancaster (1968) and its annual supplements in the *Review of the International Statistical Institute*.

Additional references can also be obtained in Thornton, Monk, and Brooke (1961), American National Library of Medicine (1967), Fitzpatrick (1957a, 1960), and Greenwood (1948).

2. GENERAL REFERENCES TO MEDICAL STATISTICS

There are many texts dealing specifically with topics in medical statistics. Of these, we can cite Armitage (1971), Benjamin (1968), Chilton (1953) on dental topics, Edge (1932), Hill (1971), Mainland (1938, 1948, 1963), Newsholme (1923), Pearl (1940), Peller (1967), UN Statistical Office (1955, 1958), von Linder (1960), and Westergaard (1881). A bibliography on vital statistics has been given by U.S. National Center for Health Statistics (1970c); it is No. 82 in the Public Health Bibliography Series. See also Institute National de la Statistique et des Études Économiques (1952, 1955) and Institut National d'Études Démographiques (1954, 1956).

For more general works on statistics, we may refer to the well-established book by Yule and Kendall (1940 and later editions) as an elementary text and to Kendall and Stuart (1969) as a general reference book (which often gives a simpler account than is implied by its title). *The Statistical Methods for Research Workers* (R. A. Fisher, 1925, and later editions) provides many well-known examples and methods that are readily applicable to medical problems; however, although it is written in concise English, it is usually found by students to be heavy reading, especially because the steps in the mathematical reasoning are omitted.

Fisher's *Design of Experiment* (1935) is rather easier reading, and its influence can be seen in the various books published under similar titles.

Of statistical and mathematical tables, we have found useful the *Biometrika Tables*, namely E. S. Pearson and Hartley (1958, 1972), Fisher and Yates (1963, and other editions), and the Chemical Rubber Tables (1962). An index to mathematical tables has been given by Greenwood and Hartley (1962). Shortened versions of such tables are also available in print.

Texts of biometry and related fields having much in common with medical statistics include Bailey (1959), Bliss (1966), de Beer (Ed., 1950), de Jonge (1960), Finney (1960), Fisher (1930, 1935), Gurland (Ed., 1964), Kempthorne (Ed., 1960), Kempthorne, Bancroft, Owen, and Lush (Eds., 1954), Olkin, Ghurye, Hoeffding, Madow, and Mann (1960), Pearl (1924), Smith (1954), and Snedecor and Cochran (1967).

For the place of statistics and mathematics in medicine and biology, the reader can refer to Dunn (1929), Hill (1947a, 1947b, 1962a, 1962b), Irwin (1959, 1963), Mainland (1960), and Rutstein, Eden, and Schützenberger (1961).

For some special topics in human development not treated in the foregoing chapters, reference can be made to Falkner (1966), Harrison, Weiner, Tanner, and Barnicott (1964), Knussman (1968), Krogman (1941), and Susser and Watson (1962).

3. THE SCOPE OF MEDICAL STATISTICS

Medical statistics can be defined as the application of the statistical theory and techniques to medical problems; but since a broadly conceived study of medicine uses the results of many other divisions of the social and natural sciences, it is difficult to place definite limits on the scope of the statistical branch. For example, the prevention of automobile accidents is a problem in preventive medicine, and so some knowledge of the theories of traffic flow and of accident proneness is relevant. We now mention some fields of study that can be said to have a peculiarly human or medical relevance.

1. *Vital statistics or medical demography.* Mortality and morbidity cannot be considered adequately in isolation from other branches of demography, in which births, marriages and economic social factors are considered in detail.

2. *Growth and normal development.* Heights, weights, blood sugar concentrations, and many other measurements are made on the developing and adult human. Such recordings must be systematized and summarized by suitable means and standard deviations or other representative measures;

normal values are to be established with a view to (*a*) detecting departures from them or (*b*) describing normal development.

3. *Epidemiology.* A search for suggestive associations between a disease and its causes is the field of epidemiology. In many investigations, statistics or statistical modes of thought are essential. There are numerous classical examples of how the statistical methods can be used, and documentary sources have often been important in the study of human diseases. In the nineteenth century, these methods often suggested preventive measures effective against the disease in the absence of exact knowledge of its etiology. There was, perhaps, a decline in standards of epidemiological investigation with the rise of clinical bacteriology after which emphasis was laid on the causative organism. However, there is more to etiology than a knowledge of the causative organism; further there are causes of disease other than infective organisms. Indeed, epidemics can, be caused by inorganic poisons such as mercury, by poisons in foods spoiled by bacteria, or by actual infections by bacteria. The epidemiology of accidents and chronic diseases can be studied by the same techniques of classical epidemiology.

4. *Clinical trials.* With the coming of effective drugs and procedures, the study of the effectiveness of therapy (principally by clinical trials) has come to dominate the attention of many medical statisticians. Here, problems in cost, organization, ethics, and law have given the conduct of clinical trials a distinctly human character, separating them from veterinary trials.

5. *Human genetics.* The long generation time in man and the absence of controlled experiment have required the development of special statistical techniques which have little counterpart in animal observations.

The five fields just enumerated can claim to have especial medical or human significance; but the same cannot be said of the control of laboratory experiments, bioassay, and other procedures, which are carried out in medical laboratories as part of the technology rather than of the science of medicine.

In the teaching of statistics to medical undergraduates in the early preclincal years, emphasis should be placed on the systematization of observations and the ideas of statistical distribution, together with elementary discussion of the control of laboratory readings. In the later years, vital statistics, epidemiology, and clinical trials might well be stressed. In present curricula, undue emphasis is often accorded to bioassay and the technological side of pharmacology.

I have tried in these pages to give due attention to the peculiarly medical side of applied statistics, especially to vital statistics, epidemiology, and clinical trials. However, it has also been my aim to indicate that, beyond the limited range of topics that can be treated in an introductory text, there are many interesting and important fields of application of statistics to medicine.

Bibliography

Acheson, E. D. 1967. *Medical record linkage.* Oxford University Press, London, New York, Toronto. xviii + 213.

Acheson, R. M. 1962. The etiology of coronary heart disease. A review from the epidemiological standpoint, *Yale J. Biol. Med.,* **35**, 143–170.

Adams, C. A. 1969. Nuclear hazards, *Advancement of Science,* **25**, 395–403.

Adams, D. P. 1950. *An index of nomograms.* Wiley, New York. ix + 174.

Ainsworth, G. C. and Sneath, P. H. A. 1962. *Microbial classification: Twelfth symposium of the Society for General Microbiology held at the Royal Institution, London, April 1962.* Cambridge University Press, Cambridge. ix + 483.

Allcock, H. J., Jones, J. R., and Michel, J. G. L. 1963. *The nomogram: The theory and practical construction of computation charts.* Pitman, London. x + 241.

American National Library of Medicine 1967. *Bibliography of the history of medicine No. 3.* Government Printing Office, Washington, D.C. 316 pp.

Andvord, K. F. 1921. Is tuberculosis to be regarded from the etiological standpoint as an acute disease of childhood? *Tubercle,* **3**, 97–116.

Antonovsky, A. 1967. Social class, life expectancy and overall mortality, *Milbank Mem. Fund Quart.,* **45**, 31–73.

Apley, J. 1964. An ecology of childhood, *Lancet,* **2**, 1–4.

Arkin, H. and Colton, R. R. 1940. *Graphs: How to make and use them.* Harper & Row, New York. xix + 236.

Arley, N. 1961. Theoretical analysis of carcinogenesis, *Proc. 4th Berkeley Symp.,* **4**, 1–18.

Armitage, P. 1959. The comparison of survival curves, *J. Roy. Statist. Soc.,* **A122**, 279–300.

Armitage, P. 1960. *Sequential medical trials.* Thomas, Springfield, Ill. viii + 105.

Armitage, P. 1971. *Statistical methods in medical research.* Wiley, New York. xv + 504.

Armitage, P. and Doll, R. 1961. Stochastic models for carcinogenesis, *Proc. 4th Berkeley Symp.,* **4**, 19–38.

Arosenius, E. 1925, 1927, 1930, 1933. Table préliminaire de mortalité et de survie pour les années 1911–1915, 1916–1920, 1921–1925, and 1926–1930, *Skand. Aktuarietidskr.,* **8**, 23–34; **10**, 36–43, **13**, 161–167; **16**, 232–240.

Aschner, B. M. and Post, R. H. 1956–1957. Modern therapy and hereditary diseases, *Acta Genet. Statist. Med.,* **6**, 362–369.

Ashburn, P. M. (Ed.). 1947. *The ranks of death, a medical history of the conquest of America.* Coward, McCann, New York. xix + 208.

Ashford, J. R. and Pearson, N. G. 1970. Who uses the health services and why? *J. Roy. Statist. Soc.,* **133**, 295–357.

Audy, J. R. (Ed.) 1964. *Public health and medical sciences in the Pacific. A forty-year review, 1920–1960. Tenth Pacific Science Congress of the Pacific Science Association, August 21st to September 6th, 1961.* University of Hawaii Press, Honolulu. x + 134.

Aycock, W. L. and Ingalls, T. H. 1946. Maternal disease as a principle in the epidemiology of congenital anomalies: with a review of rubella, *Am. J. Med. Sci.*, **212**, 366–379.

Ayers, K. N. 1969. Maritime disasters, *Advancement of Science*, **25**, 353–356.

Bachi, R. and Baron R. 1969. Confidentiality problems related to data-banks, *Bull. Int. Statist. Inst.*, **43**, 225–241.

Backer, J. 1947. Population statistics and population registration in Norway, *Popul. Stud.*, **1**, 212–226.

Backer, J. E. 1961. *Dødeligheten og dens Årsaker i Norge, 1856–1955; Trends of mortality and causes of death in Norway, 1856–1955. Samfunnsøkonomiske Studier, No. 10*, Statistik Sentralbyrä, Oslo. 246 pp.

Backer, J. E. and Angenaus, Ø. 1966. *Dødelighet blant spedbarn i Norge 1901–1963. Samfunnsok ønomiske Studier No. 17*. Statistik Sentralbyrä, Oslo. 74 pp.

Bailey, N. T. J. 1957. *The mathematical theory of epidemics*. Griffin, London. viii + 194.

Bailey, N. T. J. 1959. *Statistical methods in biology*. Wiley, New York. ix + 200.

Bailey, N. T. J. 1961. *Introduction to the mathematical theory of genetic linkage*. Clarendon Press, Oxford. x + 298.

Bailey, N. T. J. 1964. *The elements of stochastic processes*. Wiley, New York. xi + 249.

Baltazard, M. 1960. Epidemiology of plague, *WHO Chronical*, **14**, 419–426.

Barclay, G. W. 1958. *Techniques of population analysis*. Wiley, New York. xiv + 311.

Bartlett, M. S. 1956. Deterministic and stochastic models for recurrent epidemics. *Proc. 3rd Berkeley Symp.*, **4**, 81–109.

Bartlett, M. S. 1957. Measles periodicity and community size, *J. Roy. Statist. Soc.* **120A**, 48–70.

Bartlett, M. S. 1960a. Some stochastic models in ecology and epidemiology, in Olkin et al. (1960). *Contributions to probability and statistics: Essays in honor Harold Hotelling. Stanford Studies in Mathematics and Statistics, No. 2.*

Bartlett, M. S. 1960b. The critical community size for measles in the United States, *J. Roy. Statist. Soc.*, **A123**, 37–44.

Bartlett, M. S. 1961. Monte Carlo studies in ecology and epidemiology, *Proc. 4th Berkeley Symp.*, **4**, 39–55.

Bartlett, M. S. 1968. *Biomathematics: An inaugural lecture delivered before the University of Oxford on 28th May, 1968*. Clarendon Press, Oxford. 28 pp.

Beaujeu-Garnier, J. 1956. *Géographie de la population*, Vol. I. Librarie de Medicis, Paris. 435 pp.

Béhar, M. 1964. Death and disease in infants and toddlers of preindustrial countries, *Am. J. Publ. Health*, **54**, 1100–1105.

Benjamin, B. 1964. Demographic and actuarial aspects of ageing, with special reference to England and Wales, *J. Inst. Actuar.*, **90**, 211–238.

Benjamin, B. 1966. Mortality trends in the world, *J. Roy. Statist. Soc.*, **A129**, 216–221.

Benjamin, B. 1968. *Health and vital statistics*. Allen & Unwin, London. 307 pp.

Berkson, J. 1944. "Blood count error," in *Medical physics*, O. Glasser (Ed.), Vol. I, pp. 1–14. xlvi + 1744. Yearbook Publishers, Chicago.

Berkson, J. 1962. Prognosis of malignant tumors of the breast: A review of recent experience at the Mayo Clinic, *Acta Union Int. Contre Cancer*, **18**, 1003–1008.

Berkson, J., Magath, T. B., and Hurn, M. 1935. Laboratory standards in relation to chance fluctuations of the erythrocyte count as estimated with the hemocytometer, *J. Am. Statist. Assoc.*, **30**, 414–426.

Berkson, J., Magath, T. B., and Hurn, M. 1940. The error of estimate of the red blood cell as made with the hemocytometer, *Am. J. Physiol.*, **128**, 309–323.

Black, F. L. 1966. Measles endemicity in insular populations: Critical community size and its evolutionary implication, *J. Theoret. Biol.*, **11**, 207–211.

266   BIBLIOGRAPHY

Black, H. K. 1969. The conveyance of dangerous substances by road, *Advancement of Science*, **25**, 381–385.

Blake, I. 1969. Climate, survival and the second-class societies in Palestine before 3000 B.C., *Advancement of Science*, **25**, 409–421.

Blake, J. B. 1959. *Public health in the town of Boston, 1630–1822*. Harvard University Press, Cambridge, Mass. xiv + 278.

Bliss, C. J. 1966. *Statistics in biology: Statistical methods for research in the natural sciences*. McGraw-Hill, New York. xiv + 558.

Boeckh, R. 1886. *Statistisches Jahrbuch der Stadt Berlin: Statistik des Jahres 1884*. Berlin.

Boeckh, R. 1890. Die statistische Messung der ehelichen Fruchtbarkeit, *Bull. Int. Statist. Inst.*, **5**, 159–187.

Bose, S. K. and Dey, A. K. (Eds.) 1964. *Asian pediatrics. The scientific proceedings of the first all-Asian Congress of Pediatrics, New Delhi, January, 1961*. Asia Publishing House, New York. xx + 476.

Bourlière, F. 1970. *The assessment of biological age in man*. Public Health Paper, No. 37, World Health Organization, Geneva. 67 pp.

Brass, W., Coale, A. J., Demeny, P., Heisel, D. F., Lorimer, F., Romaniuk, F., and van de Walle, E. 1968. *The demography of tropical Africa*. Princeton University Press, Princeton, N.J. xxx + 539.

Brinton, W. C. 1914. *Graphic methods for presenting facts*. Engineering Magazine Co., New York. xii + 371.

Brinton, W. C. 1914–1915. Joint Committee on Standards for Graphic Presentation, *Publ. Am. Statist. Assoc.*, **14**, 790–797.

Brinton, W. C. 1915. *Preliminary report of the Joint Committee on Standards for Graphic Presentation*. American Society of Mechanical Engineers.

Brinton, W. C. 1939. *Graphic presentation*. Brinton Associates, New York. 512 pp.

British Medical Bulletin. 1971. Epidemiology of noncommunicable disease, *Brit. Med. Bull.*, **27**, No. 1.

Brockington, F. 1967. *World health*. Churchill, London. x + 373.

Bryan, W. R. 1961. Virus carcinogenesis, *Proc. 4th Berkeley Symp.*, **4**, 123–152.

Bull, J. P. 1959. The historical development of clinical therapeutic trials, *J. Chronic Dis.*, **10**, 218–248.

Bundesen, H. N., Connolly, J. I., Gorman, A. E., Hardy, A. V., McCoy, G. W., and Rawlings, I. D. 1936. *Epidemic amebic dysentery*. National Institute of Health Bulletin No. 166. Government Printing Office, Washington, D.C. xi + 187.

Burnet, (F). M. 1953. *Natural history of infectious disease*. Cambridge University Press, Cambridge. x + 356.

Butler, N. R. and Bonham, D. G. 1963. *Perinatal mortality*. Livingstone, Edinburgh. xvi + 304.

Carr-Saunders, A. M., Caradog Jones, D., and Moser, C. A. 1958. *A survey of social conditions in England and Wales as illustrated by statistics*. Clarendon Press, Oxford. xxi + 302.

Case, R. A. M. 1956. Cohort analysis of mortality rates as an historical or narrative technique, *Brit. J. Prev. Soc. Med.*, **10**, 159–171.

Case, R. A. M. 1966. Demography and the cancers, *The Scientific Basis of Medicine Annual Reviews 1966*, pp. 71–90. Athlone Press, London.

Census Library Project. 1948. *National census and vital statistics in Europe, 1918–1939: An annotated bibliography*. U.S. Library of Congress, Washington, D.C. 215 pp. 1940–1948 Supplement, 48 pp.

Central Bureau. 1952. *Social statistikkens historie i Norge gjennom 100 år (1850–1950)*. Central Bureau, Oslo. 83 pp.

Centro Interamericano de Bioestadística. 1955. *Bibliografia de obras sobre demografia en América Latina.* Santiago, Chile. 19 pp.

Chaklin, A. Y. 1962. Geographical differences in the distribution of malignant tumours: Trends in research on the etiology of human tumours, *Bull. World Health Org.,* **27**, 337–358.

Charles, E. 1953. The hour of birth, *Brit. J. Prev. Soc. Med.,* **7**, 43–59.

Chasteland, J. C. 1961. *Démographie: Bibliographie et analyse d'ouvrages et d'articles en français.* Institut National d'études, Paris. xiii + 181.

Chemical Rubber Tables. 1962. *Handbook of mathematical tables,* 1st ed. Chemical Rubber Publishing Co., Cleveland. x + 579.

Chiang, C. L. 1968. *Introduction to stochastic processes in biostatistics.* Wiley, New York. xvi + 313.

Chilton, N. W. 1953. *Analysis in dental research.* U.S. Department of Commerce, Office of Technical Service, Washington, D.C. 216 pp.

Clayson, D. B. 1962. *Chemical carcinogensis.* Churchill, London. viii + 467.

Clegg, E. J. 1968. *An introduction to human biology.* English University Press, London. viii + 212.

Clemmesen, J. 1965. *Statistical studies in the aetiology of malignant meoplasms. Review and results,* Vol. I; *Basic Tables, Denmark. 1943–1957,* Vol. II. Munksgaard, Copenhagen, 525 pp + 319 pp. Vol. III. xiv + 171 pp.

Coale, A. J. 1955. The effect of declines in mortality on age distribution, in *Trends and differentials in mortality,* Milbank Memorial Fund, New York, 125–132.

Coale, A. J. 1972. *The growth and structure of human populations.* Princeton University Press, Princeton, N.J. xviii + 228.

Coale, A. J. and Demeny, P. 1966. *Regional model life tables and stable populations.* Princeton University Press, Princeton, N.J. xiii + 871.

Cockburn, A. 1963. *The evolution and eradication of infectious diseases.* Johns Hopkins Press, Baltimore. xiii + 255.

Comfort, A. 1956. *The biology of senescence.* Routledge & Kegan Paul, London. xvi + 365.

Conference. 1968. *Viral etiology of congenital malformations: proceedings of a conference.* National Institutes of Health, Bethesda, Md. vi + 178.

Cramér, H. and Wold, H. 1935. Mortality variations in Sweden: a Study in graduation and forecasting, *Skand. Aktuarietidskr.,* **18**, 161–241.

Creighton, C. 1891, 1894. *A history of epidemics in Britain.* Cambridge University Press; reprinted, 1965, Cass. xii + 706.

Cresswell, W. L. and Froggatt, P. 1963. *The causation of bus driver accidents.* Nuffield Provincial Hospitals Trust, Oxford University Press, London. xvii + 298.

Crow, J. F. and Kimura, M. 1970. *An introduction to population genetics theory.* Harper & Row, New York. xvi + 592.

Cutler, S. J., Ederer, F., Gordon, T., Crittenden, M., and Haenszel, W. 1961. *End results and mortality trends in cancer. National Cancer Institute Monogr. No. 6.* U.S. Department of Health, Education and Welfare, Government Printing Office, Washington, D.C. 350 pp.

Cutler, S. J. and Latourette, H. B. 1959. A national cooperative program for the evaluation of end results in cancer, *J. Nat. Cancer Inst.,* **22**, 633–646.

Dainty, J. 1969. Fundamentals of water movement, *Advancement of Science,* **25**, 404–408.

Dalenius, T. 1957. *Sampling in Sweden: Contributions to the methods and theories of sample survey practice.* Almqvist and Wiksell, Stockholm. vii + 247.

Dalenius, T. 1967. Official statistics and their uses, *Bull. Int. Statist. Inst.,* **42**, 925–951.

Dalenius, T. E. 1968. Official statistics and their uses, *Rev. Int. Statist. Inst.,* **36**, 121–140.

Daric, J. 1949. Mortalité, profession et situation sociale, *Population*, **4**, 671–694.

Daric, J. 1955. L'évolution de la mortalité par suicide en France et à l'étranger, *Population*, **11**, 673–700.

Dauer, C. C., Korns, R. F., and Schuman, L. M. 1968. *Infectious diseases*. Harvard University Press, Cambridge, Mass. xviii + 262.

Davenport, C. B. 1926. Human metamorphosis, *Am. J. Phys. Anthrop.*, **9**, 205–226.

David, H. A. 1963. *The method of paired comparisons. Griffin's Statistical Monogr. and Courses No. 12*. Griffin, London. 124 pp.

Davis, D. S. 1962. *Nomography and empirical equations*, 2nd ed. Chapman & Hall, London. viii + 261.

Dean, G. 1962. Lung cancer in Australia, *Med. J. Aust.*, **1**, 1003–1006.

Dean, G. and Barnes, H. D. 1955. The inheritance of porphyria, *Brit. Med. J.*, **2**, 89–95.

Dean, G. and Barnes, H. D. 1959. Porphyria in Sweden and South Africa, *S. Afr. Med. J.*, **33**, 246–253.

de Beer, E. J. (Ed.) 1950. The place of statistical methods in biological and chemical experimentation, *Ann. N. Y. Acad. Sci.*, **52**, 789–842.

de Haas, J. H. and Rusbach, H. W. 1964. *Changing mortality patterns and cardiovascular diseases*. Bohn, Haarlem. 95 pp.

de Jonge, H. (Ed.) 1960. *Quantitative methods in pharmacology*. (Proceedings of a symposium held in Leyden, May 10–13, 1960). North Holland, Amsterdam. xx + 391.

Department of Statistics, Wellington. 1961. *Statistical* publications, 1840–1960 (mainly those produced by the Registrar General, 1853–1910, and the Government Statistician 1911–1960). Government Printer, Wellington, New Zealand. 68 pp.

Dickinson, G. C. 1963. *Statistical mapping and the presentation of statistics*. James Thin, Edinburgh. 160 pp.

Dietz, K. 1967. Epidemics and rumours: a survey, *J. Roy. Statist. Soc.*, **A130**, 505–528.

Doege, T. C. 1965. Tuberculosis mortality in the United States, 1900–1960, *J. Am. Med. Assoc.*, **192**, 1045–1048.

Doll, R. (Ed.) 1959. *Methods of geographical pathology. Report of the Study Group convened by the Council for International Organizations of Medical Sciences established under the Joint Auspices of UNESCO and WHO*. Blackwell, Oxford. 72 pp.

Doll, R. and Hill, A. B. 1950. Smoking and carcinoma of the lung, *Brit. Med. J.*, **2**, 739–748.

Doll, R. and Hill, A. B. 1964. Mortality in relation to smoking: Ten years' observations of British doctors, *Brit. Med. J.*, **1**, 1399–1410; 1460–1467.

Donovan, J. W. 1969. *Bibliography of the epidemiology of New Zealand and its island dependencies* National Health Statistics Centre, Department of Health, Wellington, New Zealand. 94 pp.

Dorn, H. F. 1944. Illness from cancer in the United States, *Public Health Reports*, **59** (2), 33–48; (3), 65–77; (4), 97–115.

Dorn, H. F. 1959. "Mortality," in Hauser and Duncan (1959), pp. 437–471.

Dorn, H. F. 1962. World population growth: An international dilemma, *Science*, **135**, 283–290.

Dorn, H. F. and Cutler, S. J. 1954. *Morbidity from cancer in the United States, Part 1. Variations in incidence by age, sex, race, marital status and geographic region*. Public Health Monograph No. 29. Government Printing Office, Washington, D.C. xi + 121.

Drummond, J. C. and Wilbraham, A. 1939. *The Englishman's food*. Jonathan Cape, London. 574 pp.

Dublin, L. I. 1948. *Health Progress, 1936–1945: A supplement to twenty-five years of health progress*. Metropolitan Life Insurance Co., New York. vii + 147.

Dublin, L. I. and Lotka, A. J. 1939. *Twenty-five years of health progress*. Metropolitan Life Insurance Co., New York.

Dublin, L. I., Lotka, A. J., and Spiegelman, M. 1949. *Length of life*, 2nd ed. Ronald Press, New York. xxv + 379.

Dubos, R. 1960. *Mirage of health: Utopias, progress and biological change*. Allen & Unwin, London 221 pp.

Dubos, R. 1961. *The dreams of reason: Science and Utopias*. Columbia University Press, New York and London. xiii + 167.

Duncan, J. M. 1871. *Fecundity, fertility, sterility, and allied topics*, 2nd ed. Black, Edinburgh.

Dunn, H. L. 1929. Application of statistical methods in physiology, *Physiol. Rev.*, **9**, 275–398.

Edge, P. G. 1932. *Vital records in the tropics*. Routledge & Kegan Paul, London. xi ± 167.

Egerton, F. N. 1968. Ancient sources for animal demography, *Isis*, **59**, 175–189.

Eisenhart, C. and Wilson, P. W. 1943. Statistical methods and control in bacteriology, *Bacteriol. Rev.*, **7**, 57–137.

Eldridge, H. T. 1959. *The materials of demography*. Publications of the International Union for the Scientific Study of Population and the Population Assoc. of America. Columbia University Press, New York. xi + 222.

Emery, A. E. H. 1970. *Modern trends in human genetics*. Butterworths, London. ix + 379.

Epstein, F. H. 1965. The epidemiology of coronary heart disease. A review, *J. Chronic Dis.*, **18**, 735–744.

Falkner, F. (Ed.) 1966. *Human development*. Saunders, Philadelphia. xx + 644.

Farr, W. 1885. *Vital statistics: A memorial volume of selections from the reports and writings of William Farr, M.D., D.C.L., C.B., F.R.S.*, N. A. Humphreys, Ed. Edward Stanford, London. xxviii + 563.

Federer, W. T. 1963. Procedures and designs useful for screening material in selection and allocation, with a bibliography, *Biometrics*, **19**, 553–587.

Feld, W. 1923. Internationale Bibliographie der Statistik der Kindersterblichkeit, *Metron*, **3** (3–4), 604–695.

Feller, W. 1940. On the logistic law of growth and its empirical verifications in biology, *Acta Biotheoret.*, *Ser. A.*, **5**, 51–66.

Feller, W. 1941. On the integral equation of renewal theory, *Ann. Math. Statist.*, **12**, 243–268.

Feller, W. 1957. *An introduction to probability theory and its applications*. Vol. I, 2nd ed. Wiley, New York. xv + 461.

Fenner, F. 1959. Recent advances in viral infections of childhood, *Med. J. Aust.*, **1**, 137–140.

Fenner, F. J. 1968. Viruses and vertebrates. Facts and speculation about the evolution of virus diseases, *Records Aust. Acad. Sci.*, **1** (2), 131–154.

Fenner, F. and Ratcliffe, F. N. 1965. *Myxomatosis*. Cambridge University Press, London. xiv + 371.

Fenner, F. and White, D. O. 1970. *Medical virology*. Academic Press, New York. xviii + 390.

Ferrero, C. 1965. Health and levels of living in Latin America, *Milbank Mem. Fund, Quart.*, **43**, 281–293.

Finney, D. J. 1960. *An introduction to the theory of experimental design*. Cambridge University Press, London. xii + 223.

Finney, D. J. 1965. Statistical techniques, medicine and computers, *Trab. Estadist.*, **16** (1) 43–61.

Fisher, R. A. 1930. *The genetical theory of natural selection*. Clarendon Press, Oxford. xiv + 272.

Fisher, R. A. 1935. *The design of experiments*. Oliver & Boyd, Edinburgh, 8th ed., 1966. xv + 248.

Fisher, R. A. 1970. *Statistical methods for Research Workers*, 14th ed. Oliver & Boyd, Edinburgh. xv + 362.

Fisher, R. A., Thornton, H. G., and MacKenzie, W. A. 1922. The accuracy of the plating method of estimating the density of bacterial populations, *Ann. Appl. Biol.,* 9, 325–359.

Fisher, R. A. and Yates, F. 1963. *Statistical tables for biological, agricultural and medical research,* 6th ed. Oliver & Boyd, Edinburgh. x + 146.

Fitzpatrick, P. J. 1957a. Statistical societies in the United States in the nineteenth century, *Am. Statist.,* 11 (5) 13–21.

Fitzpatrick, P. J. 1957b, 1958. Leading American statisticians in the nineteenth century, *J. Am. Statist. Assoc.,* 52, 301–321; 53, 689–701.

Fitzpatrick, P. J. 1960. Leading British statisticians of the nineteenth century, *J. Am. Statist. Assoc.,* 55, 38–70.

Fitzpatrick, P. J. 1962. The development of graphic presentation of statistical data in the United States, *Soc. Sci.,* 37, 203–214.

Flagle, C. D., Huggins, W. H., and Roy, R. H. 1960. *Operations research and systems engineering.* Johns Hopkins Press, Baltimore, x + 889.

Fletcher, C. M. 1963. Epidemiologist and clinical investigator, *Proc. Roy. Soc. Med.,* 56, 851–858.

Fog-Poulsen, M. 1957. Maeslingeepidemier i Grønland, *Ugeskr. Laeg.,* 119, 509–520.

Forbes, W. H. 1967. Longevity and medical costs, *New Engl. J. Med.,* 277, 71–78.

Fox, J. P., Hall, C. E., and Elveback, I. R. 1970. *Epidemiology, man and disease.* Macmillan, London. xi + 339.

Fox, T. L. 1959. The ethics of clinical trials, in *Quantitative methods in human pharmacology and therapeutics,* pp. 222–248. Pergamon Press, London.

Fraser, G. R. 1964a. Review article: Profound childhood deafness, *J. Med. Genet.,* 1, 118–151.

Fraser, G. R. 1964b. A study of causes of deafness amongst 2,355 children in special schools, in *Research into deafness in children,* L. Fisch, Ed., Blackwell Scientific Publ., 103 pp.

Frederiksen, H. 1961. Determinants and consequences of mortality trends in Ceylon, *Publ. Health Reports (Washington),* 76, 659–663.

Frost, W. H. 1941. *The papers of Wade Hampton Frost, M.D.: A contribution to epidemiological method,* K. F. Maxcy, Ed. Commonwealth Fund, New York. viii + 628.

Funkhouser, H. G. 1937. Historical development of the graphical representation of statistical data, *Osiris,* 3, 269–404.

Funkhouser, H. G. and Walker, H. M. 1935. Playfair and his charts, *Econ. Hist.,* 3, 103–109.

Gagnon, F. 1950. Contribution to the study of etiology and prevention of cancer of the cervix of the uterus, *Am. J. Obstet. Gyn.,* 60, 516–522.

Gates, R. R. 1946. *Human genetics,* Vols. I and II. Macmillan, New York.

Gille, B. 1964. *Les sources statistiques de l'histoire de France. Des enquêtes du xviieme siècle à 1870.* Minard, Paris. 228 pp.

Gille, H. 1949. The demographic history of the northern European countries in the eighteenth century, *Popul. Stud.,* 3, 3–65.

Gini, C. 1908. *Il sesso dal punto di visto statistico.* Sandron, Milan-Palermo-Naples. xix + 517.

Gini, C. 1951. Combinations and sequences of sexes in human families and mammal litters, *Acta Genet. Statist. Med.,* 2, 220–244.

Glass, D. V. 1950. Graunt's life table, *J. Inst. Actuar.,* 76, 60–64.

Glass, D. V. 1963. John Graunt and his natural and political observations, *Proc. Roy. Soc. London,* B159, 1–38.

Glass, D. V. 1964. John Graunt and his natural and political observations, *Notes Rec. Roy. Soc. London,* 19, 63–100.

Glass, D. V. and Eversley, D. E. C. 1965. *Population in history: Essays in historical demography.* Edward Arnold, London. ix + 692.

Glasser, O. (Ed.). 1944. *Medical physics.* Yearbook Publishers, Chicago. xlvi + 1744.

Goodman, R. M. 1970. *Genetic disorders of man.* Little, Brown, Boston. xviii + 1010.

Gordon, A. 1875. Official dispatch to the Secretary of State, C.1624, No. 23.

Gordon, J. E. 1966. Ecologic interplay of man, environment and health, *Am. J. Med. Sci.*, **252**, 341–356.

Gordon, J. E., Wyon, J. B., and Ascoli, W. 1967. The second year death rate in less developed countries, *Am. J. Med. Sci.*, **254**, 357–380.

Gordon, T., Crittenden, M., and Haenszel, W. 1961. Cancer mortality trends in the United States, 1930–1955. Part 2, *National Cancer Institute Monogr. No. 6*, 131–350.

Goret, P. 1966. Actualité des zoonoses infectieuses, *Bull. Inf. Minist. Aff. Sociales*, No. 1, 41–65.

Goubert, P. 1960. *Beauvais et les Beauvaisis de 1600 à 1730.* Paris, 2 vols.

Grainger, T. H. 1958. *A guide to the history of bacteriology.* Ronald Press, New York. xi + 210.

Graunt, J. 1662. *Natural and political observations made upon the bills of mortality,* W. F. Willcox, Ed., 1939. Johns Hopkins Press, Baltimore. xii + 90.

Greenwood, J. A. and Hartley, H. O. 1962. *Guide to tables in mathematical statistics.* Princeton University Press, Princeton, N.J. lxii + 1014.

Greenwood, M. 1922. Discussion on the value of life-tables in statistical research, *J. Roy. Statist. Soc.*, **85**, 537–560.

Greenwood, M. 1924. The vital statistics of Sweden and England and Wales: An essay in international comparison *J. Roy. Statist. Soc.*, **87**, 493–543.

Greenwood, M. 1926. *A report on the natural duration of cancer.* Report on Public Health and Medical Subjects, No. 33, Her Majesty's Stationery Office.

Greenwood, M. 1928. 'Laws' of mortality from the biological point of view, *J. Hyg. Camb.*, **28**, 267–294.

Greenwood, M. 1932. *Epidemiology, historical and experimental. The Herter Lectures for 1931.* Johns Hopkins Press, Baltimore. x + 80.

Greenwood, M. 1935. *Epidemics and crowd-diseases. An introduction to the study of epidemiology.* Macmillan, New York. 409 pp.

Greenwood, M. 1936a. *The medical dictator and other biographical studies.* Williams and Norgate, London. 214 pp.

Greenwood, M. 1936b. English death rates, past, present and future. A valedictory address, *J. Roy. Statist. Soc.*, **99**, 674–707.

Greenwood, M. 1942. British loss of life in the wars of 1794–1815 and in 1914–1918, *J. Roy. Statist. Soc.*, **105**, 1–16.

Greenwood, M. 1941–1943. Medical statistics from Graunt to Farr, I–IX. *Biometrika*, **32**, 101–127, 203–225; **33**, 1–24.

Greenwood, M. 1946. The statistical study of infectious diseases, *J. Roy. Statist. Soc.*, **109**, 85–110.

Greenwood, M. 1948. *Medical statistics from Graunt to Farr. The Fitzpatrick Lectures for the years 1941 and 1943.* (Reprinted from *Biometrika*.) Cambridge University Press, Cambridge. v + 73.

Greenwood, M. 1948. *Some British pioneers of social medicine.* Oxford University Press, London. ii + 118.

Greenwood, M. and Yule, G. U. 1915. The statistics of anti-typhoid and anti-cholera inoculations and the interpretation of such statistics in general, *Proc. Roy. Soc. Med.*, **8**, 113–194.

Gregg, N. M. 1941. Congenital cataract following German measles in the mother, *Trans. Ophthalmol. Soc. Aust.*, **3**, 35–46.

Gregg, N. M. 1956. Congenital anomalies due to maternal infections especially in the early months of pregnancy, *Trans. Amer. Acad. Ophthalmol. Otolaryngol.*, **60**, 199–205.

Greville, T. N. E. 1946. *United States life tables and actuarial tables, 1939–1941. Sixteenth census of the United States: 1940.* Government Printing Office, Washington, D.C. iv + 153.

Griswold, M. H., Wilder, C. S., Cutler, S. J., and Pollack, E. 1955. *Cancer in Connecticut, 1935–1951.* State Department of Health, Hartford, Conn. 141 pp.

Grove, R. D. and Hetzel, A. M. 1968. *Vital statistics rates in the United States, 1940–1960.* U.S. Department of Health, Education and Welfare, Washington, D.C. ix + 881.

Gurland, J. (Ed.) 1964. *Stochastic models in medicine and biology.* University of Wisconsin Press, Madison. xvi + 393.

Haenszel, W. (Ed.) 1966. *Epidemiological approaches to the study of cancer and other chronic diseases.* National Cancer Institute Monogr. No. 19, U.S. Department of Health, Education and Welfare, Bethesda, U.d. xi + 465.

Haight, F. A. 1967. *Handbook of the Poisson distribution.* Wiley, New York. xi + 168.

Halley, E. 1693. An estimate of the degrees of the mortality of mankind ..., *Phil. Trans. Roy. Soc. (London)*, **17**, 596–610, 654–656. (Reprinted, L. J. Reed, Ed., Johns Hopkins Press, Baltimore, 1942.)

Halliday, J. L. 1928. *An inquiry into the relationship between housing conditions and the incidence and fatality of measles.* Medical Research Council of the Privy Council, Special Report Ser. No. 120, 34 pp.

Hamer, Sir William. 1934. Health, in *New survey of London Life and Labour.* King, London, pp. 200–244.

Hammond, E. C. and Horn, D. 1958. Smoking and death rates: Report on forty-four months of follow-up of 187,783 men, *J. Am. Med. Assoc.*, **166**, 1159–1172, 1294–1308.

Harley, J. L. and Hytten, C. A. 1966. *Death rates by site, age and sex, 1911–1960 Scotland. Series I. All causes of death. Deaths from cancers at all sites. Deaths from cancer of the digestive organs.* Chester Beatty Research Institute, London. ix + 49.

Harris, E. L. and Fitzgerald, J. D. (Eds.) 1970. *The principles and practice of clinical trials: Based on a symposium organised by the association of medical advisers in the pharmaceutical industry.* Livingstone, London. 266 pp.

Harris, H. 1970. *The principles of human biochemical genetics.* North Holland, Amsterdam. xiv + 330.

Harrison, G. A., Weiner, J. S., Tanner, J. M., and Barnicot, N. A. 1964. *Human biology: An introduction to human evolution, variation and growth.* Clarendon Press, Oxford. xvi + 536.

Härting, F. H. and Hesse, W. 1879. Der Lungenkrebs, die Bergkrankheit in den Schneeberger Gruben, *Vierteljahresschr. Gerichtl. Med. Öffentl. Sanit. (N.F.)*, **30**, 296–309; **31**, 102–129, 313–337.

Hartman, C. G. et al. 1951. World population and birth control, *Ann. N.Y. Acad. Sci.*, **54**, 729–868.

Hauser, P. M. 1942. The impact of war on population and vital phenomena. *Am. J. Socl.*, **48**, 309–322. Reprinted in Spengler and Duncan (1956), pp. 207–219.

Hauser, P. M. and Duncan, O. D. (Eds.) 1959. *The study of population: An inventory and appraisal.* University of Chicago Press, Chicago. xvi + 864.

Hay, D. R. 1949. The relationship of maternal rubella to congenital deafness and other abnormalities in New Zealand, *N.Z. Med. J.*, **48**, 604–608.

Hay, D. R. 1953. Maternal rubella and congenital deafness in New Zealand, *N.Z. Med. J.*, **52**, 16–19.

Haybittle, J. L. 1963. Mortality rates from cancer and tuberculosis, *Brit. J. Prev. Soc. Med.*, **17**, 23–28.

Heady, J. A. and Heasman, M. A. 1959. *Social and biological factors in infant mortality. Studies on medical and population subjects No. 15.* Her Majesty's Stationery Office, London. viii + 195.

Heckscher, E. F. 1949. Swedish population trends before the industrial revolution, *Econ. Hist. Rev.,* **2**, (2) 266–277.

Henderson, P. 1968. Changing pattern of disease and disability in school children in England and Wales, *Brit. Med. J.,* **1**, 259–263.

Henry, L. 1948. La mortalité infantile dans les familles nombreuses. *Population,* **3**, 631–650.

Henry, L. 1956. *Anciennes Familles Génèvoises, Étude Démographique, 16me–20me Siècles.* Institut National d'Études Démographiques, Paris 234 pp.

Henry, L. 1961. La fécondité naturelle, observation-théorie-résultats, *Population,* **16**, 625–636.

Hendriks, F. 1862. On the vital statistics of Sweden, *J. Roy. Statist. Soc.,* **25**, 111–174.

Herdan, G. 1955. *Statistics of therapeutic trials.* Elsevier, London. xvi + 367.

Hermalin, A. I. 1966. The effect of changes of mortality rates on population growth and age distribution in the United States, *Milbank Mem. Fund Quart.,* **44**, 451–469.

Hewitt, R. 1957. *From earthquake, fire and flood.* Allen & Unwin, London. 215 pp.

Hill, A. B. 1947a. Statistics in medicine, *Trans. Manch. Statist. Soc.,* **1946–1947**, 1–15.

Hill, A. B. 1947b. Statistics in the medical curriculum, *Brit. Med. J.,* **2**, 366–368.

Hill, A. B. 1951. The clinical trial, *Brit. Med. Bull.,* **7**, 278–282.

Hill, A. B. 1953. Observation and experiment, *New Engl. J. Med.,* **248**, 995–1001.

Hill, A. B. 1958. The Harben Lectures, 1957. The experimental approach in preventive medicine. *J. Roy. Inst. Publ. Health Hyg.,* **21**, 177–196.

Hill, A. B. 1962a. Alfred Watson memorial lecture. The statistician in medicine, *J. Inst. Actuar.,* **88**, 178–191.

Hill, A. B. 1962b. *Statistical methods in clinical and preventive medicine.* Livingstone, Edinburgh & London. viii + 610.

Hill, A. B. 1963. Medical ethics and controlled trials, *Brit. Med. J.,* **1**, 1043–1049.

Hill, A. B. 1971. *Principles of medical statistics,* 9th ed. The Lancet, London. ix + 390.

Hill, A. B. and Knowelden, J. 1950. Inoculation and poliomyelitis: A statistical investigation in England and Wales in 1949, *Brit. Med. J.,* **2**, 1–6.

Hirsch, A. 1883. *Handbook of geographical and historical pathology,* 3 vols. New Sydenham Society, London.

Hirst, L. F. 1953. *The conquest of plague: A study of the evolution of epidemiology.* Clarendon Press, Oxford. xvi + 478.

Historisk Statistik för Sverige. 1955. *Historical statistics of Sweden, Vol. I. Population, 1720–1950.* Statistika Centralbyrån, Stockholm.

Hollingsworth, T. H. 1959. Using an electronic computer in a problem of medical diagnosis, *J. Roy. Statist. Soc.,* **A122**, 221–231.

Hollingsworth, T. H. 1957. A demographic study of the British ducal families, *Popul. Stud.,* **11**, 4–26.

Hollingsworth, T. H. 1965. *The demography of the British peerage.* Population Investigation Council, London, 108 pp. (Also *Popul. Stud., Suppl.,* Vol. XVIII.)

Honohan, W. A. 1960. The population of Ireland, *J. Inst. Actuar.,* **86**, 30–68.

Hope-Simpson, R. E. 1954. Studies on shingles. Is the virus ordinary chickenpox virus? *Lancet,* **2**, 1299–1302.

Hope-Simpson, R. E. 1965. The nature of *herpes zoster*: A long-term study and a new hypothesis, *Proc. Roy. Soc. Med.,* **58**, 9–20.

Hopkins, L. A. 1946. Congenital deafness and other defects following German measles in the mother, *Am. J. Dis. Child.,* **72**, 377–381.

Hopkins, L. A. 1949. Rubella-deafened infants, *Am. J. Dis. Child.,* **78**, 182–200.

Hotelling, H. and Hotelling, F. 1932. A new analysis of pregnancy data, *Am. J. Obstet. Gyn.*, **23**, 643–657.

Hueper, W. C. 1950. *A methodology for environmental and occupational cancer surveys.* Public Health Technical Monograph, No. 1, Federal Security Agency, Washington. D.C. ii + 37.

Hueper, W. C. 1961. Carcinogens in the human environment, *Arch. Pathol.*, **71**, 237–267, 355–380.

Hueper, W. C. 1962. Symposium on chemical carcinogenesis. Part. I. Environmental and occupational cancer hazards, *Clin. Pharmacol. Ther.*, **3**, 776–813.

Hueper, W. C. 1966. *Occupational and environmental cancer of the respiratory system.* Springer-Verlag, Heidelberg, New York. xi + 214.

Hull, C. H. 1899. *The economic writings of Sir William Petty, together with the observations upon the bills of mortality more probably by Captain John Graunt*, Vol. 2, pp. 315–435. Cambridge University Press. Cambridge.

Hull, T. G. (Ed.) 1963. *Diseases transmitted from animals to man.* Thomas, Springfield, Ill. 990 pp.

Humphreys, N. A. 1883. The recent decline in the English death rate, *J. Roy. Statist. Soc.*, **46**, 189–224.

Ingalls, T. H. Babbott, F. L., Hampson, K. W., and Gordon, J. E. 1960. Rubella: Its epidemiology and teratology, *Am. J. Med. Sci.*, **239**, 363–383.

Institut National de la Statistique et des Études Économiques. 1952. *Bibliographie sur la méthode statistique et ses applications: Listes des principaux ouvrages en langue francaise.* 49 pp.

Institut National de la Statistique et des Études Économiques. 1955. *Bibliographie sur la méthode statistique appliqué à la médicine et aux sciences anthropologiques: Liste d'ouvrages et d'articles en langue francaise.* 34 pp. Institut National de la Statistique et des Études Économiques et Faculté de Médecine de Paris, Paris.

Institut National d'Études Demographiques. 1954. *Études européennes de population—main— d'oeuvre, emploi, migrations. Situation et perspectives.* Institut National d'Études Demographiques Paris. 440 pp.

Institut National d'Études Demographiques. 1956. *Economie et population. Les doctrines françaises avant 1800. Bibliographie générale commentée.* Institut National d'Études Demographiques Paris. 680 pp.

Irwin, J. O. 1959. Biometric method, past, present and future, *Biometrics*, **15**, 363–375.

Irwin, J. O. 1963. The place of mathematics in medical and biological statistics. The inaugural address of the President (with proceedings), *J. Roy. Statist. Soc.*, **126** (1), 1–45.

Irwin, J. O. 1964. The personal factor in accidents—a review article, *J. Roy. Statist. Soc.*, **A127** 438–451.

Jacobson, P. H. 1964. Cohort survival for generations since 1840, *Milbank Mem. Fund Quart.*, **42**, 36–53.

James, G. and Rosenthal, T. 1962. *Tobacco and health.* Thomas, Springfield, Ill. xv + 408.

James, W. H. 1963. Estimates of fecundability, *Popul. Stud.*, **17**, 57–65.

Johnson, G. W. 1964. Health conditions in rural and urban areas of developing countries, *Popul. Stud.*, **17**, 293–307.

Jonsson, S. 1844. Sóttarfar og sjúkdómar á Íslandi 1400–1800 (Epidemics in Iceland, 1400–1800). Bókmentapelagió, Reykjavik.

Joslin, E. P., Root, H. F., White, P., and Marble, A. 1959. *The treatment of diabetes mellitus*, 10th ed. Henry Kempton, London. 798 pp.

Kartman, L. 1967. Human ecology and public health, *Am. J. Publ. Health*, **57**, 737–750.

Kempthorne, O. 1952. *The design and analysis of experiments.* Wiley, New York. xix + 631.

Kempthorne, O, 1955. The theoretical values of correlations between relatives in random mating populations, *Genetics*, **40**, 153–167.

Kempthorne, O. 1957. *Introduction to genetic statistics.* Wiley, New York. xvii + 545.

Kempthorne, O. (Ed.) 1960. *Biometrical genetics. Proceedings of an Internation Symposium held at Ottawa, August, 1958. Int. Union Biolog. Sci.*, ser. B, Colloquia no. 38, Pergamon Press, London. viii + 234.

Kempthorne, O., Bancroft, T. A., Owen, J. W. G., and Lush, J. L. 1954. *Statistics and mathematics in biology.* Iowa State College Press, Ames, Iowa. ix + 632.

Kendall, M. G. and Stuart, A. 1961. *The advanced theory of statistics*, Vol. 2. Griffin, London. ix + 676.

Kendall, M. G. and Stuart, A. 1969. *The advanced theory of statistics*, 3rd ed, Vol. I. Griffin, London. xii + 439.

Kendall, N. 1958. Neonatal mortality in Philadelphia, *Trans. Studies Coll. Physicians (Philadelphia)*, **26**, 76–79.

Kennaway, E. L. and Waller, R. E. 1953. Studies on cancer of the lung, in *Cancer of the lung (endemiology)*. C.I.O.M.S. Louvain, Belgium, Reprinted from *Acta Union Int. conf. Cancer*, **9**, 485–494.

Kermack, W. O., McKendrick, A. G., and McKinlay, P. L. 1934a. Death rates in Great Britain and Sweden. Some general regularities and their significance, *Lancet*, **1**, 698–703.

Kermack, W. O. McKendrick, A. G., and McKinlay, P. L. 1934b. Death rates in Great Britain and Sweden: Expression of specific mortality rates as products of two factors and some consequences thereof. *J. Hyg. Camb.*, **34**, 433–457.

Kessler, E. I. and Levin, M. L. (Eds.). 1970. *The community as an epidemiologic laboratory: A casebook of community studies.* Johns Hopkins Press, Baltimore. xiv + 326.

Keyfitz, N. 1968. *Introduction to the mathematics of population.* Addison-Wesley, Reading, Mass. xiv + 450.

Keyfitz, N. and Flieger, W. 1968. *World population: An analysis of vital data.* University of Chicago Press, Chicago. xi + 672.

Knussmann, R. 1968. Körperbautypologie als biometrische Aufgabe, *Biometr. Z.*, **10**, 199–218.

Koren, J. 1918. *The history of statistics: Their development and progress in many countries.* Macmillan, New York. xii + 773.

Kottler, F. 1950. The distribution of particle sizes: I, The facts; II, The probability graphs, *J. Franklin Inst.*, **250**, 339–356, 419–441.

Kramer, M. 1969. *Applications of mental health statistics.* World Health Organization, Geneva. 112 pp.

Krogman, W. M. 1941. *A bibliography of human morphology, 1914–1939.* University of Chicago Press, Chicago. xxxi + 385.

Ku, H. H. (Ed.) 1969. *Precision measurement and calibration: Selected NBS papers on statistical concepts and procedures.* National Bureau of Statistics Spec. Publ. 300, Vol. I., Government Printing Office, Washington, D.C. x + 436.

Kuczynski, R. R. 1928. *The balance of births and deaths*: Vol. I, *Western and Northern Europe*. Macmillan, New York, ix + 140. Vol. II, *Eastern and Southern Europe*. The Brookings Institution, Washington, D.C. xii + 170.

Kuczynski, R. R. 1948–1953. *Demographic survey of the British Colonial Empire.* Vol. I, *West Africa*. vii + 821, Vol. II, *South and East Africa*. x + 983, Vol. III, *West Indian and American Territories*. xiii + 498. Oxford University Press, London.

Kuller, L. 1966. Sudden and unexpected non-traumatic death in adults: A review of epidemiological and clinical studies, *J. Chronic Dis.*, **19**, 1165–1192.

Lancaster, H. O. 1950a. Tuberculosis mortality in Australia, 1908–1945, *Med. J. Austl.*, **1**, 655–662.

Lancaster, H. O. 1950b. The theory of amoebic surveys, *J. Hyg. Camb.*, **48**, 257–276.

Lancaster, H. O. 1950c. Statistical control in haematology, *J. Hyg. Camb.*, **48**, 402–417.

Lancaster, H. O. 1950d. The sex ratios in sibships with special reference to Geissler's data, *Ann. Eugen.* (*London*), **15**, 153–158.

Lancaster H. O. 1951a. Deafness as an epidemic disease in Australia: A note on census and institutional data, *Brit. Med. J.*, **2**, 1429–1432.

Lancaster, H. O. 1951b. The measurement of mortality in Australia, *Med. J. Austl.*, **1**, 389–399.

Lancaster, H. O. 1951c. Australian life tables from a medical point of view, *Med. J. Aust.*, **2**, 251–258.

Lancaster, H. O. 1952a. The mortality in Australia from acute infective disease, *Med. J. Aust.*, **1**, 175–180.

Lancaster, H. O. 1952b. The mortality in Australia from measles, scarlatina and diphtheria, *Med. J. Aust.*, **2**, 272–276.

Lancaster, H. O. 1953a. The mortality in Australia from typhus, typhoid fever and infections of the bowel, *Med. J. Aust.*, **1**, 576–579.

Lancaster, H. O. 1953b. Accuracy of blood cell counting, *Austl. J. Exp. Biol. Med. Sci.*, **31**, 603–606.

Lancaster, H. O. 1954a. The epidemiology of deafness due to maternal rubella, *Acta Genet. Statist. Med.*, **5**, 12–24.

Lancaster, H. O. 1954b. The mortality in Australia from infective disease (concluded), *Med. J. Aust.*, **1**, 506–510.

Lancaster, H. O. 1957. Generation death-rates and tuberculosis, *Lancet*, **273**, 391–392.

Lancaster, H. O. 1960. Mortality at young adult ages—a relative maximum, *Aust. J. Statist.*, **2**, 93–96.

Lancaster, H. O. 1962. An early statistician—John Graunt (1620–1674), *Med. J. Aust.*, **2**, 734–738.

Lancaster, H. O. 1963. Vital statistics as human ecology, *Aust. J. Sci.*, **25**, 445–453.

Lancaster, H. O. 1964a. Bibliography of vital statistics in Australia and New Zealand, *Aust. J. Statist.*, **6**, 33–99.

Lancaster, H. O. 1964b. Rubella deafness, *Brit. Med. J.*, **1**, 1046.

Lancaster, H. O. 1965. Aging of the population in Australia, *Gerontologist*, **5**, 252–253.

Lancaster, H. O. 1967. The infections and population size in Australia, *Bull. Int. Statist. Inst.*, **42**, 459–471.

Lancaster, H. O. 1968. *Bibliography of statistical bibliographies*. Oliver & Boyd, Edinburgh. ix + 103.

Lancaster, H. O. 1969. *The chi-squared distribution*. Wiley, New York. xiv + 356.

Lancaster, H. O. 1970. Problems in the bibliography of statistics, *J. Roy. Statist. Soc.*, **133A**, 409–441.

Lancaster, H. O. 1973. Bibliography of vital statistics in Australia. A second list, *Aust. J. Statist.*, **15**, 1, 1–26.

Lancaster, H. O. and Donovan, J. W. 1966. A study in New Zealand mortality. 1. Population data, *N. Z. Med. J.*, **65**, 946–953.

Lancaster, H. O. and Nelson, J. 1957. Sunlight as a cause of melanoma: A clinical survey, *Med. J. Aust.*, **1**, 452–456.

Lancaster, H. O. and Pickering, H. 1952. The incidence of births of the deaf in New Zealand, *N. Z. Med. J.* **51**, 184–189.

Lancaster, H. O. and Willcocks, W. J. 1950. Mortality in Australia: Population and mortality data, *Med. J. Aust.*, **1**, 613–619.

Landry, A. 1945. *Traité de démographie*. Payot, Paris. 651 pp.

Langmuir, A. D. 1963. The surveillance of communicable diseases of national importance, *N. Engl. J. Med.*, **268**, 182–192.

Larsson, T. 1965. Mortality in Sweden. *Acta Genet. Statist. Med.*, Suppl. 15. 143 pp.

Latter, J. H. 1969. Natural disasters, *Advancement of Science*, **25**, 362–380.

Learmonth, A. T. A. 1965. *Health in the Indian subcontinent 1955–1964. A geographer's review of some medical literature*. Australian National University, Canberra. i + 80.

Ledley, R. S. 1962. *Programming and utilizing digital computers*. McGraw–Hill, New York. 592 pp.

Ledley, R. S. and Lusted, L. B. 1960. The use of electronic computers in medical data processing, *IRE Trans. Med. Electron.*, **ME7**, 31–47.

Lerner, M. and Anderson, O. W. 1963. *Health progress in the United States 1900–1960. A report of the health information foundation*, University of Chicago Press, Chicago. xvi + 354.

Levens, A. S. 1948. *Nomography*, 2nd ed. Wiley, New York. viii + 296.

Li, C. C. 1955. *Population genetics*. Cambridge University Press, for University of Chicago Press. xi + 366.

Li, C. C. 1967. Genetic equilibrium under selection, *Biometrics*, **23** (3), 397–484.

Linder, F. E. 1949. A case study of the international collection of demographic statistics, *Milbank Mem. Fund Quart.*, **27**, 154–178.

Linder, F. E. 1958. National health survey, *Science*, **127**, 1275–1280.

Linder, F. E. 1962. Some principles of statistical organization underlying the United States National Center for Health Statistics, *Rev. Inst. Int. Statist.*, **30** (1), 33–41.

Linder, F. E. and Grove, R. D. 1943. *Vital statistics rates in the United States 1900–1940*. Government Printing Office, Washington, D.C. vii + 1051.

Lloyd, C. and Coulter, J. L. S. 1961 & 1963. *Medicine and the Navy 1200–1900*, Vol. III, *1714–1815*, xiii + 402; Vol. IV, *1815–1900*, xi + 300. Livingstone, Edinburgh & London.

Logan, W. P. D. 1950. Mortality in England and Wales from 1848 to 1947, *Popul. Stud.*, **4**, 132–178.

Logan, W. P. D. 1951. *The census explained*. Her Majesty's Stationery Office, London.

Logan, W. P. D. 1952. The use of general practice records in studying morbidity, *Monogr. Bull. Min. Health. Publ. Health Lab. Ser.*, **11**, 224–226.

Logie, H. B. 1933. *A standard classified nomenclature of disease compiled by the National Conference on Nomenclature of Disease*. Commonwealth Fund, New York. 870 pp.

Lorenz, E. 1944. Radioactivity and lung cancer; a critical review of lung cancers in miners of Schneeberg and Joachimsthal, *J. Nat. Cancer Inst.*, **5**, 1–15.

Lotka, A. J. 1931. Orphanhood in relation to demographic factors. A study in population analysis, *Metron*, **9** (2), 37–110.

Lundström, R. 1962. Rubella in pregnancy, *Acta Paediat. Suppl.*, **133**, 1–110.

McArthur, N. 1967. *Island populations of the Pacific*. Australian National University Press, Canberra, xiv + 381.

McCloskey, B. P. 1950. The relation of prophylactic inoculations to the onset of poliomyelitis, *Lancet*, **1**, 659–663.

McGovern, V. J. 1952. Melanoblastoma, *Med. J. Aust.*, **1**, 139–142.

McGovern, V. J. and Lane, M. M. 1969. *The nature of melanoma*. Thomas, Springfield, Ill. 196 pp.

McKendrick, A. G. 1926. Applications of mathematics to medical problems, *Proc. Edinb. Math. Soc.*, **44**, 98–130.

McKenzie, A., Case, R. A. M., and Pearson, J. T. 1957. *Cancer statistics for England and Wales, 1901–1955, Studies in Medical and Population Subjects, No. 13*. Her Majesty's Stationery Office, London. 99 pp.

McKeown, T. 1961. The next forty years of public health, *Milbank Mem. Fund Quart*, **39**, 594–630.

McKeown, T. 1966. *An introduction to social medicine*. Blackwell, Oxford. xiii + 327.

McKeown, T. and Record, R. G. 1962. Reason for the decline in mortality in England and Wales during the nineteenth century, *Popul. Stud.*, **16**, 94–122.

McMullan, J. J. 1963. The Brackenbury Prize Essay, British Medical Association, 1960, The problem of the ageing population, *Postgrad. Med. J.*, **39**, 382–393.

Mackie, B. S. and McGovern, V. J. 1958. The mechanism of solar carcinogensis: A study of the role of collagen degeneration of the dermis in the production of skin cancer, *Arch. Dermatol.*, **78**, 218–244.

Mackintosh, J. M. 1964. The relevance of western experience to the needs of cities in developing countries, *Popul. Stud.*, **17**, 311–320.

Magath, T. B., Berkson, J., and Hurn, M. 1936. The error of determination of the erythrocyte count, *Am. J. Clin. Pathol.*, **6**, 568–579.

Mainland, D. 1938. *The treatment of clinical and laboratory data*. Oliver & Boyd, Edinburgh. xi + 340.

Mainland, D. 1948. Statistical methods in medical research. I. Qualitative statistics (enumeration data), *Can. J. Res.*, **E26**, 1–166.

Mainland, D. 1960. The use and misuse of statistics in medical publications, *Clin. Pharmacol. Therap.*, **1**, 411–422.

Mainland, D. 1963. *Elementary medical statistics*, 2nd ed. Saunders, London. xiii + 381.

Manson, M. M., Logan, W. P. D., and Loy, R. M. 1960. *Rubella and other virus infections during pregnancy*. Reports on Public Health and Medical Subjects No. 101, Her Majesty's Stationery Office, London.

Mantel, N. and Haenszel, W. 1959. Statistical aspects of the analysis of data from retrospective studies of disease, *J. Nat. Cancer Inst.*, **22**, 719–748.

Martin, W. J. 1960. The trend of mortality since 1840, *Med. Officer*, **104**, 273–280.

Mathiessen, P. C. 1965. *Infant mortality in Denmark, 1931–1960*. Statistical Department, Copenhagen. 100 pp.

May, J. M. (Ed.) 1961. *Studies in disease ecology*. Hafner, New York. xx + 613.

Medawar, P. B. (Ed.) 1945. *Essays on growth and form presented to d'Arcy Wentworth Thompson*. Clarendon Press, Oxford. viii + 408.

Medical Research Council. 1965. *Mathematics and computer science in biology and medicine. Proceedings of conference held by Medical Research Council with the Health Departments, Oxford 1964*. Her Majesty's Stationery Office, London. ix + 317.

Mendel, G. 1965. *Experiments in plant hybridization (Mendel's original paper translated with a commentary by Sir Ronald Fisher and a reprint of a biographical note by W. Bateson.)* Oliver & Boyd, Edinburgh. ix + 95.

Milbank Memorial Fund. 1955. *Catalogue of publications 1905–1955*. Milbank Memorial Fund, New York. 65 pp.

Milbank Memorial Fund. 1956. *Trends and differentials in mortality papers presented at the 1955 Annual Conference of the Milbank Memorial Fund, New York*. Milbank Memorial Fund. 165 pp.

Milbank Memorial Fund. 1959. *Thirty years of research in human fertility: Retrospect and prospect*. Milbank Memorial Fund, New York. 157 pp.

Mills, F. C. 1955. *Statistical methods*, 3 ed. Pitman, London. xviii + 842.

Monkhouse, F. J. and Wilkinson, H. R. 1971. *Maps and diagrams: Their compilation and construction*. Methuen, London. xxii + 522.

Moran, P. A. P. 1962. *The statistical processes of evolutionary theory*. Clarendon Press, Oxford. vii + 200.

Moran, P. A. P. 1969. Statistical methods in psychiatric research, *J. Roy, Statist. Soc.*, **132**, 484–524.

Moriyama, I. M. and Guralnick. L. 1956. *Occupational social class differences in mortality*, in Milbank Memorial Fund (1956), pp. 61–73.

Morris, J. N. 1957. *Uses of epidemiology*. Livingstone, Edinburgh and London. viii + 135.

Mudd, S. (Ed.) 1964. *The population crisis and the use of world resources*. Jup, The Hague. xix + 563.

Mullett, C. F. 1956. *The bubonic plague and England: An essay in the history of preventive medicine*. University of Kentucky Press, Lexington. ix + 401.

Mueller, F. H. 1939. Tabakmissbrauch und Lungencarcinom, *Zeitschr. f. Krebsforschung* **49** (1), 57–85.

Myers, R. J. 1963. An instance of the pitfalls prevalent in graveyard research, *Biometrics*, **19**, 638–650.

Naraghi, E. 1960. *L'étude des populations dans les pays à statistique incomplète: Contribution méthodologique*. Mouton, Paris. 137 pp.

News and Comment. 1964. Human experimentation: Cancer studies at Sloan-Kettering stir public debate on medical ethics, *Science*, **143**, 551–553.

Newsholme, A. 1923. *The elements of vital statistics*. Swan Sonnenschein, London. 623 pp.

Nixon, J. W. 1960. *A history of the International Statistical Institute, 1885–1960*. International Statistical Institute. The Hague. viii + 188.

Nixon, J. W. 1964. *Official statistics*. Oliver & Boyd, Edinburgh. 160 pp.

Norman, L. G. 1962. *Road traffic accidents*: Epidemiology, control and prevention. Public Health Organization, Geneva. 110 pp.

Norman-Taylor, W. 1964. Public health in the South Pacific, *Am. J. Publ. Health*, **54**, 780–790.

Office of Health Economics. 1966. *Disorders which shorten life. A review of mortality trends for those between the ages of 15–44*. Office of Health Economics, London. 33 pp.

Olkin, I., Ghurye, S. G., Hoeffding, W., Madow, W. G., and Mann, H. B. 1960. *Contributions to probability and statistics: Essays in honor of Harold Hotelling*. Stanford studies in mathematics and statics, No. 2. ix + 517.

Ovenall, L. 1965. A select bibliography of epidemiological literature since 1894, in Charles Creighton, *A history of epidemics in Britain*. Reprinted 1965 by F. Cass & Co., London, pp. 139–166.

Panse, V. G. 1940. A statistical study of quantitative inheritance, *Ann. Eugen. (Camb.)* **10**, 76–105.

Panum, P. L. 1846. *Iagttagelser, anstillende under Maeslinge-Epidemien paa Faerøerne i Aaret 1846*. Abstracted as "Beobachtungen über das Maserncontagium," in *Virchows Arch. Pathol. Med.*, **1** (1847) 491–512. Translated as *Observations made upon the epidemic of measles in the Faroe Islands in the year 1846*, by A. S. Hatcher, with a biographical memoir by J. J. Petersen (trans. by J. Dimont). Delta Omega Society and American Public Health Association, New York. xxxviii + 111.

Parsons, H. F. 1899–1900. On the comparative mortality of English districts, *Trans. Epidemiol. Soc. (London)*, **19**, 1–24.

Pascua, M. 1948. Diversity of stillbirth definitions and some statistical repercussion, *WHO Epidemiol. Vital statist Rept*. **1** (March), 210–220.

Pascua, M. 1952. Evolution of mortality in Europe during the twentieth century, cancer mortality, *WHO Epidemiol. Vital statist. Rept*, **4**, 36–137.

Paul, J. R. 1955. *Epidemiology of Poliomyelitis*, In World Health Organization Monograph Series, No. 26–29, 9–29. 408 pp.

Paul, J. R. 1966. *Clinical epidemiology*. University of Chicago Press, Chicago. xix + 305.

Pavlovsky, Y. N. (Ed.) 1963. *Human diseases with natural foci*. (trans. from Russian). Foreign Languages Publishing House, Moscow. 346 pp.

Pearl, R. 1924. *Studies in human biology*. Williams & Wilkins, Baltimore. 653 pp.

Pearl, R. 1927. The growth of populations, *Quart. Rev. Biol.*, **2**, 532–548.

Pearl, R. 1940. *Introduction to medical biometry and statistics*, 3rd ed. revised and Enlarged. Saunders, Philadelphia. xvi + 537.

Pearson, E. S. and Hartley, H. O. 1958. *Biometrika tables for statisticians*, Vol. I. Cambridge University Press, Cambridge. 240 pp. Vol. 2, 1972, xviii + 385.

Pearson, K. 1900. On a criterion that a given system of deviations from the probable in the case of a correlated system of variables is such that it can be reasonably supposed to have arisen from random sampling, *Phil. Mag.*, **50** (5), 157–175.

Peart, A. F. W. and Nagler, F. P. 1954. Measles in the Canadian Arctic, *Can. J. Publ. Health*, **45**, 146–156.

Pedersen, E. B. and Moodie, P. M. 1966. *The health of Australian aborigines. An annotated bibliography with classification by subject matter and locality*. School of Public Health and Tropical Medicine Sydney. 155 pp. (mimeo).

Peller, S. 1943. Studies on mortality since the Renaissance, *Bull. Hist. Med.*, **13**, 427–461.

Peller, S. 1944. Studies on mortality since the Renaissance, *Bull. Hist. Med.*, **16**, 362–381.

Peller, S. 1947. Studies on mortality since the Renaissance, *Bull. Hist. Med.*, **21**, 51–101.

Peller, S. 1948. Mortality, past and future, *Popul. Stud.*, **1**, 405–456. (A revised version of these papers is given in Glass and Eversley, 1965.)

Peller, S. 1967. *Quantitative research in human biology and medicine*. Wright, Bristol. xi + 422.

Penrose, L. S. 1959. *Outline of human genetics*. Wiley, New York. 146 pp.

Penrose, L. S. 1963. Limitations of eugenics, *Proc. Roy. Inst.*, **39**, 506–519.

Pfanzagl, J. 1968. *Theory of measurement*. Physica-Verlag, Würzburg-Vienna; Wiley, New York. 235 pp.

Pickles, W. N. 1939. *Epidemiology in country practice*. Wright, Bristol. viii + 110.

Pike, E. R. 1966. *Human documents of the Industrial Revolution in Britain*. Allen & Unwin, London. 368 pp.

Pollard, G. N. and Pollard, A. H. 1966. Fertility in Australia, *Trans. Instit. Actuar. (Aust. and N.Z.)*, **17**, 19–46.

Pollitzer, R. 1954. *Plague*. World Health Organization, Monograph Series No. 22, WHO, Geneva. 698 pp.

Pollitzer, R. 1959. *Cholera: With a chapter on world incidence by S. Swaroop and a chapter on problems of immunology by W. Burrows*. WHO, Geneva. 1019 pp.

Population Division. 1954. The past and future population of the world and its continents, *World Population Conference, United Nations*. Reprinted in Spengler and Duncan (1956), pp. 26–33.

Powell, N. P. 1947. *Summary of international vital statistics 1937–1944*. U.S. National Office of Vital Statistics. Government Printing Office, Washington, D.C. v + 299.

Pratt, R. T. C. 1967. *The genetics of neurological disorders*. Oxford monographs on medical genetics. Oxford University Press, London. vii + 310.

Ptukha, M. V. 1937. John Graunt, fondateur de la démographie (1620–1674), *Congrès International de la Population*, Institut International de Statistique, Paris, 61–74.

Rahn, O. 1939. *Mathematics in bacteriology*. Burgess, Minneapolis, Minn., 63 pp.

Ransome, A. 1877. Losses and gains in the death-toll of England and Wales during the last thirty years, *Lit. Phil. Soc. Proc.* (Manch.), **16**, 194–208; also in *Memoirs*, **7**, (1879), 126–140.

Ransome, A. 1880. On epidemic cycles, *Proc. Lit. Phil. Soc.* (Manch.), **19**, 75–95.

Record, R. G. 1952. Relative frequencies and sex distributions of human multiple births, *Brit. J. Prev. soc. Med.*, **6**, 192–196.

Rees, M. S. 1969. The inflation of National Health Service Registers of patients and its effect on the remuneration of general practitioners, *J. Roy. Statist. Soc.*, **132**, 526–542.

Registrar-General. 1957. *Registrar-General's decennial supplement, England and Wales, 1951 life tables*. Her Majesty's Stationery Office, London. 38 pp.

Registrar-General. 1958. *Registrar-General's decennial supplement, England and Wales, 1951 occupation mortality Part II*. Vols. I and II. Her Majesty's Stationery Office, London.

Registrar-General. 1959. *Census 1951. England and Wales fertility report.* Her Majesty's Stationery Office, London. cxi + 251.

Reid, D. D. 1957. Records and research in occupational medicine, *J. Roy. Soc. Promot. Health*, **77**, 675–680.

Reid, D. D. 1960. *Epidemiological methods in the study of mental disorders.* Publ. Health Paper No. 2., WHO, Geneva. 79 pp.

Reinhard, M. R. 1961. *Etude de la population pendant la Révolution et l'Empire.* Ministère de l'Education Nationale, Paris, 72 pp.

Reinhard, M. R. and Armengaud, A. 1961. *Histoire générale de la population mondiale.* Éditions Montchrestien, Paris. v + 597.

Renold, A. E. and Cahill, G. F. 1960. Diabetes mellitus, in Stanbury, Wyngaarden, and Fredrickson (1960), pp. 65–120.

Reports on Public Health and Medical Subjects No. 94. 1949. *Neonatal mortalty and morbidity.* Her Majesty's Stationery Office, London. 90 pp.

Riordan, J. 1958. *An introduction to combinatorial analysis.* Wiley, New York. x + 242.

Robb-Smith, A. H. T. 1967. *The enigma of coronary heart disease.* Lloyd-Luke (Medical Books), London. ix + 150.

Robens of Woldingham, Lord. 1969. Mine disasters, *Advancement of Science*, **25**, 391–394.

Roberts, E., Dawson, W. M., and Madden, M. 1939. Observed and theoretical ratios in Mendelian inheritance, *Biometrika*, **31**, 56–66.

Robertson, D. F. 1968. Solar ultraviolet radiation in relation to sunburn and skin cancer, *Med. J. Aust.*, **2**, 1123–1132.

Robertson, D. F. 1968. Long-term field measurements of erythemally effective natural ultra-violet radiation, in Urbach (1968). *The biologic effects of ultraviolet radiation.* Pergamon Press, Oxford. 650 pp.

Roe, R. F. C. and Lancaster, M. C. 1964. Natural, metallic and other substances as carcinogens, *Brit. Med. J.*, **2**, 127–133.

Rogers, E. S. 1960. *Human ecology and health: An introduction for administrators.* Macmillan, New York. xviii + 334.

Rolleston, J. D. 1937. *History of the acute exanthemata.* Heineman, London. x + 114.

Rosenberg, C. E. 1962. *The cholera years; the United States in 1832, 1849 and 1866.* University of Chicago Press, Chicago. x + 257.

Rouquette, C. and Corone, J. 1965. Evolution récente de la mortalité chez les enfants de 1 à 14 ans, *Bull. Inst. Nat. Santé Rech. Med.*, **20**, 183–202.

Rowntree, S. 1901. *Poverty, a study of town life.* Macmillan, London. xviii + 437.

Royal Commission on Population. 1949. Vol. I, *Family limitation;* Vol. II, *Reports and selected papers of the Statistics Committee;* Vol. III, *Report of the Economics Committee;* Vol. IV, *Reports of the Biological and Medical Committees;* Vol. V, *Memoranda presented to the Royal Commission, Papers: Report-command paper 7695.* Her Majesty's Stationery Office, London.

Royston, E. 1956. Studies in the history of probability and statistics. III. A note on the history of the graphical presentation of data, *Biometrika*, **43**, 241–247.

Rudd, J. 1962. The statistics of accidents collected by Her Majesty's Factory Inspectorate, Ministry of Labour, *J. Roy. Statist. Soc.* **A125**, 144–150.

Russell, J. C. 1937. Length of life in England, 1250–1348, *Hum. Biol.*, **9**, 528–541.

Russell, J. C. 1941. The ecclesiastical age: A demographic interpretation of the period, A.D. 200–900, *Rev. Relig.*, **5**, 137–147.

Russell, J. C. 1945. Late medieval population pattern, *Speculum*, **20**, 157–171.

Russell, J. C. 1948. *Medieval British population.* University of New Mexico Press, Albuquerque. xvi + 389.

Rutstein, D. D., Eden, M., and Schützenberger, M. P. 1961. Report on mathematics in the medical sciences, *N. Engl. med. J.*, **265**, 172–175.

Rutstein, D. D., Nickerson, R. J., and Heald, F. P. 1952. Seasonal incidence of patent ductus arteriosus and maternal rubella, *Am. J. Dis. Child.*, **84**, 199–213.

Ryder, N. B. 1955. The influence of declining mortality on Swedish reproductivity, *Milbank Mem. Fund Conf., 1955*, 65–81.

Ryle, J. A. 1948. *The natural history of disease*, Oxford University Press, London. xiv + 484.

Ryser, H. J. 1963. *Combinatorial mathematics*. Carus Mathematical Monograp. No. 14. Wiley, New York. xi + 154.

Sackett, D. L. and Winkelstein, W., Jr. 1965. The epidemiology of aortic and peripheral atherosclerosis. A selective review, *J. Chronic Dis.*, **18**, 775–795.

Sainsbury, P. 1955. *Suicide in London: an ecological study*. Chapman & Hall, London. 116 pp.

Salaman, R. N. 1949. *The history and social influence of the potato*. Cambridge University Press, Cambridge. xxiv + 685.

Sauvy, A. 1954*a*. *Théorie générale de la population*, 2 vols. Presse Universitaire de France, Paris.

Sauvy, A. 1954*b*. Le vieillissement des populations et l'allongement de la vie. *Population*, **9**, 675–682.

Sauvy, A. 1969. *General theory of population*. (transl. by C. Campos.) Weidenfeld & Nicholson, London. xii + 551.

Schleisner, P. A. 1851. Vital statistics of Iceland, *J. Roy. Statist. Soc.*, **14**, 1–10.

Schmid, C. F. 1954. *Handbook of graphic presentation*. Ronald Press, New York. vii + 316.

Schuman, L. M. 1965. The epidemiology of thromboembolic disorders. A review, *J. Chronic Dis.*, **18**, 815–845.

Schwartz, D. and Lazar, P. H. 1961. Taux de mortalité par une cause donnée de décès en tenant compte d'autres causes de décès ou de disparition, *Rev. Inst. Int. Statist.*, **29** (3), 44–56.

Scotch, N. A. and Geiger, H. J. 1962. The epidemiology of rheumatoid arthritis. A review with special attention to social factors, *J. Chronic Dis.*, **15**, 1037–1067.

Scott, D. 1965. *Epidemic disease in Ghana, 1901–1960*. Oxford University Press, London. 208 pp.

Secretary General of the United Nations. 1961. Review of international statistics. A report by the Secretary General of the United Nations, *Rev. Inst. Int. Statist.*, **29** (1), 32–80.

Selmer, E. S. 1967. Registration numbers in Norway: Some applied number theory and psychology, *J. roy. Statist. Soc.*, **143**, 225–231.

Serfling, R. E. 1952. Historical review of epidemic theory, *Hum. Biol.*, **24**, 145–166.

Shapiro, S. and Moriyama, I. M. 1963. International trends in infant mortality and their implications for the United States, *Am. J. Publ. Health*, **53**, 747–760.

Shapiro, S., Ross, L. J., and Levine, H. S. 1965. Relationship of selected prenatal factors to pregnancy outcome and congenital anomalies, *Am. J. Publ. Health*, **55**, 268–282.

Shapiro, S., Schlesinger, E. R., and Nesbitt, R. E. L. 1968. *Infant, perinatal, maternal, and childhood mortality in the United States*. Harvard University Press, Cambridge, Mass. xix + 388.

Sheldon, J. H. 1948. *The social medicine of old age: Report of an enquiry at Wolverhampton*. Oxford University Press, London. x + 239.

Sheldon, J. H. 1960. Problems of an ageing population, *Brit. Med. J.*, **1**, 1223–1226.

Sheps, M. C. 1958. Shall we count the living or the dead? *N. Engl. Med. J.*, **259**, 1210–1214.

Sheps, M. C. 1971. A review of models for population change, *Rev. Int. Statist. Inst.*, **39**, 185–196.

Sheps, M. C. and Ridley, J. C. (Eds.) 1966. *Public health and population change*. University of Pittsburgh Press, Pittsburgh, Pa. xvii + 557.

Shimkin, M. B., Guttentag, O. E., Kidd, A. M., and Johnson, W. H. 1953. The problem of experimentation on human beings, *Science*, **117** 205–215.

Shrewsbury, J. F. D. 1970. *A history of bubonic plague in the British Isles*. Cambridge University Press, Cambridge. xi + 661.

Shubik, M. 1960. Bibliography on simulation, gaming, artificial intelligence and allied topics, *J. Am. Statist. Assoc.*, **55**, 736–751.

Siegel, M., Fuerst, H. T., and Peress, N. S. 1966. Comparative fetal mortality in maternal virus diseases. A prospective study on rubella, measles, mumps, chickenpox and hepatitis, *N. Engl. Med. J.*, **274**, 768–771.

Siegel, M. and Fuerst, H. T. 1966. Low birth weight and maternal virus diseases. A prospective study of rubella, measles, mumps, chickenpox and hepatitis, *J. Am. Med. Assoc.*, **197**, 680–684.

Sigurdsson, S. and Tomasson, B. 1968. Public health in Iceland, *World Med. J.*, **15**, 97–100.

Sigurjonsson, J. 1961. Rubella and congenital deafness, *Am. J. Med. Sci.*, **242**, 712–720.

Sigurjonsson, J. 1962. Rubella and congenital cataract blindness, *Med. J. Aust.*, **1**, 588–590.

Simon, H. J. 1968. Mortality among medical students, 1947–1967, *J. Med. Educ.*, **43**, 1175–1182.

Smart, J. (Ed.) 1961. Symposium on chronic bronchitis, *Brit. J. Clin. Pract.*, **15**, 405–471.

Smith, C. A. B. 1954. *Biomathematics. The principles of mathematics for students of biological science*. Griffin, London. xv + 712.

Smith, F. C. 1948. The force of mortality function, *Am. Math. Mon.*, **55**, 277–284.

Snedecor, G. W. and Cochran, W. G. 1967. *Statistical methods*, 6th ed. Iowa State University Press, Ames, Iowa. xiv + 593.

Snyder, L. H. 1959. Fifty years of medical genetics, *Science*, **129**, 7–13.

Sokal, R. R. and Sneath, P. H. A. 1963. *The principles of numerical taxonomy*. Freeman, London. xvi + 359.

Solomons, B. 1958. The history of infant welfare, *J. Pediatr. (St. Louis)*, **53**, 360–377.

Speizer, F. E., Doll, R., and Heaf, P. 1968. Observations on the recent increase in mortality from asthma, *Brit. Med. J.*, **1**, 335–339.

Spengler, J. J. and Duncan, O. D. (Eds.). 1956. *Population theory and policy*. Free Press, Chicago. 522 pp.

Spiegelman, M. 1955. *Introduction to demography*. Society of Actuaries, Chicago. xxi + 309.

Spiegelman, M. 1956. Recent trends and determinants of mortality in highly developed countries, in Milbank Memorial Fund (1956) pp. 51–60.

Springett, V. H. 1950. A comparative study of tuberculosis mortality rates, *J. Hyg. Camb.*, **48**, 361–395.

Squire, W. 1875–1877. On measles in Fiji, *Trans. Epidemiol. Soc.*, **4**, 72–74.

Stallones, R. A. 1965. Epidemiology of cerebrovascular disease. A review, *J. Chronic Dis.*, **18**, 859–872.

Stanbury, J. B., Wyngaarden, J. B., and Fredrickson, D. S. 1960. *The metabolic basis of inherited disease*. McGraw-Hill, New York. xiv + 1477.

Standing Committee. 1971. Dietary fat and coronary heart disease: A review. Prepared by a standing subcommittee appointed by the National Heart Foundation of Australia, *Med. J. Aust.* **1**, 1155–1160.

Stark, J. 1851. Contribution to the vital statistics of Scotland, *J. Roy. Statist. Soc.*, **14**, 48–87.

Stavem, P. 1964. The distribution of erythrocytes and reticulocytes in blood smears, *Acta Med. Scand.*, **175**, Suppl. **409**, 1–111.

Stearman, R. L. 1955. Statistical concepts in microbiology, *Bacteriol. Rev.*, **19**, 160–215.

Steinberg, A. G. 1959. The genetics of diabetes: A review, *Ann. N. Y. Acad. Sci.*, **82**, 197–207.

Steiner, P. E. 1954. *Cancer: Race and geography*. Williams & Wilkins, Baltimore. xiii + 363.

Stevens, P. J. 1970. *Fatal civil aircraft accidents: Their medical and pathological investigation.* Wright, New York, 218 pp.

Stevenson, A. C. and Cheeseman, E. A. 1956. Hereditary deaf mutism with particular reference to Northern Ireland, *Ann. Hum. Genet.,* **20**, 177–207.

Stevenson, A. C., Johnston, H. A., Stewart, M. I. P., and Golding, D. R. 1966. *Congenital malformations. A report of a study of consecutive births in 14 centres.* Bulletin of the World Health Organization, 34 Suppl. 127 pp.

Stevenson, T. H. C. 1921. The incidence of mortality upon the rich and poor districts of Paris and London, *J. Roy. Statist. Soc.,* **84**, 90–99.

Stevenson, T. H. C. 1928. The vital statistics of wealth and poverty, *J. Roy. Statist. Soc.,* **91**, 207–230.

Stewart, H. L. and Herrold, K. M. 1961. A critique of experiments on attempts to induce cancer with tobacco derivatives, *Bull. Int. Statist. Inst.,* **39** (3), 457–477.

Stocks, P. 1938. The effects of occupation and its accompanying environment on mortality, *J. Roy. Statist. Soc.,* **101**, 668–708.

Stocks, P. 1942. Measles and whooping-cough incidence before and during the dispersal of 1939–1941, *J. Roy. Statist. Soc.,* **105**, 259–291.

Stocks, P. 1944. Diabetes mortality in 1861–1942 and some of the factors affecting it, *J. Hyg. Camb.,* **43**, 242–247.

Stocks, P. 1950. Fifty years of progress as shown by vital statistics, *Brit. Med. J.,* **1**, 54–57.

Stocks, P. 1953. Studies of cancer death rates at different ages in England and Wales in 1921 to 1940: Uterus, breast and lung, *Brit. J. Cancer,* **7**, 283–302.

Stolnitz, G. J. 1955. A century of international mortality trends, *Popul. Stud.,* **9**, 24–55.

Stolnitz, G. J. 1956a. *Life tables from limited data: A demographic approach.* Office of Population Research, Princeton University Press, Princeton, N.J. xii + 164.

Stolnitz, G. J. 1956b. Comparison between some recent mortality trends in underdeveloped areas and historical trends in the West, in Milbank Memorial Fund (1956). pp. 26–34.

Stolnitz, G. J. 1957. A century of international mortality trends: II, *Popul. Stud,* **10**, 17–42.

Stowman, K. 1947. Epidemiological and vital statistics report, *United Nations/WHO,* August, 1947, 38–45.

Stowman, K. 1949. World health statistics, *Milbank Mem. Fund Quart.,* **27**, 179–187.

Strandskov, H. H. 1942. On the variance of human live birth sex ratios, *Hum. Biol.,* **14**, 85–94.

Strauss, E. 1954. *Sir William Petty, portrait of a genius.* Bodley Head, London. 260 pp.

Studies in Official Statistics No. 4. 1959. *The length of working life of males in Great Britain.* Studies in Official Statistics, No. 4, Min. Lab. Nat. Serv. Her Majesty's Stationery Office, London.

Sundbärg, G. 1906. Fortsatta bidrag till en svensk befölkningsstatistik för åren 1750–1900. Parts I–IV, 169–1906; V, VI, 179–1907; VII–IX, 175–1908; X, 175–1909. *Statistisk Tidskrift* (Stockholm).

Susser, M. W. and Watson, W. 1962. *Sociology in medicine.* Oxford University Press, London. xii + 338.

Süssmilch, J. P. 1742. *Die göttliche Ordnung in den Veränderungen des menschlichen Geschlechts aus der Geburt, dem Tode, und der Fortpflanzung desselben Erwiesen,* 2 vols. Berlin. 2nd ed., 1761–1762.

Sutherland, I. 1963. John Graunt: A tercentenary tribute, *J. Roy. Statist. Soc.,* **A126**, 537–556.

Sutter, J. 1950. *L'eugénique.* Institut National d'Études Demographiques, Paris, 256 pp.

Sutter, J. 1958. The relation of human genetics to demography, *Eugen. Quart.,* **5**, 131–136.

Sutter, J. and Tabah, L. 1950. Le problème de la mortalité génétique périnatale, *Population,* **5**, 311–332.

Sutter, J. and Tabah, L. 1952. La mortalité, phénomène biométrique, *Population*, **7**, 69–94.

Sutton, D. H. 1945. Gestation period, *Med. J. Aust.*, **1**, 611–613.

Swan, C., Tostevin, A. L., Moore, B., Mayo, H., and Black, G. H. B. 1943. Congenital defects in infants following infectious diseases during pregnancy, *Med. J. Aust.* **2**, 201–210.

Swan, C., Tostevin, A. L., and Black, G. H. B. 1946. Final observations on congenital defects in infants following infectious diseases during pregnancy, with special reference to rubella, *Med. J. Aust.*, **2**, 889–908.

Sydenstricker, E. and Notestein, F. W. 1930. Differential fertility according to social class: A study of 69,620 native white married women under forty-five years of age based upon the United States Census returns of 1910, *J. Am. Statist., Assoc.*, **25**, 9–32.

Sydenstricker, E., Dublin, L. I., and Lotka, A. J. 1934. The history of longevity in the United States, *Hum. Biol.*, **6**, 43–86.

Symposium. 1961. Trends in infant mortality in Asia and Oceania. A symposium, *J. Philipp. Med. Assoc.*, **37**, 581–613.

Tabah, L. and Sutter, J. 1948. Influence respective de l'age maternel et du rang de naissance sur la mortinatalité. La notion de létalité, *Population*, **3**, 63–92.

Taeuber, C. and Taeuber, I. B. 1958. *The changing population of the United States*. Wiley, New York. xi + 357.

Taeuber, K. E., Haenszel, W., and Sirken, M. G. 1961. Residence histories and exposure residences for the United States population, *J. Am. Statist., Assoc.*, **56**, 824–834.

Tandy, E. 1935. *Comparability of maternal mortality rates*. Children's Bureau, U.S. Department of Labor, Bull. No. 229.

Taylor, C. E. and Hall, M. F. 1967. Health, population and economic development, *Science*, **157**, 651–657.

Taylor, I. and Knowleden, J. 1964. *Principles of epidemiology*. Churchill, London. vii + 366.

Taylor, W. 1951. Changing mortality from 1841 to 1947 measured by the life table, *Brit. J. Prev. Soc. Med.*, **5**, 162–176.

Taylor, W. F. 1961. On the methodology of studying aging in humans, *Proc. 4th Berkeley Symp.*, **4**, 347–368.

Thomas, D. S. 1941. *Social and economic aspects of Swedish population movements, 1750–1933*. Macmillan, New York. xxiii + 487.

Thompson, E. T. and Slaughter, D. P. 1957. Standard nomenclature in approved cancer clinics, *J. Am. Med. Assoc.*, **163**, 1131–1134.

Thompson, E. T. and Hayden, A. C. 1961. *Standard nomenclature of diseases and operations*. 5th ed. McGraw-Hill, New York. 980 pp.

Thompson, W. S. 1959. *Population and progress in the Far East*. University of Chicago Press, Chicago, 445 pp.

Thornton, J. L., Monk, A. J., and Brooke, E. S. 1961. *A select bibliography of medical biography*. The Library Association, London. 112 pp.

Topley, W. W. C. 1942. *Authority, observation and experiment in medicine*. The Linacre Lecture, 1940. Cambridge University Press, Cambridge. 45 pp.

Topley, W. W. C. and Wilson, G. S. 1936. *The principles of bacteriology and immunity*, 2nd ed. Edward Arnold, London. xv + 1645.

Toutain, J. C. 1963. *La population de la France de 1700 à 1958*. Cahiers de l'Institut de Science Économique Appliquée, Ser. A.F.3. 264 pp.

Tromp, S. W. (Ed.) 1963. *Medical biometeorology: Weather climate and the living organism*. Elsevier, Amsterdam. xxvii + 991.

Tromp, S. W. (Ed.) 1963. *Biometereology: Proceedings of the Second International Bio-climatological Congress*. Pergamon Press, London. xxxii + 687.

Twaddle, A. C. 1968. Aging, population growth and chronic illness. A projection, United States, 1960–1985, *J. Chronic Dis.*, **21**, 417–422.

UN Handbook. 1955. *Handbook of vital statistics methods.* United Nations, New York, Ser. F. No. 7. 258 pp.

UN Population Studies No. 4. 1949. *Population census methods.* Department of Social Affairs, United Nations, New York. xii + 197.

UN Population Studies No. 5. 1949. *Problems of migration statistics.* Department of Social Affairs, United Nations, New York. vii + 65.

UN Population Studies No. 6. 1949. *Fertility data in population censuses.* Department of Social Affairs, United Nations, New York. iii + 31.

UN Population Studies No. 7. 1949. *Methods of using census statistics for the calculation of life tables and other demographic measures.* Department of Social Affairs, United Nations, New York. v + 60.

UN Population Studies No. 8. 1950. *Data on urban and rural population in recent censuses.* Department of Social Affairs, United Nations, New York. vi + 27.

UN Population Studies No. 9. 1951. *Application of international standards to census data on the economically active population.* Department of Social Affairs, United Nations, New York. x + 139.

UN Population Studies No. 13. 1954. *Foetal, infant and early childhood mortality.* Vol. I. *The Statistics.* Vol. II. *Biological, social and economic factors.* Department of Social Affairs, United Nations, New York. vi + 137 and 44 pp.

UN Population Studies No. 17. 1953. *The determinants and consequences of population trends.* Department of Social Affairs, United Nations, New York. xii + 404.

UN Population Studies No. 18. 1953. *Training in techniques of demographic analysis.* Department of Social Affairs, United Nations, New York. iv + 17.

UN Population Studies No. 20. 1954. *Population growth and the standard of living in under-developed countries.* Department of Social Affairs, United Nations, New York. iii + 9.

UN Population Studies No. 22. 1955. *Age and sex patterns of mortality. Model life-tables for under-developed countries.* Department of Social Affairs, United Nations, New York. iv + 28 + tables.

UN Population Studies No. 24. 1955. *Analytical bibliography of internation migration statistics, 1925–1950.* Department of Economic and Social Affairs, United Nations, New York. v + 195.

UN Population Studies No. 25. 1956. *Methods for population projections by sex and age.* Department of Economic and Social Affairs, United Nations, New York. v + 81.

UN Population Studies No. 26. 1956. *The aging of populations and its economic and social implications.* Department of Economic and Social Affairs, United Nations, New York. vii + 168.

UN Statistical Office. 1955. *Handbook of vital statistics methods.* Studies in methods, Ser. F, No. 7. United Nations, New York. vi + 163.

UN Statistical Office. 1958. *Handbook of population census methods.* Vol. I. *General aspects of a population census.* Statistical Office of the UN, United Nations, New York. vi + 163.

UN Statistical Papers. 1954. *Bibliography of recent official demographic statistics.* Statistical Papers Ser. M, No. 18, United Nations, New York. 80 pp.

UN Studies in Methods. 1958–1959. *Handbook of population census methods.* Studies in methods, Ser. F. No. 5, Rev. 1, United Nations, New York. 3 vols.

UN/WHO Joint Committee 1970. *Programmes of analysis of mortality, trends and levels: Report of a joint UN/WHO meeting.* Technical Report Series, No. 440, WHO, Geneva. 36 pp.

Underwood, E. A. (Ed.) 1953. *Science, medicine and history.* Oxford University Press, London. Vol. I, xxxii + 563. Vol. II, viii + 646.

Urbach, F. 1968. *The biologic effects of ultraviolet radiation.* Pergamon Press, Oxford. 650 pp.

Urlanis, B. Ts. 1960. *Wars and population in Europe. Losses of human lives in the armed forces and European countries during the last three and a half centuries.* Social Economic and Literary Publishers, Moscow. 567 pp.

Urquhart, M. C. (Ed.) and Buckley, K. A. H. (Asst. Ed.) 1965. *Historical statistics of Canada.* Cambridge University Press, Cambridge. xv + 672.

U.S. Bureau of the Census. 1911, 1924, 1931, 1940. *Manual of the international list of the causes of death.* 2nd, 3rd, 4th, and 5th revisions. Government Printing Office, Washington, D.C.

U.S. Bureau of the Census. 1960. *Historical statistics of the United States, Colonial times to 1957: A statistical abstract supplement.* Bureau of the Census, Washington, D.C. xi + 789.

U.S. Department of Labor. 1962. *Implications of automation and other technological developments: A selected bibliography.* Bulletin 1319, U.S. Department of Labor, Washington, D.C. 136 pp.

Usher, A. P. 1930. History of population and settlement in Eurasia, *Geograph. Rev.,* **20,** 110–132. Reprinted in Spengler and Duncan (1956), pp. 3–25.

U.S. National Center for Health Statistics. 1964a. *The change in mortality trend in the United States.* Ser. 3, No. 1, National Center for Health Statistics. 43 pp.

U.S. National Center for Health Statistics. 1964b. *Recent mortality trends in Chile.* Ser. 3, No. 2, National Center for Health Statistics. 34 pp.

U.S. National Center for Health Statistics. 1965a. *Infant and perinatal mortality in the United States.* Ser. 3, No. 4, National Center Health Statistics. iv + 87.

U.S. National Center for Health Statistics. 1965b. *Infant mortality trends, United States and each state, 1930–1964.* Ser. 20, No. 1, National Center for Health Statistics. ii + 70.

U.S. National Center for Health Statistics. 1965c. *Weight at birth and survival of the newborn in the United States, early 1950.* Ser. 21, No. 3, National Center Health Statistics. 33 pp.

U.S. National Center for Health Statistics. 1965d. *Weight at birth and survival of the newborn by age of mother and total birth order, United States, early 1950.* Ser. 21, No. 5, National Center for Health Statistics, pp. 21–73.

U.S. National Center for Health Statistics. 1965e. *Weight at birth and cause of death in the neonatal period, United States, early 1950.* Ser. 21, No. 6, National Center for Health Statistics, pp. 223–299.

U.S. National Center for Health Statistics. 1965f. *Changes in mortality trends in England and Wales 1931–1961.* (Hubert Campbell). Ser. 3, No. 3, National Center for Health Statistics. 49 pp.

U.S. National Center for Health Statistics. 1965g. *An index of health: Mathematical models.* (C. L. Chiang). Ser. 2, No. 5, National Center for Health Statistics. iii + 19.

U.S. National Center for Health Statistics. 1966a. *Infant, fetal, and maternal mortality United States—1963.* Ser. 20, No. 3, National Center for Health Statistics. vi + 64.

U.S. National Center for Health Statistics. 1966b. *Infant and perinatal mortality in Scotland.* (Charlotte A. Douglas) Ser. 3, No. 5, National Center for Health Statistics. 44 pp.

U.S. National Center for Health Statistics. 1966c. *Mortality trends in the United States, 1954–1963.* Ser. 20, No. 2, National Center for Health Statistics. vi + 57.

U.S. National Center for Health Statistics. 1967a. *Multiple births United States—1964.* Ser. 21, No. 14, National Center for Health Statistics. ii + 49.

U.S. National Center for Health Statistics. 1967b. *International comparison of perinatal and infant mortality.* (Helen C. Chase). Ser. 3, No. 6, National Center for Health Statistics. 97 pp.

U.S. National Center for Health Statistics. 1968a. *Migration, vital, and health statistics.* Ser. 4, No. 9, National Center for Health Statistics. vi + 17.

U.S. National Center for Health Statistics. 1968b. *Recent retardation of mortality trends in Japan.* Ser. 3, No. 10, National Center for Health Statistics. vi + 28.

U.S. National Center for Health Statistics. 1969a. *The 1970 census and vital and health statistics.* Ser. 4, No. 10, National Center for Health Statistics. viii + 14.

288   BIBLIOGRAPHY

U.S. National Center for Health Statistics. 1969b. *Mortality trends in Czechoslovakia*. Ser. 3, No. 13, National Center for Health Statistics. ii + 26.

U.S. National Center for Health Statistics. 1970a. *Needs for national studies of population dynamics: A report of the United States National Committee on Vital and Health Statistics*. Ser. 4, No. 12, National Center for Health Statistics. viii + 31.

U.S. National Center for Health Statistics. 1970b. *Natality statistics analysis United States, 1965–1967*. Ser. 21 No. 19, National Center for Health Statistics. viii + 38.

U.S. National Center for Health Statistics. 1970c. *Annotated bibliography on vital and health statistics*. Public Health Service Publ. No. 2094, Health Services and Mental Health Administration. vii + 143.

U.S. National Center for Health Statistics. 1971. *Current estimates from the Health Interview Survey, United States, 1969*. Ser. 10, No. 63. U.S. Department of Health, Education and Welfare, Washington, D.C. vi + 57.

U.S. National Health Survey. 1958a. *Health statistics from the U.S. National Health Survey: Concepts and definitions in the health household—interview survey*. U.S. Public Health Service, Ser. A3. 29 pp.

U.S. National Health Survey. 1958b. *Health statistics from the U.S. National Health Survey*. Ser. A3. U.S. Public Health Service Ser. No. 584. 29 pp.

U.S. National Health Survey. 1959a. *Health statistics from the U.S. National Health Survey. Impairments by type, age and sex, United States, July, 1957–June, 1958*. Ser. B9, U.S. Public Health Service, No. 684. 28 pp.

U.S. National Health Survey. 1959b. *Health statistics from the U.S. National Health Survey. Disability days: United States, July, 1957–June, 1958*. Ser. B10, No. 584. 68 pp. U.S. Department of Health, Education and Welfare, Public Health Service, Washington, D.C.

U.S. Public Health Service. 1956. *Health and demography. Charts on population trends in the United States*. Washington, D.C. 94 pp.

U.S. Public Health Service 1971. *The health consequences of smoking: a Report of the Surgeon-General*. U.S. Department of Health, Education, and Welfare. 459 pp.

U.S. Public Health Service Publication. 1960. *Survival experience of patients with malignant neoplasms*. U.S. Public Health Service Publ. No. 789, Government Printing Office, Washington, D.C. 119 pp.

Valaoras, V. G. 1956. Standard age and sex patterns of mortality, pp. 133–149 in *Trends and differentials in mortality*. Milbank Memorial Fund, New York.

Vance, R. B. and Madigan, F. C. 1956. Differential mortality and the style of life of men and women: A research design, in *Trends and differentials in mortality*. Milbank Memorial Fund, New York.

Vickery, B. C. 1958. *Classification and indexing in science*. Butterworths, London, xvii + 185.

Von Linder, A 1960. *Statistische Methoden für Naturwissenschafter, Mediziner und Ingenieure*, 2nd ed. Verlag Birkhauser, Basel. 484 pp.

Walsh, R. J., Arnold, B. J., Lancaster, H. O., Coote, M. A., and Cotter, H. 1953. *A study of haemoglobin values in New South Wales*. Special Report Series, No. 5, National Health and Medical Research Council, Canberra. 84 pp.

Warkany, J. and Kalter, H. 1961. Congenital malformations. *N. Engl. J. Med.*, **265**, 993–1001, 1046–1052.

Westergaard, H. 1880. Mortality in remote corners of the world, *J. Roy. Statist. Soc.*, **43**, 509–520.

Westergaard, H. 1881. *Die Lehre von der Mortalität und Morbilität, anthropologisch-statistische Untersuchungen*. G. Fischer, Jena, 703 pp. 2nd ed., 1901.

Whelpton, P. K. 1947. *Forecasts of the population of the United States, 1945–1975*. U.S. Bureau of the Census, Government Printing Office, Washington, D.C. 111 pp.

Whitworth, W. A. 1948. *Choice and chance: With one thousand exercises*, ... 5th ed., 1901, Deighton Bell, London, viii + 342. Reprinted by Hafner, New York.

WHO. 1970. *Mortality from malignant neoplasms 1955–1965*. (Bilingual publication—English and French). 1147 pp.

WHO Bibliography. 1958. *Publications of the World Health Organization, 1947–1957*. 128 pp.

WHO Bibliography. 1964. *Publications of the World Health Organization, 1958–1962*. 125 pp.

WHO Bibliography. 1969. *Publications of the World Health Organization, 1963–1967: A bibliography*. 152 pp.

WHO Bibliography on Cancer. 1963. *Bibliography on the epidemiology of cancer, 1946–1960*. 168 pp.

WHO Committee on Health Statistics. 1959. *Sixth report, including the third report of the sub-committee on cancer statistics*. WHO Technical Report Series, No. 164. 43 pp.

WHO Director-General. 1970. *The work of WHO, 1970: Annual report of the Director-General to the World Health Assembly and to the United Nations*. xvii + 306.

WHO Epidemiological Report. 1964. *Infant and child mortality in selected countries, 1951–1962*. Epidemiological and vital statistics report, Vol. 17, pp. 536–642.

WHO Expert Committee. 1966. *Sampling methods in morbidity surveys and public health investigations: tenth report of the WHO Expert Committee on health statistics*. WHO. Technical Report Services, No. 336. 29 pp.

WHO Expert Committee. 1967. *National health planning in developing countries. Report of a WHO Expert Committee*. WHO Technical Report Series, No. 350. 40 pp.

WHO Expert Committee. 1968. *Morbidity statistics: Twelfth report of the WHO Expert Committee on Health Statistics*. WHO Technical Report series, No. 389. 29 pp.

WHO Expert Committee. 1969. *Statistics of health services and of their activities: Thirteenth report of WHO Expert Committee on health statistics*. WHO Technical report Series, No. 429. 36 pp.

WHO Expert Committee. 1970. *Report of the WHO Expert Committee on the prevention of perinatal mortality and morbidity*. WHO Technical Report Series, No. 457. 60 pp.

WHO Expert Committee on Human Genetics. 1964. *Second report: Human genetics and public health*. WHO. Technical Report Series, No. 282, WHO, Geneva. 38 pp.

WHO Manual. 1948–1955. *International statistical classification of diseases, injuries, and causes of death*. Sixth Revision of the International Lists of Diseases and Causes of Death as adopted, 1948. Vol. I, 1948. Vol. II, *Alphabetical Index*, 1949; *Index Alphabeticus*, 1955. WHO, Geneva.

WHO Manual, 1967, 1969. *International classification of diseases*. Eighth Revision of the International Statistical Classification of Diseases, Injuries and Causes of Death 1965. Vol. I. xxxiii + 478. Vol. II. xiv + 616.

WHO Scientific Group. 1964. *Research in population genetics of primitive groups: Report of a WHO scientific group*. WHO Technical Report Series, No. 279, WHO, Geneva. 26 pp.

WHO Scientific Group. 1966. *Principles for preclinical testing of drug safety: Report of a WHO scientific group*. WHO Technical Report Series, No. 341, WHO, Geneva. 22 pp.

WHO Scientific Group. 1967. *Research on human population genetics. Report of a WHO scientific group, Geneva, 3–7 July, 1967*. WHO, Geneva, 32 pp.

WHO Scientific Group. 1970. *Genetic factors in congenital malformations, Report of a WHO scientific group*, WHO Technical Report Series, No. 438, Geneva. 42 pp.

WHO Scientific Group. 1971. *Methodology for family studies of genetic factors: Report of a WHO scientific group*. WHO Technical Report Series, No. 466. 37 pp.

WHO Seminar. 1962. *The use of vital and health statistics for genetic and radiation studies*. UN Publications, New York. xi + 260.

WHO Study Group. 1957. *Measurement of levels of health. Report of a study group*. WHO Technical Report Series, No. 137. WHO, Geneva. 29 pp.

WHO Study Group. 1957. Report of study group on atherosclerosis and ischaemic heart disease. WHO Technical Report Series, No. 117, 10 pp.

WHO Study Group. 1960. Epidemiology of cancer of the lung: Report of a study group: WHO Technical Report Series, No. 185, 32 pp.

WHO (various authors). 1965. *Trends in the study of morbidity and mortality*. Public Health Papers, No. 27, WHO, Geneva. 196 pp.

Wickens, C. H. 1930. Australian mortality, *J. Inst. Actuar.*, **61**, 165–213.

Willcox, W. F. 1923. Population and the world war: A preliminary survey, *J. Am. Statist. Assoc.*, **18**, 699–712.

Willcox, W. F. 1937. The founder of statistics, *Rev. Inst. Int. Statist.*, year 5, Pt. 4, 321–328.

Wilson, E. B. 1952. *An introduction to scientific research*. McGraw-Hill, New York. xiii + 375.

Witts, L. J. (Ed.) 1959. *Medical surveys and clinical trials*. Oxford University Press, Oxford. 336 pp.

Wolfbein, S. L. 1949. The length of working life, *Popul. Stud.*, **3**, 286–294.

Wolfenden, H. H. 1954. *Population statistics and their compilation* (with an appendix by W. E. Deming). University of Chicago Press, Chicago. xxii + 258.

World Health Organization: see WHO.

Wright, C. D. and Hunt, W. C. 1900. *History and growth of the United States census*. (Prepared for the U.S. Senate Committee on the Census.) Government Printing Office, Washington, D.C. 967 pp. (Johnson Reprint Corp., 1966).

Wynder, E. L. and Graham, E. A. 1950. Tobacco smoking as a possible etiologic factor in bronchiogenic carcinoma, *J. Amer. Med. Assoc.*, **143**, 329–336.

Yates, F. 1960. *Sampling methods for censuses and surveys*, 3rd ed. Griffin, London. xvi + 440.

Yntema, L. 1952. *Mathematical modes of demographic analysis*, Groen, Leyden. viii + 78.

Young, M. and Russell, W. T. 1927. Historical expectation of life: A study of the longevity of males at different periods in the history of Great Britain and Ireland from the sixteenth to the beginning of the nineteenth century, based on data from the *Dictionary of National Biography* and *Burke's Peerage and Baronetage*, *J. Hyg. Camb.*, **25**, 256–272.

Yule, G. U. 1934. On some points relating to vital statistics, more especially statistics of occupational mortality, *J. Roy. Statist. Soc.*, **97**, 1–84.

Yule, G. U. and Kendall, M. G. 1940. *An introduction to the theory of statistics*. Griffin, London. xiii + 570.

Zelinsky, W. 1962. *A bibliographic guide to population geography*. Research Paper No. 80, Department of Geography, University of Chicago Press, Chicago. xxx + 257.

Zinsser, H. 1935. *Rats, lice and history*. Routledge & Kegan Paul, London. xii + 301.

Appendix

Table A.1

ORDINATES OF THE NORMAL
DISTRIBUTION[a]

x	$g(x)$	x	$g(x)$
0	0.3989	2.0	0.0540
0.1	0.3970	2.1	0.0440
0.2	0.3910	2.2	0.0355
0.3	0.3814	2.3	0.0283
0.4	0.3683	2.4	0.0224
0.5	0.3521	2.5	0.0175
0.6	0.3332	2.6	0.0136
0.7	0.3123	2.7	0.0104
0.8	0.2897	2.8	0.0079
0.9	0.2661	2.9	0.0060
1.0	0.2420	3.0	0.0044
1.1	0.2179	3.1	0.0033
1.2	0.1942	3.2	0.0024
1.3	0.1714	3.3	0.0017
1.4	0.1497	3.4	0.0012
1.5	0.1295	3.5	0.0009
1.6	0.1109	3.6	0.0006
1.7	0.0940	3.7	0.0004
1.8	0.0790	3.8	0.0003
1.9	0.0656	3.9	0.0002

[a] In columns 2 and 4,

$$g(x) = (2\pi)^{-1/2} \exp[-\tfrac{1}{2}x^2].$$

Note: $g(-x) = g(x)$.

Table A.2

Percentage $= 100P$	One-Way Test x	Two-Way Test y
0.1	3.090	3.291
0.5	2.576	2.807
1	2.326	2.576
5	1.645	1.960
10	1.282	1.645
20	0.842	1.282
30	0.524	1.036
40	0.253	0.842
50	0.000	0.674
60	−0.253	0.524
70	−0.524	0.385
80	−0.842	0.253
90	−1.282	0.126
95	−1.645	0.063
99	−2.326	0.012
99.5	−2.576	0.006
99.9	−3.090	0.001
100	−∞	0

[a] In the one-way test, the probability that the standard normal variable X should be greater than the x shown in the second column is given by the entry in the first column.
In the two-way test, the probability that $|X|$ should be greater than y is given by the entry in the first column.

TABLE A.3

Some Percentage Points of χ^2 and of Student's t[a]

Degrees of Freedom	χ^2 (%)		Student's t (%)			
	5	1	10	5	2	1
1	3.841	6.635	6.314	12.706	31.821	63.657
2	5.991	9.210	2.920	4.303	6.965	9.925
3	7.815	11.345	2.353	3.182	4.541	5.841
4	9.488	13.277	2.132	2.776	3.747	4.604
5	11.070	15.086	2.015	2.571	3.365	4.032
6	12.592	16.812	1.943	2.447	3.143	3.707
7	14.067	18.475	1.895	2.365·	2.998	3.499
8	15.507	20.090	1.860	2.306	2.896	3.355
9	16.919	21.666	1.833	2.262	2.821	3.250
10	18.307	23.209	1.812	2.228	2.764	3.169
11	19.675	24.725	1.796	2.201	2.718	3.106
12	21.026	26.217	1.782	2.179	2.681	3.055
13	22.362	27.688	1.771	2.160	2.650	3.012
14	23.685	29.141	1.761	2.145	2.624	2.977
15	24.996	30.578	1.753	2.131	2.602	2.947
16	26.296	32.000	1.746	2.120	2.583	2.921
17	27.587	33.409	1.740	2.110	2.567	2.898
18	28.869	34.805	1.734	2.101	2.552	2.878
19	30.144	36.191	1.729	2.093	2.539	2.861
20	31.410	37.566	1.725	2.086	2.528	2.845
21	32.671	38.932	1.721	2.080	2.518	2.831
22	33.924	40.289	1.717	2.074	2.508	2.819
23	35.172	41.638	1.714	2.069	2.500	2.807
24	36.415	42.980	1.711	2.064	2.492	2.797
25	37.652	44.314	1.708	2.060	2.485	2.787
26	38.885	45.642	1.706	2.056	2.479	2.779
27	40.113	46.963	1.703	2.052	2.473	2.771
28	41.337	48.278	1.701	2.048	2.467	2.763
29	42.557	49.588	1.699	2.045	2.462	2.756
30	43.773	50.892	1.697	2.042	2.457	2.750

[a] The χ^2-test is a one-way or single tailed test. The Student's t are given as two-way or two-tailed tests.
The percentage points of the single-tailed Student's t at 5 and 1% are identical with those of the two-tailed test at 10 and 2%, respectively.

TABLE A.4

TABLE OF χ^2

Values of P

n	0.99	0.98	0.95	0.90	0.80	0.70	0.50	0.30	0.20	0.10	0.05	0.02	0.01
1	0.000157	0.000628	0.00393	0.0158	0.0642	0.148	0.455	1.074	1.642	2.706	3.841	5.412	6.635
2	0.0201	0.0404	0.103	0.211	0.446	0.713	1.386	2.408	3.219	4.605	5.991	7.824	9.210
3	0.115	0.185	0.352	0.584	1.005	1.424	2.366	3.665	4.642	6.251	7.815	9.837	11.345
4	0.297	0.429	0.711	1.064	1.649	2.195	3.357	4.878	5.989	7.779	9.488	11.668	13.277
5	0.554	0.752	1.145	1.610	2.343	3.000	4.351	6.064	7.289	9.236	11.070	13.388	15.086
6	0.872	1.134	1.635	2.204	3.070	3.828	5.348	7.231	8.558	10.645	12.592	15.033	16.812
7	1.239	1.564	2.167	2.833	3.822	4.671	6.346	8.383	9.803	12.017	14.067	16.622	18.475
8	1.646	2.032	2.733	3.490	4.594	5.527	7.344	9.524	11.030	13.362	15.507	18.168	20.090
9	2.088	2.532	3.325	4.168	5.380	6.393	8.343	10.656	12.242	14.684	16.919	19.679	21.666
10	2.558	3.059	3.940	4.865	6.179	7.267	9.342	11.781	13.442	15.987	18.307	21.161	23.209

Table A.5

RANDOM SAMPLING NUMBER[a]

PI = 3.+

```
1415926535  8979323846  2643383279  5028841971  6939937510  5820974944  5923078164  0628620899  8628034825  3421170679
8214808651  3282306647  0938446095  5058223172  5359408128  4811174502  8410270193  8521105559  6446229489  5493038196
4428810975  6659334461  2847564823  3786783165  2712019091  4564856692  3460348610  4543266482  1339360726  0249141273
7245870066  0631558817  4881520920  9628292540  9171536436  7892590360  0113305305  4882046652  1384146951  9415116094
3305727036  5759591953  0921861173  8193261179  3105118548  0744623799  6274956735  1885752724  8912279381  8301194912
9833673362  4406566430  8602139494  6395224737  1907021798  6094370277  0539217176  2931767523  8467481846  7669405132
0005681271  4526356082  7785771342  7577896091  7363717872  1468440901  2249534301  4654958537  1050792279  6892589235
4201995611  2129021960  8640344181  5981362977  4771309960  5187072113  4999999837  2978049951  0597317328  1609631859
5024459455  3469083026  4252230825  3344685035  2619311881  7101000313  7838752886  5875332083  8142061717  7669147303
5982534904  2875546873  1159562863  8823537875  9375195778  1857780532  1712268066  1300192787  6611195909  2164201989

3809525720  1065485863  2788659361  5338182796  8230301952  0353018529  6899577362  2599413891  2497217752  8347913151
5574857242  4541506959  5082953311  8861727855  8890750983  8175463746  4939319255  0604009277  0167113900  9848824012
8583616035  6370766010  4710181942  9555961989  4676783744  9448255379  7747268471  0404753464  6208046684  2590694912
9331367702  8989152104  7521620569  6602405803  8150193511  2533824300  3558764024  7496473263  7411992726  0426992279
6782354781  6360093417  2164121992  4586315030  2861829745  5570674983  8505494588  5869269956  9092721079  7509302955
3211653449  8720275596  0236480665  4991198818  3479775356  6369807426  5425278625  5181841757  4672890977  7727938000
8164706001  1451249192  1732172147  7235014144  1973568548  1613611573  5255213347  5741849468  4385233239  0739414333
4547762416  8625189835  6948556209  9219206407  7885561271  5688034856  0494601653  4668049886  2723279178  6085784383
8279679766  8145410095  3883786360  9506800642  2512520511  7392984896  0841284886  2694560424  1965285022  2106611863
0674427862  2039194945  0471237137  8696095636  4371917287  4677646575  7396241389  0865832645  9951309004  7802759009

9465764078  9512694683  9835259570  9825822620  5224894077  2671947826  8482601476  9909026401  3639443745  5305068203
4962524517  4939965143  1429809190  6592509372  2169646151  5709858387  4105978859  5977297549  8930161753  9284681382
6868386894  2774155991  8559252459  5395997700  9972524680  8459872736  4469584865  3836736222  6260991246  0805124388
4390451244  1365497627  8079771569  1435997700  1296160894  4169486855  5848406353  4220722258  2848864815  8460285036
0168427394  5226746767  8895252138  5225499546  6672782398  6456596116  3548862305  7745649803  5936345681  1743241125
1507606947  9451096596  0940252288  7971089314  5669136867  2287489405  6010101330  8617926680  9208747609  1782493858
9009714909  6759852613  6554978189  3129784821  6829989487  2265880485  7564014270  4775551323  7964145152  3746234364
5428584447  9526586782  1051141354  7357395231  1342716610  2155969536  2314429524  8493718711  0145765403  5902799344
0374200731  0578539062  1983874478  0847848968  3321445713  8687519435  0643021845  3191048481  0053706146  8067491927
8191197939  9520614196  6342875444  0643745123  7181921799  9839101591  9561814675  1426912397  4894090718  6494231961
```

295

```
5679452080 9514655022 5231603881 9301420937 6213785595 6638937787 0830390697 9207734672 2182562599 6615014215
0306803844 7734549202 6054146659 2520149744 2850732518 6660021324 3408819071 0486331734 6496514539 0579626856
1005508106 6587969981 6357473638 4052571459 1028970641 4011097120 6280439039 7595156771 5770042033 7869936007
2305587631 7635942187 3125147120 5322281918 2618612586 7321579198 4148488291 6447060957 5270695722 0917567116
7229109816 9091528017 3506712748 5833228718 3520935396 5725121083 5791513698 8209144421 0067510334 6711031412
6711136990 8658516398 3150197016 5151168517 1437657618 3515565088 4909989859 9823873455 2833163550 7647918535
8932261854 8963213293 3089857064 2046752590 7091548141 6549859461 6371802709 8199430992 4488957571 2829805923
2332609729 9712084433 5732654893 8239119325 9746366730 5836041428 1388303203 8249037589 8524374417 0291327656
1809377344 4030707469 2112019130 2033038019 7621101100 4492932151 6084244485 9637669838 9522868478 3123552658
2131449576 8572624334 4189303968 6426243410 7732269780 2807318915 4411010446 8232527162 0105265227 2111660396

6655730925 4711055785 3763466820 6531098965 2691062056 4793125700 5863566201 8558100729 3606598764 8611791045
3348850346 1136576867 5324094166 8039626059 7877185650 8455296541 2665408530 6143444318 5867697511 5661406800
7002378776 5913440171 2749470420 5622305389 9456131407 1127000407 8547332699 3908145466 4645880797 2708266830
6343285878 5698305235 8069330657 5740049545 7163775254 2021149957 6158140025 0126228594 1302164715 5097925923
0990796567 3761255176 5675135571 7829666454 7791745011 2914803903 0463994713 2962107340 4375189573 5961458901
9389713111 7904297828 5647503203 1986915140 2870808599 0480109412 1472213179 4764777262 2414254854 5403321571
8530614228 8137585043 6633217518 2997866223 7172159160 7716692547 4873898665 4949450114 6540628433 6639379003
9769265672 1463853067 3609657120 0680763832 7166416274 8888007869 2560090228 4721040317 2118608204 1900042296
6171196377 9213375751 1495950156 6049631862 9472654736 4252308177 0367515906 7350235072 8354056704 0867743513
6222247715 8915049530 9844489333 0963408780 7693259939 7805419341 4473774418 4263129860 8099888687 4132604721
```

```
5695162396 5864573021 6315981931 9516735381 2974167729 4786724229 2465436680 0980676928 2382806899 6400482435
4037014163 1496589794 0924323789 6907069779 4223625082 2168899738 3798623001 5937764716 5122893578 6015881617
5578297352 3344604281 5126272037 3431465319 7777414031 9906655418 7639792933 4419521541 3418994854 4473456738
3162499341 9131814809 2777710386 3877343177 2075456545 3220777092 1201905166 0962804909 2636019759 8828161332
3166636528 6193266863 3606273567 6303544776 2803504507 7723554710 5855948072 7908143562 4014517180 6246463267
9456127531 8134078330 3362542327 8394497538 2437205835 3114771199 2606381334 6776879695 9703098339 1307710987
0408591337 4641442822 7726346594 0694115528 7787201927 7152807317 6790770715 7213444730 6057007334 9243693113
8350493163 1284042512 1925651798 0338507224 0131470130 7781643788 5185290908 5452011658 3934196562 1349143415
9562586586 5570552690 4965209858 0338507224 2648293972 8584783163 0577775606 8887644624 8246857926 0395353273
4803048029 0058760758 2510474709 1643961362 6760449256 2740420283 2085661190 6254543372 1315359584 5068724460

2901618766 7952406163 4252257719 5429162991 9306455377 9914037340 4328752628 8896399587 9475729174 6426357455
2540790974 5135711136 9410911939 3251910760 2082520261 8798531887 7058429971 9167781314 9690090019 2116971737
2784768472 6860849003 3770242429 1651300500 5168323364 3503895170 2989392233 4517220138 1280696501 1784408747
1960121228 5993716231 3017114448 4640903890 6449544400 6198690754 8516026327 5052983491 8740786680 8818838510
2283345085 0486082503 9302133219 7155184306 3545500766 8829844683 1377656527 3975175461 3953984683 3936383047
4611996653 8581538420 5685338621 8672523340 2830871123 2827892125 0771262946 3229563989 8989358211 6745627010
2183564622 0134967151 8819097303 8119800497 3407239610 3685406643 1939509790 1906996395 5245300545 0580686501
9567302292 1913933918 5680344903 9820595510 0226335336 4004199447 4553859381 0234395544 9597783779 0237420617
2711172364 3435439478 2218185286 2408514006 6604433258 8556986705 4315470696 5747458550 3323233421 0730154594
0516553790 6866273337 9958511562 5784322988 8757141595 8757141595 7811196358 3300594087 3068121602 8764962867
```

```
4460477464 9159950549 7374256269 0104903778 1986835938 1465741268 0492564879 8556145372 3478673303 9046883834
3634655379 4986419270 5638729317 4872332083 7601123029 9113679386 2708943879 9362016295 1541337142 4892830722
0126901475 4668476535 7616477379 4675200490 7571555278 1965362132 3926406160 1363581559 0742202020 3187277605
2772190055 6148425551 8792530343 5139844253 2234157623 3610642506 3904975008 6562710953 5919465897 5141310348
2276930624 7435363256 9160781547 8181152843 6679570611 0861533150 4452127473 9245449454 2368288606 1340841486
3776700961 2071512491 4043027253 8607648236 3414334623 5189757664 5216413767 9690314950 1910857598 4423919862
9164219399 4907236234 6468441173 9403265918 4044378051 3338967257 4239950829 6591228508 5558215725 0310712570
1266830240 2929525220 1187267675 6220415420 5161841634 8475651699 9811614101 0029960783 8690929160 3028840026
9104140792 8862150784 2451670908 7000699282 1206604183 7180653556 7252532567 5328612910 4248776182 5829765157
9598947036 2226293486 0034158772 9805349896 5022629171 8788202734 2092222453 3985626476 6914905562 8425039127

5771028402 7998066365 8254889264 8802545661 0172967026 6407655904 2909945681 5065265305 3718294127 0336931378
5178600040 7086667149 6558343434 7693385781 7113864558 7367812301 4587687126 6034891390 9562009939 3610310291
6161528813 8437909904 2317473363 9480457593 1493140529 7634757481 1935670911 0137751721 0080315590 2485309066
9203767192 2033229094 3346768514 2214477379 3937517034 4366199104 0337511173 5471918550 4644902636 5512816228
8244265759 1633303910 7225383742 1821408835 0865739177 1509682887 4782656995 9957449066 1758344137 5223970968
3408005355 9849175417 3818839994 4697486762 6551658276 5843858845 3142775687 9002909517 0283529716 3446521296
4043523117 6006651012 4120065975 5851276178 5838292041 9748442360 8007193045 7618932349 2292796501 9875187212
7267507981 2554709589 0455635792 1210033346 6974992356 3025494780 2490111195 2123828153 0911407907 3860251522
7429958180 7247162591 6685451333 1239480494 7079119153 2673430282 4418601142 6363954800 0448002670 4926482017
9289647669 7583183271 3142517029 6923488962 7668440323 2609275249 6035799646 9256504936 8183609003 2380929345

9588970695 3653494060 3402166544 3755890045 6328822505 4525564056 4482465151 8754711962 1814396582 5337543885
6909411303 1509526179 3780029741 2076651479 3942590298 9695949695 5657612186 5619673378 6236256125 2163208628
6922210327 4889218854 3648022967 8070576561 5144632046 9279068212 0738837781 4233562823 6089632080 6822246801
2248261177 1858963814 0918390367 5432228088 3215137556 0037279839 4004152970 0287830766 7094447456 0134556417
2543700069 7939612257 1928994581 5435784687 8861444581 2314593571 9849225284 7160504922 1242470141 2147805734
5510500801 9086996033 0276347870 8108175450 1193071412 2339086639 3833952942 5786905076 4310063835 1983438934
1596131854 3475464955 2054274648 3097164651 4384070070 7360411237 3599834452 2516105070 2705623526 6012764848
3080476118 3013052793 6540360367 4532865105 7065874882 2569815793 6789766974 6789766974 2205750596 8344086973
5020140020 6723585020 0724522563 2651341055 9240109274 2162484391 4035998953 5394590944 0704691209 1409387001
2645600162 3742880210 9276457931 0657922955 2498872758 4610126483 6999892256 9596881592 0560010165 5256375678
```

a The table is reproduced from D. Shanks and J. W. Wrench, "Calculation of π to 100,000 decimals," *Mathematics of Computation*, **16** (1962), 76–99. Reprinted with permission of the publisher The American Mathematical Society, from *Mathematics of Computation*, copyright © 1962, Volume 16, pp. 80 and 81.

Author Index

Abbe, E., 219

Bayes, T., 257
Bernoulli, D., 260
Bertillon, J., 69, 259
Bienamyé, I. J., 260
Boltzmann, H., 219
Booth, C., 260
Brown, R., 244

Davenant, C., 260
de Witt, J., 259
Domagk, G., 117, 220

Ehrlich, P., 117, 220
Einstein, A., 244
Euler, L., 260

Farr, W., 69, 88, 259
Finlaison, J., 259
Fisher, R. A., 221, 261
Fourier, J. B. J., 260

Galton, F., 199, 221, 260
Gavarret, L. D. J., 221, 260
Gosset, W. S., 198, 219
Graunt, J., 12, 68, 99, 259
Greenwood, M., 260
Gregg, N. M., 11

Halley, E., 99, 259
Hill, A. B., 222

Kermack, W. O., 247
King, G., 260

Laplace, P. S., 260
Lister, J., 220
Lotka, A. J., 260
Louis, P. C. A., 221, 260

McKendrick, A. G., 247
Malthus, T. R., 260
Mendel, G., 55, 154, 261

Nightingale, F., 260

Pascal, B., 46
Pearson, K., 221, 261
Petty, W., 69, 259
Pott, P., 229
Prinzing, F., 260
Price, R., 260

Quetelet, L. A. J., 260

Ross, R., 246

"Student," see Gosset, W. S.
Suessmilch, J. P., 260

Wargentin, P. W., 259
Weldon, W. F. R., 261
Westergaard, H., 260

Subject Index

Abscissa, 13
Absolute value, 36
Accidents, *see* Violence
Accuracy, 27, 210
Africa, 123
After-effects, 187
Age, at census, 57
  mortality by, adult life, 104
  childhood, 73, 102, 126
  infancy, 126
  old age, 104, 126
  young adulthood, 76, 103
Age distribution, stable, 131, 139
Age-specific, 74
Aging of population, 143, 149
Alastrim, 170
Alleles, 152
Amebiasis, 205, 240, 242
America, Latin, 123
Ancient times, 126
Antibiotics, 117
Approximation, normal, 53
Arithmetic mean, 5
Asia, 123
Asthma, 125
Attributes, 8
Australia, 1, 65, 80, 84, 92, 96, 113, 123,
  128, 129, 130, 132, 134, 248, 250
Automation, 243
Automobiles, 103
Autosomes, 151
Average, 5, 32
Axes, 13
Axioms, 174

Bacteriology, 203, 219, 251, 255
Bar diagram, 16
Bayesian, 257
Best in the least squares sense, 200
Bias, 210
  unbiasedness, 27, 181, 210, 211
Bills of mortality, 68
Binomial probability theorem, 49
Biometry, 262

Birth, 60, 128
  hour of, 202
  live, 71, 72
  twin, 50, 168
Birthrate, crude, 129
Blood type, 27, 245
Bronchiectasis and bronchitis, 147
Business, 61

Calculus, 22
Calendar analysis of death rates, 76
Calibration, 213
Canada, 100, 123
Cancer, 58, 77, 79, 104, 112, 117, 125, 205
  lung, 58, 77, 111, 125, 229, 230
  lung and smoking, 230
  registries, 95, 238
Canvasser, 56
Card systems, 11, 236
Care, statistics of medical, 62
Carrier, 241
Cataract, congenital, 1
Census, 26, 56, 65
  de facto, 56
  de jure, 56
  medical, 59
Centers of location, 28, 36. *See also* Mean;
  Median; and Mode
Chance events, 183. *See also* Random;
  Variables
Check on computations, 5, 33, 34
Chemotherapy, 117, 220
Chi-squared, 189, 204
Childhood, 73, 102, 126
Chile, 123
Choice and chance, 55
Cholera, 124, 207, 229
Chromosomes, 151
Class, positive, 253
  ultimate, 253
Class frequencies, 11
Class intervals, 8
Classification, 8, 252, 258
  exhaustive, 9, 47, 253

hierarchical, 254
  mutually exclusive, 9, 47, 253
  principles of, 8
  set theoretically independent, 254
Coefficient of variation, 39
Cohort analysis, 77, 88, 110, 112
Combination, 43
Combinatorics, 209
Comparisons, multiple, 11, 180
Complement, *see* Sets
Computers, 232, 233, 243, 256, 258
Confidentiality, 60
Conjugal, 58
Consanguineity, 59, 159, 163
Contingency tables, 10, 11, 194, 195, 204
Continuous, 6, 8, 31
Contour diagram, 18
Control, quality, 213, 215, 216, 234
Convergence, 51
Correlation, 199, 234
Co-ordinates, cartesian, 13
  polar, 14, 16
Cosine, 14
Counting, 5, 30, 33, 187, 192, 203, 213,
    218, 219
Criminal records, 61
Critical region, 177
Cyclic diagram, 18
Cure, criteria of, 226
Czechoslovakia, 123

Data banks, 60, 61
Data-linkage, 60
Deafness and deaf-mutism, 1, 2, 59, 173,
    249, 251
Death, 160
  definitions of, 71
  fetal, 72, 101
Deaths at age x years, number of, 90
Death certificate, 70
Death rate, crude, 77
Defects, congenital, 11, 101, 125, 249, 251.
    See also Deafness; and Cataract
Degrees of freedom, 189
Demography, 67, 173, 262
Demonstrability, 242, 258
Denmark, 123
Dependency, invalid, 147
Design of experiments, 175, 225, 230
Deterministic model, 246
Development, 262
Deviation, 35
  mean, 35
  standard, 36
Diabetes, 63, 125, 170, 173
Diagnosis, 252, 255

Diagram, 16
  bar, 16
  contour, 18
  cyclic, 18
  logarithmic, 19
  semi-logarithmic, 19
  spot, 18
Dichotomy, 253
Directories, professional, 60
Disability, 59
Discrete, 5, 8
Disease, 59, 252
Diseases, classes of, cardiovascular, 70, 104,
    125
  genito-urinary, 70, 104, 125
  ill-defined, 70, 104
  nervous, 70, 105
Dispersion, measures of, 28; *see also* Var-
    iance
Distribution, binomial, 44, 47, 50, 53, 178,
    181, 192
  chi-squared, 189, 204
  multinomial, 188, 190, 202
  normal, 51, 52, 178, 179, 181, 193, 197,
    198
  bivariate, 198
  Poisson, 179, 181, 186, 191, 202
  rectangular, 211
  Student's-*t*, 197, 208
  symmetrical, 41
  theory, 183
Dominant, 152, 193, 203
Drugs and antibiotics, 117, 231
Duration of illness, 63

Ecology, 251
Educational records, 61
Effects, random, 175
Electoral, 60
Elite, *see* Select Tables of mortality
Endocrine therapy, 118
Enumerator, 56
Epidemiology, 3, 176, 228, 240, 244, 248,
    250, 263
Equally likely, 46
Equilibrium of genotypes, 156
Equivalent average death rate, 79
Equation, integral, of population growth,
    134
  linear, 21
Error, 36
Errors, accidental, 212
  of first kind, 179
  probable, 35
  of second kind, 179
  standard of the mean, 197

systematic, 212, 216
Estimation, 181, 182, 210
  unbiased, 27, 211
Ethics of experimentation, 221, 227, 231
Ethnic data in the census, 58
Etiology, 263
Eugenics, 173
Events, equally likely, 46
Evolutionary aspects of mortality, 169, 173
Exponential function, 51
Extreme values, 31

Factorial n, 42
Famine, 68
Fecundity, 128
Fertility, 128, 150
Fertility rate, 129, 150
Fever, 255
Field investigations, special, 63
Follow-up, 95, 230, 238, 239, 243
Foot, 32
Forecasting the mortality rates, 83
France, 65, 88, 123, 144
Frequency distributions, empirical, 26
  cumulative, 28, 41
Frequency polygon, 17
Frequency table, 1
Function, 22
  generating, 46

Gamete, 151
  female (=ovum), 151
  male (=spermatozoon), 151
Genealogy, 159
Generation death rates, 77, 88, 105, 112, 126
Generation effect, 133
Genes, 151
  frequency of, 157, 245
  independent segregation of, 50, 156, 192, 203
  major, 160
  sex-linked, 165
Genetic correlation, 173
Genetical control of diseases, 118
Genetical influences on mortality, 110, 169
Genotype, 152, 173
Genotypes, equilibrium of, 156
Genetics, human, 263
Geographical, 58, 251
Germany, 68, 88, 123
Glossina morsitans, 40
Graph theory, 25
Graphical representation, 13, 16
Greenland, 123
Grids, 1, 2, 19, 23

Grid, semilogarithmic, 23
Growth of individual, 262

Halothane, 237
Health, measurement of, 67
Heart defects, congenital, 11
Heights, 6, 23, 24, 28
Hematocrit, 212, 217
Hemizygous, 165
Hemocytometer, 4, 5, 203
Hemoglobin, 6, 193
Hemophilia, 165, 170
Herpes, 249, 251
Heterozygotes, 153
Hierarchical, 254
Histogram, 17
History, 88, 126, 259
Homozygosity, 153, 245
Hospital records and statistics, 61, 62, 239
Householder, 56
Hybrid, 155
Hypothesis, alternative, 177
  falsification, 1
  null, 176, 225
  simple, 177

Iceland, 124, 250
Immunology, 118
Incidence rate, 63
Income tax, 60
Indefinite causes, 104
Independence, 185
Index, vital, 142
India, 124
Induction, mathematical, 46
Infant mortality, 68, 71, 100, 126, 207
Infections, 101, 102, 251
  population size, 245, 251
Inference, 174, 176
Inflection, 53
Information, 252, 258
Information retrieval, 252, 258
Inheritance, polygenic, 160
Input, 234
Insect vectors, 118
Insurance, medical, 61
Intercept, 21
International Classification of Causes of Death, 69, 104, 123
Internation Statistical Congress, 56
International Statistical Institute, 64
Interpolation, 24
Intersection (of sets), 252
Invalid dependency, 147
Ireland, 124
Isolation, 58, 115

Italy, 124

Japan, 65, 124, 140

Laboratory measurements, 210
Law, Gompertz-Makeham, 77
    Hardy-Weinberg, 157
Laws, 174
Least squares, linear regression, 202
Legend, 19
Legitimacy, 60
Life table, 87
    assumptions, 89
Life table construction, 91, 175
Life table functions, d_x (deaths), 90
$\overset{o}{e}_x$ (expectation of life), 91, 96
    l_x (survivors), 89
    m_x (mortality), 74, 75, 90
    p_x (probability of survival), 89
    q_x (probability of dying), 74, 90
    u_x (force of mortality), 91
Life table, select, 88
Life table methodology, 167, 243
Life table population, stable, 139
    stationary, 139
Likelihood ratio, 178
List, International, 69
Literacy, 56, 59
Live-births, 71
Loci, 151

Malformations, congenital, 101, 125
Masculinity, 102, 103
Maternal, 68, 101, 125
Maximum, local in death rates, 103
Mean, arithmetic, 32
    geometric, 35
    harmonic, 34
Measles, 59, 171, 245, 248, 249, 251
Measurement procedures, 210, 212
Median, 32
Medical, care, 62, 67
    demography, 262
    services, 67
Medical statistics, history of, 259
    scope, 262
Medicolegal requirements, 239
Meiosis, 151
Melanoma, 125, 230, 237
Memory, 234
Meteorology, 126
Mice, 95
Migration, 58, 149
Mitosis, 151
Mixture, 31
Mode, 30, 31

Models, mathematical, 87, 133, 138, 157,
        166, 175, 183, 214, 232, 234, 246
    for sampling, unrestricted bivariate, 195
        comparative trial, 195
Moment, about the origin, 39
    about the mean, 39
Morbidity, 61, 67, 240
Mortality, see Age
    age specific rates of, 74, 75, 76
    analysis of rates, 76
    comparisons, 100, 123
    crude rate of, 77
    declines in rates of, 115, 169
    fetal, 101
    force of, 91
    general, 100, 122
    infant, 100
    measurement of, 68
    neonatal, 101
    standardized rates of, 79, 81
Motion, Brownian, 244
Multifactorial inheritance, 160
Municipal services, 118
Mutations, 161
Myxoma virus, 170

Nationality, 59
Navy, 126
Neonatal period, 101
New Zealand, 65, 124, 250
Noble families, 68, 88, 126
Nomography, 25
Norway, 65, 124
Notification rates, 62
Nutrition, 126

Observations, 11, 174, 220, 228, 230, 231
Oceania, 124
Occupation, 59, 126
Official statistics, 59, 60
Operations research, 232, 243
Orderliness, 187
Ordinate, 13
Origin, 13
    arbitrary, 33
Orphanhood, 146
Output, 234
Ovum, 151

Panmixia, 156
Papua, 7
Parameter, 52, 174, 186
Pascal's triangle, 44, 46
Pathognomonic, 256
Patients, 235
Pedigree, 159

Percentile, 32
Permutation, 42, 224
Person-years, 73
Pertussis, vaccines against, 229
   and sex, 57
Phenotype, 152
Plague, 124, 229
Pneumococcus, 223
Poliomyelitis, 124, 229
Polymorphism, 160
Population, 26, 149
   at census, 57
   dynamics, 127, 128, 134, 175
   integral equation of growth, 134, 150
   intrinsic rate of increase, 142
   register, 60
   at risk, 73
   sex, 57
   size, 245
Porphyria, 173
Power (of tests), 177
Powers (of variable), 44
Precision, 181, 210
Pregnancy, length of, 150
Prematurity, 71, 72, 101
Prevalence, 59
   point rate, 63
   period rate, 63
Probability, conditional, 185
   unconditional, 185
Profession, 60
Property registers, 61
Prospective, 230
Pseudo-random numbers, 184
Psychiatry, 125
Pure lines, 154

Quadrants, 13
Qualitative, 8
Quality control, 213, 215
Quantitative, 8
Quartile, 32

Radiation, 125, 187
Radiotherapy, 118
Random effects, 175
Randomization, 224, 225
Randomness, 184
Random sampling numbers, 26, 39, 40, 183
Range, 31, 35
   semi-interquartile, 32, 35
Rank correlation coefficient, 43
Rat, 249
Rate, crude birth, 128
   of increase, intrinsic, 142
Ratio chart, 19

Recessive inheritance, 59, 152, 162
Records, criminal, 61
   health, 61, 67
   hospital, 61, 67, 243
Recurrence relation, 44
Registers and registries, business, 61
   cancer, 238
   electoral, 60
   patients, 61, 62
   social insurance, 60
   social welfare, 61
   telephone, 60
Regression, linear, 200, 207
Relations between variables, 20
Remote areas, 126
Representation of data, 13
Reproduction rates, 131, 133, 142
Research, clinical, 236
Retrospective, 230
Rheumatic diseases, 125
Risk, the populations at, 63
Rubella, 1, 176, 228, 249, 251

Sample, 27
Sample survey, 26, 57, 67
Sampling, simple random, 26
   cluster, 27
   unrestricted (bivariate), 195
Schedule (of rates), 87
Scotland, 124
Scientific method, 174
Sedimentation rate, 24, 218
Select tables of mortality, 68, 88, 101, 126,
   260
Senility, 104
Sets, complementary, 252
   empty (=null), 252
   exhaustive, 47, 253
   improper, 252
   intersection, 252
   mutually exclusive, 9, 47, 253
   null (= empty), 252
   union, 252
Set Theoretically independent, 254
Sex, 50, 57, 114, 127
Sex chromosomes, 151
Sex-ratio, 20, 104
Sex-specific, 74
Sibs, full, 160
Sibs, half-, 160
Sickling, 160
Sigmoid, 30
Significance, level of, 53, 177, 209
Simulation, 234, 243, 248
Sine, 14
Size of particle, 219

Slope, 20
Smallpox, 171
Social factors, 59, 103, 118, 127, 149, 238
Social insurance, 60
Social problems, 146
Social security data, 60, 62
Social welfare registers, 61
Sorting, 11
Spermatozoon, 151
Spot diagram, 18
Standardization of the death rates, direct, 79
  equivalent average, 79
  indirect, 81
Stable age distribution, 131, 139
Stationary age distribution, 139
Statistics and mathematics, 262
Statistics, health, 61
Statistics, official, 56, 60
Stillborn, 71, 100
Stochastic processes, 187, 244, 251
Stratification, 27, 225
Students, 126
Student's-*t*, 197, 208
Subset, 252
Success, 48
Summation, 5
Surgery, 116
Surveillance, 251
Survival for one year, probability of, 89
Survivors (in life table), 89
Syndromes, 252
Syphilis, 104
Sweden, 65, 68, 79, 124, 144, 245

Table, contingency, 10, 194, 195
  fourfold, 194, 223
Tabulation, 1
Taxon, 252
Taxonomy, 252, 255
Telephone directories, 60
Tests of hypothesis, single-tailed, 178
  two-tailed, 178
Thalidomide, 63
Theorem, binomial, 44
  central limit, 198, 211
Therapy, effects of, 103, 104, 105, 115
  magna therapia sterilans, 117

Total, grand, 5
Trauma, birth, 101
Trials, clinical, 220, 222, 230, 235, 263
  alternatives to, 227
  comparative, 195
Trypanosomes, 24, 33, 34, 36, 38, 40
Tuberculosis, 27, 68, 77, 101, 102, 103, 105, 124, 194, 204, 206, 257
Twinning, 50, 167
Typhoid, 206
Typhus, 125

Unbiased, 27, 181, 210, 211
Underdeveloped countries, 124
Undermining, 144
Union, 252
United Kingdom, 66, 68, 69, 82, 84, 88, 96, 99, 123, 245, 250
United States of America, 66, 78, 83, 96, 97, 98, 99, 119, 124, 146, 168, 169, 240
Urban-rural differences, 127

Value, absolute, 36
  intermediate, 9
Variables, continuous, 6, 8, 31
  discrete, 5, 8
  nonnegative, 36
  random, 46, 48, 183
Variance, 36
Variation, coefficient of, 39
Varicella, 249
Vectors (insect) of disease, 118
Violence, 57, 68, 103, 114, 116, 125, 235
Virus, 125
Vital events, 60
Vital index, 142
Vitamins, 118
Volunteers, 27

War, 103, 125
Weights, 24
Widowhood, 147
World Health Organization, 64
World population, 150

Zoonoses, 126
Zygote, 151

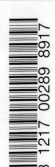

Applied Probability and Statistics (Continued)

SEAL · Stochastic Theory of a Risk Business
SEARLE · Linear Models
THOMAS · An Introduction to Applied Probability and Random
   Processes
WHITTLE · Optimization under Constraints
WILLIAMS · Regression Analysis
WONNACOTT and WONNACOTT · Econometrics
YOUDEN · Statistical Methods for Chemists
ZELLNER · An Introduction to Bayesian Inference in Econometrics

Tracts on Probability and Statistics

BILLINGSLEY · Ergodic Theory and Information
BILLINGSLEY · Convergence of Probability Measures
CRAMER and LEADBETTER · Stationary and Related Stochastic
   Processes
JARDINE and SIBSON · Mathematical Taxonomy
KINGMAN · Regenerative Phenomena
RIORDAN · Combinatorial Identities
TAKACS · Combinatorial Methods in the Theory of Stochastic
   Processes